TOXIC

RECALL SERIES EDITOR

Lorne H. Blackbourne, MD, FACS
Trauma, Burn, and Critical Care Surgeon
San Antonio, Texas

TOXICOLOGY RECALL

EDITORS

CHRISTOPHER P. HOLSTEGE, MD
Director
Division of Medical Toxicology
Associate Professor
Departments of Emergency Medicine & Pediatrics
University of Virginia School of Medicine
Charlottesville, Virginia

MATTHEW P. BORLOZ
Medical Student, Class of 2008
University of Virginia School of Medicine
Charlottesville, Virginia

JOHN P. BENNER, NREMT-P
Lieutenant
Madison County EMS
Madison, Virginia

ASSOCIATE EDITORS

DAVID T. LAWRENCE, DO
Assistant Professor
Division of Medical Toxicology
Department of Emergency Medicine
University of Virginia School of Medicine
Charlottesville, Virginia

NATHAN P. CHARLTON, MD
Medical Toxicology Fellow
Division of Medical Toxicology
Department of Emergency Medicine
University of Virginia School of Medicine
Charlottesville, Virginia

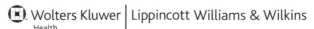 Wolters Kluwer | Lippincott Williams & Wilkins
Health
Philadelphia · Baltimore · New York · London
Buenos Aires · Hong Kong · Sydney · Tokyo

Acquisitions Editor: Charles W. Mitchell
Managing Editor: Kelley A. Squazzo
Marketing Manager: Emilie Moyer
Compositor: Maryland Composition/ASI

351 West Camden Street   530 Walnut Street
Baltimore, MD 21201   Philadelphia, PA 19106

Printed in China

9 8 7 6 5 4 3 2 1

Library of Congress Cataloging-in-Publication Data

Toxicology recall / editors, Christopher P. Holstege, Matthew P. Borloz, John P. Benner ; associate editors, David T. Lawrence, Nathan P. Charlton.
   p. ; cm.
Includes bibliographical references and index.
ISBN 978-0-7817-9089-5
1. Toxicology—Handbooks, manuals, etc. I. Holstege, Christopher P.
[DNLM: 1. Toxicology—Examination Questions. 2. Poisoning—diagnosis—Examination Questions. 3. Poisoning—therapy—Examination Questions. 4. Poisons—Examination Questions. QV 18.2 T7545 2009]
  RA1215.T697 2009
  615.9—dc22

                                      2008029897

DISCLAIMER

Care has been taken to confirm the accuracy of the information present and to describe generally accepted practices. However, the authors, editors, and publisher are not responsible for errors or omissions or for any consequences from application of the information in this book and make no warranty, expressed or implied, with respect to the currency, completeness, or accuracy of the contents of the publication. Application of this information in a particular situation remains the professional responsibility of the practitioner; the clinical treatments described and recommended may not be considered absolute and universal recommendations.

The authors, editors, and publisher have exerted every effort to ensure that drug selection and dosage set forth in this text are in accordance with the current recommendations and practice at the time of publication. However, in view of ongoing research, changes in government regulations, and the constant flow of information relating to drug therapy and drug reactions, the reader is urged to check the package insert for each drug for any change in indications and dosage and for added warnings and precautions. This is particularly important when the recommended agent is a new or infrequently employed drug.

Some drugs and medical devices presented in this publication have Food and Drug Administration (FDA) clearance for limited use in restricted research settings. It is the responsibility of the health care provider to ascertain the FDA status of each drug or device planned for use in their clinical practice.

To purchase additional copies of this book, call our customer service department at (800) 638-3030 or fax orders to (301) 223-2320. International customers should call (301) 223-2300.

Visit Lippincott Williams & Wilkins on the Internet: http://www.lww.com. Lippincott Williams & Wilkins customer service representatives are available from 8:30 am to 6:00 pm, EST.

CCS1208

We dedicate this book to all students, residents, and fellows from the schools of medicine, nursing, and pharmacy who strive to become the best caretakers of their patients. We hope this book will aid you in your quest for excellence.

Acknowledgments

We wish to acknowledge our spectacular Administrative Assistants, Heather Collier and Janet Mussleman (deceased), for their tireless support of our work. We also wish to acknowledge our Managing Director, Steve Dobmeier, who continually provides the tools necessary for all the work we set to accomplish.

Contributors

Seth Althoff, MD
University of Virginia Department of
  Emergency Medicine
Resident, Class of 2009
Charlottesville, Virginia

D. Steele Beasley, MD
University of Virginia Department of
  Emergency Medicine
Chief Resident, Class of 2008
Charlottesville, Virginia

Ashley L. Blair, PhD
Charlottesville-Albemarle Rescue
  Squad
Charlottesville, Virginia

William J. Brady, MD
University of Virginia Department of
  Emergency Medicine
Professor & Vice-Chair of
  Emergency Medicine
Charlottesville, Virginia

William E. Brooks
Jefferson Medical College
Class of 2009
Philadelphia, Pennsylvania

Christina M. Burger, MD
University of Virginia Department of
  Emergency Medicine
Resident, Class of 2009
Charlottesville, Virginia

Brian T. Fengler, MD
University of Virginia Department of
  Emergency Medicine
Resident, Class of 2008
Charlottesville, Virginia

**Jeffrey D. Ferguson, MD,
  NREMT-P**
East Carolina University Department
  of Emergency Medicine
Assistant Professor of Emergency
  Medicine
Greenville, North Carolina

F. J. Fernandez, MD
University of Cincinnati Department
  of Emergency Medicine
Resident, Class of 2010
Cincinnati, Ohio

Geoffrey Froehlich
Charlottesville-Albemarle Rescue
  Squad
Charlottesville, Virginia

Rachel Garvin, MD
University of Cincinnati Department
  of Emergency Medicine
Resident, Class of 2010
Cincinnati, Ohio

Ashley E. Gunnell, NREMT-I
Charlottesville-Albemarle Rescue
  Squad
Charlottesville, Virginia

Todd Hansen, NREMT-I
Charlottesville-Albemarle Rescue
  Squad
Charlottesville, Virginia

Nicholas D. Hartman
University of Virginia School of
  Medicine
Class of 2008
Charlottesville, Virginia

Joshua Hilton, MD
Northwestern University Department
of Emergency Medicine
Resident, Class of 2009
Chicago, Illinois

Brian B. Hughley
University of Virginia School of
Medicine
Class of 2009
Charlottesville, Virginia

Jason A. Inofuentes
Charlottesville-Albemarle Rescue
Squad
Charlottesville, Virginia

Anand Jain
Drexel University College of
Medicine
Class of 2008
Philadelphia, Pennsylvania

Anthony E. Judkins, NREMT-I
Madison County EMS
Charlottesville, Virginia

Erin S. Kalan
Charlottesville-Albemarle Rescue
Squad
Charlottesville, Virginia

Brian J. Kipe
University of Virginia School of
Medicine
Class of 2008
Charlottesville, Virginia

Michael C. Kurz, MD, MS-HES
Virginia Commonwealth University
Department of Emergency
Medicine
Assistant Professor of Emergency
Medicine
Richmond, Virginia

Todd Larson
University of Virginia School of
Medicine
Class of 2008
Charlottesville, Virginia

Richard M. Law
The Ohio State University College
of Medicine
Class of 2008
Columbus, Ohio

Benjamin J. Lehman, MD
University of Virginia Department of
Emergency Medicine
Resident, Class of 2008
Charlottesville, Virginia

Pauline E. Meekins, MD
Medical University of South Carolina
Division of Emergency Medicine
Clinical Faculty
Charleston, South Carolina

Christopher A. Mitchell
The Ohio State University College
of Medicine
Class of 2008
Columbus, Ohio

Lisa J. Mitchell
Charlottesville-Albemarle Rescue
Squad
Charlottesville, Virginia

J.V. Nable
University of Virginia School of
Medicine
Class of 2009
Charlottesville, Virginia

Christopher Pitotti
University of Virginia School of
Medicine
Class of 2008
Charlottesville, Virginia

James Platts-Mills
University of Virginia School of
    Medicine
Class of 2009
Charlottesville, Virginia

Timothy F. Platts-Mills, MD
University of North Carolina at
    Chapel Hill Department of
    Emergency Medicine
Assistant Professor of Emergency
    Medicine
Chapel Hill, North Carolina

Michelle A. Ramos
University of Virginia School of
    Medicine
Class of 2008
Charlottesville, Virginia

Amy Schutt
Texas Tech University Health
    Sciences Center School of
    Medicine
Class of 2009
Lubbock, Texas

Robert Schutt III
Texas Tech University Health
    Sciences Center School of
    Medicine
Class of 2009
Lubbock, Texas

Landon Smith
University of Virginia School of
    Medicine
Class of 2008
Charlottesville, Virginia

Jeffrey St. Amant, MD
University of Virginia Department of
    Emergency Medicine
Resident, Class of 2009
Charlottesville, Virginia

Stephen Stacey
Eastern Virginia Medical School
Class of 2010
Norfolk, Virginia

Stephen Thornton, MD
University of Kansas Hospital
Clinical Associate Professor
Leakwood, Kansas

Sara Naomi Tsuchitani, MD
Eastern Virginia Medical School
    Department of Emergency
    Medicine
Resident, Class of 2010
Norfolk, Virginia

Amber Turner
University of Virginia School of
    Medicine
Class of 2010
Charlottesville, Virginia

Edward Walsh, MD
Mary Washington Hospital
    Department of Emergency
    Medicine
Attending Physician
Fredericksburg, Virginia

Michael J. Ward, MD, MBA
University of Cincinnati Department
    of Emergency Medicine
Resident, Class of 2010
Cincinnati, Ohio

Elisabeth B. Wright
University of Virginia School of
    Medicine
Medical Simulation Technology
    Specialist
Charlottesville, Virginia

Contents

Dedication v
Acknowledgments vii
Contributors ix
Preface xxi

1 Evaluation of the Poisoned Patient 1
Introduction 1
Clinical Evaluation 1
Testing in Poisoning 3
Management 10
Conclusion 15

2 Medications 17
Acetaminophen 17
Amantadine 20
Anesthetics 21
  Central 21
  Local 23
Angiotensin-Converting Enzyme Inhibitors 25
Angiotensin Receptor Blockers 26
Antibacterial Agents 27
Anticholinergics 30
Anticonvulsants 32
Antidepressants 33
  Cyclic 33
  Monoamine Oxidase Inhibitors 37
  Selective Serotonin Reuptake Inhibitors 39
  Other 41
Antidiarrheal Agents 43
Antiemetic Agents 44
Antifungal Agents 45
Antihistamines 47
Antihyperlipidemia Agents 49
Antimalarial Agents 51
Antipsychotic Agents 52
Antiviral and Antiretroviral Agents 54
Barbiturates 55
Benzodiazepines 56
Beta 2-Adrenergic Agonists 58

Botulin (Botulism) 59
Caffeine 60
Camphor and Other Essential (Volatile) Oils 62
Carbamazepine 64
Chemotherapeutic Agents 65
Chloroquine and Other Aminoquinolines 67
Clonidine and Related Agents 68
Colchicine 69
Dapsone 70
Decongestants 72
Digoxin 73
Disulfiram 76
Diuretics 77
Ergot Derivatives 78
Heparin 80
Hypoglycemic Agents 81
    Insulin 81
    Metformin 84
    Sulfonylureas 84
    Other 86
Immunosuppressants 88
Ipecac Syrup 89
Isoniazid (INH) 91
Ketamine 92
Lithium 95
Magnesium 96
Neuromuscular Blockers 98
Nitrates 100
Nitrites 101
Nitroprusside 102
Nitrous Oxide 103
Nonsteroidal Anti-inflammatory Drugs 104
Opioids 105
Phenytoin 107
Rauwolfia Alkaloids 109
Salicylates 110
Sedative-Hypnotic Agents 113
Skeletal Muscle Relaxants 114
Theophylline 115
Thyroid Hormones 117
Type I Antidysrhythmic Agents 118
Type II Antidysrhythmic Agents 121
Type III Antidysrhythmic Agents 122
Type IV Antidysrhythmic Agents 123

Valproic Acid 124
Vasodilators 125
Vitamins 126
Warfarin 129

3   Drugs of Abuse **132**
Amphetamines 132
Cocaine 133
Designer Drugs 135
Dextromethorphan 138
Ethanol 139
Gamma-hydroxybutyrate (GHB) 141
Hallucinogens 142
Inhalants 144
Marijuana 146
Mescaline 147
Nicotine 149
Opioids 150
Phencyclidine (PCP) 152

4   Environmental and Industrial Toxins **154**
Acids 154
Ammonia 156
Antiseptics and Disinfectants 158
Asbestos 161
Azide 162
Benzene 163
Boric Acid, Borates, and Boron 165
Bromates 166
Bromides 167
Camphor 169
Carbon Disulfide 170
Carbon Monoxide 172
Carbon Tetrachloride 174
Caustics 176
Chlorates 178
Chlorine 179
Chloroform 181
Cyanide 183
Detergents 185
Dimethyl Sulfoxide (DMSO) 187
Dioxins 188
Disk Batteries 190
Ethylene Dibromide 191
Ethylene Glycol 192

Ethylene Oxide 195
Fluorides 197
Fluoroacetate 200
Formaldehyde 201
Freons and Halons 202
Gases (Irritant) 204
Glycol Ethers 206
Hydrocarbons 207
Hydrogen Sulfide 210
Iodine 211
Isocyanates 213
Isopropanol 214
Metaldehyde 215
Methanol 216
Methemoglobinemia Inducers 218
Methyl Bromide 220
Methylene Chloride 222
Mothballs 223
Nitrites 224
Nitrogen Oxides 225
Nontoxic and Minimally Toxic Household Products 228
Oxalic Acid 229
Pentachlorophenol and Dinitrophenol 231
Perchloroethylene 232
Phenol 234
Phosphine & Phosphides 236
Phosphorus 237
Phthalates 238
Polychlorinated Biphenyls (PCBs) 239
Radiation (Ionizing) 240
Smoke Inhalation 248
Strychnine 249
Sulfur Dioxide 251
Toluene 252
Trichloroethane and Trichloroethylene 254

5 **Heavy Metals** **256**
Aluminum 256
Antimony and Stibine 258
Arsenic and Arsine 262
Barium 265
Beryllium 267
Bismuth 269
Cadmium 270

Chromium 272
Cobalt 274
Copper 276
Gallium 279
Germanium 280
Gold 281
Iron 282
Lead 285
Lithium 288
Manganese 291
Mercury 292
Molybdenum 295
Nickel 296
Platinum 298
Rare Earths 299
Selenium 300
Silver 302
Thallium 303
Tin 305
Vanadium 306
Zinc 307
Metal Fume Fever 309

6   Pesticides **311**
Fungicides 311
Herbicides 313
   Chlorophenoxy 313
   Diquat 314
   Paraquat 316
   Other 318
Insecticides 321
   Carbamates 321
   Organochlorines 322
   Organophosphates 324
   Pyrethrins & Pyrethroids 327
   Other 329
Rodenticides 331
   Alpha-naphthylthiourea (ANTU) 331
   Anticoagulants 331
   Cholecalciferol 333
   Sodium Monofluoroacetate (1080) 334
   Strychnine 335
   Vacor (PNU) 337
   Other 338

7   Chemical Agents of Terrorism **342**
   Botulinum Toxin 342
   Incapacitating Agents 344
   Incendiary Agents 345
   Irritants 346
   Nerve Agents 347
   Phosgene 353
   3-Quinuclidinyl Benzilate 355
   Ricin 356
   Trichothecene Mycotoxins 359
   Vesicants 360
   Vomiting Agents 363
   Other 364

8   Natural Toxins **366**
   Amphibians 366
   Arthropods 367
      Black Widow Spiders 367
      Brown Recluse Spiders 369
      Scorpions 371
      Ticks 372
      Other 378
   Botulism 381
   Essential Oils 385
   Food Poisoning, Bacterial 386
   Herbal Products 389
   Marine 392
      Ingested 392
      Invertebrates 398
      Vertebrates 400
   Mushrooms 402
      Coprine Group 402
      Cortinarius Group 403
      Cyclopeptide Group 404
      Gastrointestinal Irritant Group 406
      Hallucinogen Group 407
      Ibotenic/Muscimol Group 408
      Monomethylhydrazines Group 409
      Muscarine Group 411
   Mycotoxins 412
   Plants 415
      Anticholinergic 415
      Cardiac Glycosides 417
      Cyanogenic Glycosides 418
      Dermatitis-Producing 420

Gastrointestinal Irritants 422
Nicotinics 423
Oxalates 424
Sodium Channel Openers 425
Solanine 427
Toxalbumins 428
Other 430
Reptiles 432
Snakes 432
Elapidae 432
Viperidae 434
Other 437
Tetanus 439

9   Therapies **444**
Acetylcysteine (*N*-acetylcysteine, NAC) 444
Antivenom 446
Black Widow 446
Scorpion 447
Snake 448
Atropine and Glycopyrrolate 450
Barbiturates 451
Benzodiazepines 453
Benztropine 454
Bicarbonate 454
Botulinum Antitoxin 456
Bromocriptine 457
Calcium 458
Calcium Disodium Ethylenediaminetetraacetic
    Acid (CaNa$_2$EDTA) 460
L-Carnitine 461
Charcoal (Activated) 462
Cyproheptadine 463
Cyanide Antidote Package 465
Dantrolene 467
Deferoxamine 467
Dialysis 469
Dimercaptopropanesulfonic Acid (DMPS) 470
Diethyldithiocarbamate 471
Digoxin Immune Fab 471
Dimercaprol 473
Dimethyl-P-Aminophenol (DMAP) 474
Diphenhydramine 476
Ethanol 477
Flumazenil 478

Folic Acid 479
Fomepizole (4-Methylpyrazole, 4-MP) 480
Glucagon 481
Glucose 483
Haloperidol and Droperidol 484
Histamine-2 Receptor Antagonists (H_2 Blockers) 486
Hydroxocobalamin 487
Hyperbaric Oxygen 488
Inamrinone (previously Amrinone) 491
Insulin 492
Iodide 494
Ipecac Syrup 495
Isoproterenol 496
Leucovorin 497
Lidocaine 498
Magnesium 499
Methylene Blue 500
Naloxone, Naltrexone, and Nalmefene 502
Neuromuscular Blockers 503
Octreotide 505
Penicillamine 506
Phentolamine 507
Phenytoin and Fosphenytoin 508
Physostigmine and Neostigmine 509
Pralidoxime (2-PAM) and Other Oximes 510
Propofol 512
Propranolol 514
Protamine 515
Prussian Blue 516
Pyridoxine (Vitamin B_6) 517
Silibinin or Milk Thistle (*Silybum marianum*) 518
Succimer (DMSA) 519
Thiamine (Vitamin B_1) 519
Vasopressors 521
Vitamin K_1 (Phytonadione) 525
Other 527

10 Visual Diagnosis in Medical Toxicology **531**

Abbreviations 551

Index **554**

Preface

Throughout the world each year, millions of people are evaluated by health care professionals following a poisoning. There are innumerable potential toxins that can inflict harm to humans, including pharmaceuticals, herbals, household products, environmental agents, occupational chemicals, drugs of abuse, and chemical terrorism threats. The Centers for Disease Control reported that poisoning (both intentional and unintentional) was one of the top ten causes of injury-related death in the United States in all adult age groups. From the beginnings of written history, poisons and their effects have been well-described. Paracelsus (1493–1541) correctly noted that "All substances are poisons; there is none which is not a poison. The right dose differentiates a poison . . . ." As life in the modern era has become more complex, so has the study of toxicology.

This book is intended to assist the reader in learning the pertinent toxicities of various agents seen in clinical practice. It has become increasingly difficult for healthcare providers to learn these facts with the emergence of numerous and vastly different pharmaceuticals, abused drugs, chemicals within the work place, and agents of terrorism. As the editors, we considered numerous topics for inclusion in this book. It is our hope that this book will provide both a rapid insight into specific toxins for medical personnel caring for potentially poisoned patients and a valuable resource for students pursuing their education.

Chapter 1

Evaluation of the Poisoned Patient

INTRODUCTION

Toxicologic emergencies are commonly encountered in the practice of medicine. Patients can be exposed to potential toxins either by accident (e.g., workplace incidents or drug interactions) or intention (e.g., drug abuse or suicide attempt). The outcome following a poisoning depends on numerous factors, such as the dose taken, the time before presentation to the healthcare facility, and the preexisting health status of the patient. If a poisoning is recognized early and appropriate supportive care is initiated quickly, the majority of patient outcomes will be good.

CLINICAL EVALUATION

When evaluating a patient who has presented with a potential poisoning, it is important not to limit the differential diagnosis. A comatose patient who smells of alcohol may be harboring an intracranial hemorrhage or an agitated patient who appears anticholinergic may actually be encephalopathic from an infectious etiology. Patients must be thoroughly assessed and appropriately stabilized. There is often no specific antidote or treatment for a poisoned patient and careful supportive care is the most important intervention.

All patients presenting with toxicity or potential toxicity should be aggressively managed. The patient's airway should be patent and adequate ventilation ensured. If necessary, endotracheal intubation should be performed. Too often, healthcare providers are lulled into a false sense of security when a patient's oxygen saturations are adequate on high flow oxygen. If the patient has either inadequate ventilation or a poor gag reflex, then the patient may be at risk for subsequent CO_2 narcosis with worsening acidosis or aspiration. The initial treatment of hypotension consists of intravenous fluids. Close monitoring of the patient's pulmonary status should be performed to ensure that pulmonary edema does not develop as fluids are infused. The healthcare providers should place the patient on continuous cardiac monitoring with pulse oximetry and make frequent neurological checks. In all patients with altered mental status, blood glucose should be checked. Poisoned patients should receive a large-bore peripheral intravenous line, and all symptomatic patients should have a second line placed in either the peripheral or central venous system. Placement of a urinary catheter should be considered early in the care of hemodynamically unstable poisoned patients to monitor urinary output, as this is one of the best indicators of adequate perfusion.

Many toxins can potentially cause seizures. In general, toxin-induced seizures are treated in a similar fashion to other seizures. Clinicians should ensure the patient maintains a patent airway, and the blood glucose should be measured. Most toxin-induced seizures will be self-limiting. However, for seizures requiring treatment, the first-line agent should be parenteral benzodiazepines. If benzodiazepines are not effective at controlling seizures, a second-line agent such as phenobarbital should be employed. In rare cases, such as isoniazid poisoning, pyridoxine should be administered. In cases of toxin-induced seizures, phenytoin is generally not recommended as it is usually ineffective and may add to the underlying toxicity of some agents. If a poisoned patient requires intubation, it is important to avoid the use of long-acting paralytic agents, as these agents may mask seizures if they develop.

TOXIDROMES

Toxidromes are toxic syndromes or the constellation of signs and symptoms associated with a class of poisons. Rapid recognition of a toxidrome, if present, can help determine whether a poison is involved in a patient's condition and can help determine the class of toxin involved. Table 1-1 lists selected

Table 1-1.   Toxidromes

Toxidrome	Signs and Symptoms
Anticholinergic	Mydriasis, dry skin, dry mucous membranes, decreased bowel sounds, sedation, altered mental status, hallucinations, dysarthria, urinary retention
Cholinergic	Miosis, lacrimation, diaphoresis, bronchospasm, bronchorrhea, vomiting, diarrhea, bradycardia
Opioid	Sedation, miosis, decreased bowel sounds, decreased respirations
Sedative-hypnotic	Sedation, decreased respirations, normal pupil size, normal vital signs
Serotonin syndrome	Altered mental status, tachycardia, hypertension, hyperreflexia, clonus, hyperthermia
Sympathomimetic	Agitation, mydriasis, tachycardia, hypertension, hyperthermia, diaphoresis

toxidromes and their characteristics. It is important to note that patients may not present with every component of a toxidrome and that toxidromes can be clouded in mixed ingestions.

Certain aspects of a toxidrome can have great significance. For example, noting dry axillae may be the only way of differentiating an anticholinergic patient from a sympathomimetic patient, and miosis may distinguish opioid toxicity from a benzodiazepine overdose. There are several notable exceptions to the recognized toxidromes. For example, some opioid agents do not cause miosis (e.g., meperidine, tramadol). In most cases, a toxidrome will not indicate a specific poison but rather a class of poisons. Several poisons have unique toxidromes which make their presence virtually diagnostic. An example is botulinum toxin. A patient with bulbar palsy, dry mouth, mydriasis, and diplopia with intact sensation is almost certain to have botulism.

TESTING IN POISONING

When evaluating the intoxicated patient, there is no substitute for a thorough history and physical exam. On today's television programming, numerous medical shows depict a universal *toxicology screen* that automatically determines the agent causing a patient's symptoms. Unfortunately, samples cannot be simply "sent to the lab" with the correct diagnosis to a clinical mystery returning on a computer printout. Clues from a patient's physical exam are generally more likely to be helpful than a "shotgun" laboratory approach that involves indiscriminate testing of blood or urine for multiple agents.

When used appropriately, diagnostic tests may be of help in the management of the intoxicated patient. When a specific toxin or even class of toxins is suspected, requesting qualitative or quantitative levels may be appropriate. In the suicidal patient whose history is generally unreliable, or in the unresponsive patient where no history is available, the clinician may gain further clues as to the etiology of a poisoning by responsible diagnostic testing.

ANION GAP

Obtaining a basic metabolic panel from all poisoned patients is generally recommended. When low serum bicarbonate is discovered on a metabolic panel, the clinician should determine if an elevated anion gap exists. The formula most commonly used for the anion gap calculation is:

$$\text{Anion gap} = [Na^+] - [Cl^- + HCO_3^-]$$

This equation allows one to determine if serum electroneutrality is being maintained. The primary cation (sodium) and anions (chloride and bicarbonate) are represented in the equation. There are other contributors to this equation that are "unmeasured." Other serum cations are not commonly included in this calculation because either their concentrations are relatively low (e.g., potassium), or assigning a number to represent their respective contribution is difficult (e.g., magnesium, calcium). Similarly, there is a multitude of other serum anions (e.g., sulfate, phosphate, organic anions) that are also difficult to measure in the serum and quantify in an equation. These "unmeasured" ions represent the anion gap calculated using the equation above. The normal range for this anion gap is accepted to be 8 to 16 mEq/L. Practically speaking, an increase in the anion gap beyond an accepted normal range, accompanied by a metabolic acidosis, represents an increase in unmeasured endogenous (e.g., lactate) or exogenous (e.g., salicylates) anions. A list of the more common causes of this phenomenon is organized in the classic MUDILES mnemonic:

Methanol
Uremia
Diabetic ketoacidosis
Iron, **I**nhalants (e.g., carbon monoxide, cyanide, toluene), **I**soniazid,
    Ibuprofen
Lactic acidosis
Ethylene glycol, **E**thanol ketoacidosis
Salicylates, **S**tarvation ketoacidosis, **S**ympathomimetics

It is imperative that clinicians who admit poisoned patients initially presenting with an increased anion gap metabolic acidosis investigate the etiology of that acidosis. Many symptomatic poisoned patients may have an initial mild metabolic acidosis upon presentation due to the processes resulting in the elevation of serum lactate. However, with adequate supportive care including hydration and oxygenation, the anion gap acidosis should improve. If, despite adequate supportive care, an anion gap metabolic acidosis worsens in a poisoned patient, the clinician should consider either toxins that form acidic metabolites (e.g., ethylene glycol, methanol, ibuprofen) or toxins which cause lactic acidosis by interfering with aerobic energy production (e.g., cyanide, iron).

OSMOL GAP

The serum osmol gap is a common laboratory test that may be useful when evaluating poisoned patients. This test is most often discussed in the context of evaluating the patient suspected of toxic alcohol (i.e., ethylene glycol, methanol, isopropanol) intoxication. Though this test may have utility in such situations, it has many pitfalls and limitations.

Osmotic concentrations are themselves expressed both in terms of osmolality [milliosmoles/kg of solvent (mOsm/kg)] and osmolarity [milliosmoles/liter of solution (mOsm/L)]. This concentration can be measured by use of an osmometer, a tool that most often utilizes the technique of freezing point depression and yields values expressed as osmolality (Osm_m). A calculated serum osmolarity (Osm_c) may be obtained by any of a number of equations involving the patient's glucose, sodium, and urea which contribute almost all of the normally measured osmolality. One of the most commonly used of these calculations is expressed below:

$$Osm_c = 2\,[Na^+] + \frac{[BUN]}{2.8} + \frac{[glucose]}{18}$$

The correction factors in the equation are based on the relative osmotic activity of the substance in question. Assuming serum neutrality, sodium as the predominant serum cation is doubled to account for the corresponding anions. Finding the osmolarity contribution of any other osmotically active substances reported in mg/dL (like BUN and glucose) is accomplished by dividing by one-tenth their molecular weight (MW) in daltons. For BUN this conversion factor is 2.8, and for glucose it is 18. Similar conversion factors may be added to this equation in an attempt to account for ethanol and the various toxic alcohols as shown below:

$$Osm_c = 2\,[Na^+] + \frac{[BUN]}{2.8} + \frac{[glucose]}{18} + \frac{[ethanol]}{4.6} + \frac{[methanol]}{3.2}$$

$$+ \frac{[ethylene\ glycol]}{6.6} + \frac{[isopropanol]}{6.0}$$

The difference between the measured (Osm_m) and calculated (Osm_c) is the osmol gap (OG) and is depicted by the equation below:

$$OG = Osm_m - Osm_c$$

If a significant osmol gap is discovered, the difference in the two values may indicate the presence of foreign substances in the blood. A list of possible causes of an elevated osmol gap is provided in Table 1-2. Unfortunately, what constitutes a normal osmol gap is widely debated. Traditionally, a normal gap has been defined as ≤ 10 mOsm/kg. Analytical variance alone may account for the variation found in patients' osmol gaps. This concern that even small errors in the measurement of sodium can result in large variations in the osmol gap has been voiced by other researchers. Overall, the clinician should recognize that there is likely significant variability in a patient's baseline osmol gap.

The osmol gap should be used with caution as an adjunct to clinical decision making and not as a primary determinant to rule out toxic alcohol

Table 1-2.   Toxins Causing Elevated Osmol Gap

Acetone
Ethanol
Ethyl ether
Ethylene glycol
Glycerol
Isoniazid
Isopropanol
Mannitol
Methanol
Osmotic contrast dyes
Propylene glycol
Trichloroethane

ingestion. If the osmol gap obtained is particularly large, it suggests that an agent from Table 1-2 may be present. A "normal" osmol gap should be interpreted with caution; a negative study may, in fact, not rule out the presence of such an ingestion. As with any test result, this must be interpreted within the context of the clinical presentation.

URINE DRUG SCREENING

Many clinicians regularly obtain urine drug screening on "altered" patients or on those suspected of ingestion. Such routine urine drug testing, however, is of questionable benefit. The effect of such routine screening on management is low because most of the therapy is supportive and directed at the clinical scenario (i.e., mental status, cardiovascular function, respiratory condition). Interpretation of the results can be difficult even when the objective for ordering a comprehensive urine screen is adequately defined. Most assays rely on antibody identification of drug metabolites, with some drugs remaining positive days after use, and thus provide information potentially unrelated to the patient's current clinical picture. The positive identification of drug metabolites is likewise influenced by chronicity of ingestion, fat solubility, and co-ingestions. Conversely, many drugs of abuse (e.g., ketamine, fentanyl) are not detected on most urine drug screens.

The ordering of urine drug screens is fraught with significant testing limitations, including false-positive and false-negative results. Many authors have shown that the test results rarely affect management decisions. Routine drug screening of those with altered mental status, abnormal vital signs, or suspected ingestion is not warranted and rarely guides patient treatment or disposition.

ELECTROCARDIOGRAM

The interpretation of the electrocardiogram (ECG) in the poisoned patient can challenge even the most experienced clinician. Numerous drugs can cause ECG changes. The incidence of ECG changes in the poisoned patient is unclear, and the significance of various changes may be difficult to define. Despite the fact that drugs have widely varying indications for therapeutic use, many unrelated drugs share common cardiac electrocardiographic effects if taken in overdose. Potential toxins can be placed into broad classes based on their cardiac effects. Two such classes, agents that block the cardiac potassium efflux channels and agents that block cardiac fast sodium channels, can lead to characteristic changes in cardiac indices, consisting of QT prolongation and QRS prolongation, respectively. The recognition of specific ECG changes associated with other clinical data (e.g., toxidromes) can potentially be life-saving.

Studies suggest that approximately 3% of all noncardiac prescriptions are associated with the potential for QT prolongation. Myocardial repolarization is driven predominantly by outward movement of potassium ions. Drug-induced blockade of these outward potassium currents prolongs the action potential. This results in QT-interval prolongation and the potential emergence of T or U wave abnormalities on the ECG. This prolonged repolarization causes the myocardial cell to have less charge difference across its membrane, which may result in the activation of the inward depolarization current (early after-depolarization) and promote triggered activity. These changes may lead to re-entry and subsequent polymorphic ventricular tachycardia, most often as the torsade de pointes. The QT interval is simply measured from the beginning of the QRS complex to the end of the T wave. Within any ECG tracing, there is lead-to-lead variation of the QT interval. In general, the longest measurable QT interval on an ECG is regarded as the overall QT interval for a given tracing. The QT interval is influenced by the patient's heart rate. Several formulas have been developed to correct the QT interval for the effect of heart rate (QT_C) using the RR interval (RR), with Bazett's formula utilized most commonly:

$$QT_c = \frac{QT}{\sqrt{RR}}$$

QT prolongation is considered to occur when the corrected QT interval (QT_C) is greater than 440 msec in men and 460 msec in women. Arrhythmias are most commonly associated with values greater than 500 msec. The potential for an arrhythmia at a given QT interval will vary, however, from drug to drug and patient to patient. Drugs associated with QT prolongation are listed in Table 1-3. Other etiologies with the potential to cause prolongation of the QT interval include congenital long QT syndrome, mitral valve prolapse, hypokalemia, hypocalcemia, hypomagnesemia, hypothermia, myocardial ischemia, neurological catastrophes, and hypothyroidism.

The ability of drugs to induce cardiac sodium channel blockade and thereby prolong the QRS complex has been well described in numerous literature reports. This sodium channel blockade activity has been described as *a membrane stabilizing effect, a local anesthetic effect*, or *a quinidine-like effect*. Cardiac voltage-gated sodium channels reside in the cell membrane and open in conjunction with cell depolarization. Sodium channel blockers bind to the transmembrane sodium channels and thereby decrease the number available for depolarization. This creates a delay of Na^+ entry into the cardiac myocyte during phase 0 of depolarization. As a result, the upslope of depolarization is slowed and the QRS complex widens. In some cases, the QRS complex may take the pattern of recognized bundle branch blocks. In the most severe cases, QRS prolongation becomes so profound that it is difficult to distinguish between ventricular and supraventricular rhythms. Continued prolongation of the QRS may result in a sine wave pattern and eventual asystole. It has been theorized that sodium channel blockers can cause slowed intraventricular conduction, unidirectional block, development of a re-entrant circuit, and ultimately ventricular tachycardia. This can then degenerate into ventricular fibrillation. Differentiating toxic versus nontoxic etiologies for a prolonged QRS can be difficult. Rightward axis deviation of the terminal 40 msec of the QRS complex has been associated with tricyclic antidepressant poisoning; however, the occurrence of this finding with other sodium channel blocking agents is unknown. Myocardial sodium channel blocking drugs comprise a diverse group of pharmaceutical agents (Table 1-4). Patients poisoned with these agents will have a variety of clinical presentations. For example, sodium channel blocking medications such as diphenhydramine, propoxyphene, and cocaine may also yield anticholinergic, opioid, and sympathomimetic syndromes, respectively. In addition, specific drugs may affect not only the myocardial sodium channels, but also the calcium influx and potassium efflux channels. This may result in ECG changes and rhythm disturbances not related entirely to the drug's sodium channel blocking activity. All of the agents listed in Table 1-4, however, are similar in that they may induce myocardial sodium channel blockade *and* may respond to therapy with hypertonic saline or sodium bicarbonate. In patients with a prolonged QRS interval, particularly those with hemodynamic instability, it is therefore reasonable to

Table 1-3. Potassium Efflux Channel Blocking Drugs

Antihistamines	Class III antidysrhythmics
Astemizole	Amiodarone
Clarithromycin	Dofetilide
Diphenhydramine	Ibutilide
Loratadine	Sotalol
Terfenadine	
	Cyclic Antidepressants
Antipsychotics	Amitriptyline
Chlorpromazine	Amoxapine
Droperidol	Desipramine
Haloperidol	Doxepin
Mesoridazine	Imipramine
Pimozide	Maprotiline
Quetiapine	Nortriptyline
Risperidone	
Thioridazine	Erythromycin
Ziprasidone	
	Fluoroquinolones
Arsenic trioxide	Ciprofloxacin
	Gatifloxacin
Bepridil	Levofloxacin
	Moxifloxacin
Chloroquine	Sparfloxacin
Cisapride	Halofantrine
Citalopram	Hydroxychloroquine
Clarithromycin	Levomethadyl
Class IA antidysrhythmics	Methadone
Disopyramide	
Procainamide	Pentamidine
Quinidine	
	Quinine
Class IC antidysrhythmics	
Encainide	Tacrolimus
Flecainide	
Moricizine	Venlafaxine
Propafenone	

Table 1-4.   Sodium Channel Blocking Drugs

Amantadine	Diltiazem
Carbamazepine	Diphenhydramine
Chloroquine	Hydroxychloroquine
Citalopram	Loxapine

Class IA antidysrhythmics
  Disopyramide
  Procainamide
  Quinidine
	Orphenadrine

	Phenothiazines
	  Mesoridazine
	  Thioridazine

Class IC antidysrhythmics
  Encainide
  Flecainide
  Propafenone
	Propoxyphene

	Propranolol
Cocaine	Quinine
Cyclic antidepressants	Verapamil

treat empirically with 1-2 mEq/kg of sodium bicarbonate. A post-treatment shortening of the QRS duration can confirm the presence of a sodium channel blocking agent. In addition, sodium bicarbonate can improve inotropy and help prevent arrhythmias.

There are multiple agents that can result in human cardiotoxicity and resultant ECG changes, from those noted above to others, such as bradycardia and tachycardia. Physicians managing patients who have overdosed on medications should be aware of the various electrocardiographic changes that may occur in this setting.

MANAGEMENT

After initial evaluation and stabilization of the poisoned patient, it is time to initiate specific therapies if appropriate. Decontamination should be considered. Also, several poisons have specific antidotes which, if utilized in a timely and appropriate manner, can be of great benefit. Lastly, the final disposition of the patient must be determined. Most patients may be discharged home or to a psychiatric facility after a short observation period; however, a number will need admission due to their clinical condition or potential for deterioration.

DECONTAMINATING THE POISONED PATIENT

Approximately 80% of all poisonings occur by ingestion, and the most common type of subsequent decontamination performed is gastrointestinal decontamination, using a variety of techniques including emesis, gastric lavage, activated charcoal, cathartics, and whole bowel irrigation. Poisonings may also occur by dermal and ocular routes, both of which necessitate external decontamination. Significant controversy exists concerning the need for routine gastric emptying in the poisoned patient. Current available evidence dissuades the routine use of gastric decontamination, though it may be considered in select cases and specific scenarios. Before performing gastrointestinal decontamination techniques, the clinician responsible for the care of the poisoned patient must clearly understand that these procedures are not without hazards and that any decision regarding their use must consider whether the benefits outweigh any potential harm.

Dermal Decontamination

Patients with dermal contamination who present to healthcare facilities pose a potential risk to healthcare personnel. As a result, contaminated patients should not gain entrance into the healthcare facility prior to decontamination. Personnel involved in the dermal decontamination may need to don personal protective equipment (PPE). Most chemical exposures do not pose a risk of secondary exposure. In general, patients exposed to gas or vapor do not require decontamination; removal from the site should be sufficient. However, contaminated clothing should be removed and sealed within plastic bags to avoid potential off gassing.

Patients exposed to toxic liquids, aerosols, or solids will require dermal decontamination. Moving from head to toe, irrigate the exposed skin and hair for 10 to 15 minutes and scrub with a soft surgical sponge, being careful not to abrade the skin. Patient privacy should be respected if possible, and warm water should be used to avoid hypothermia. Irrigate wounds for an additional 5 to 10 minutes with water or saline. Clean beneath the nails with a brush. Stiff brushes and abrasives should be avoided, as they may enhance dermal absorption of the toxin and can produce skin lesions that may be mistaken for chemical injuries. Sponges and disposable towels are effective alternatives.

Ocular Decontamination

Ocular irrigation should be performed immediately by instillation of a gentle stream of irrigation fluid into the affected eye(s). The contiguous skin should also be irrigated. In cases of minor ocular toxicity, this procedure can be conducted in the home. If irritation persists following home irrigation, referral to an emergency department may be necessary. In the emergency department, the patient should undergo ocular irrigation with sterile normal saline or lactated Ringer's solution for a period of at least 15 to 30 minutes. Tap water is acceptable if it is the only available solution; however, due to its hypotonicity relative to the stroma, tap water may facilitate penetration of corrosive substances into the cornea and worsen the outcome. Lactated Ringer's solution may be a preferable irrigant due its buffering capacity and neutral pH. Instillation of tetracaine or another ocular anesthetic agent will reduce pain and facilitate irrigation. Irrigation of the eyes should be directed away from the medial canthus to avoid forcing contaminants into the lacrimal duct. Longer irrigation times may be needed with specific substances, and the endpoint of irrigation should be determined by normalization of the ocular pH. If the pH does not normalize with copious irrigation, it may be necessary to invert the lids to search for retained material.

Gastrointestinal Decontamination

Emesis, gastric lavage, activated charcoal, cathartics, and whole bowel irrigation are the available means of gastrointestinal decontamination. As a result of emerging evidence, gastric lavage and syrup of ipecac-induced emesis are rarely being utilized to decontaminate the poisoned patient. At the present time, the documented risks associated with these procedures should be carefully weighed in light of the rare indications. Activated charcoal as the sole means of gastric decontamination is increasing in popularity, but its efficacy has specific limitations. The major issue currently facing the clinician is the choice of gastrointestinal (GI) decontamination in the significantly poisoned patient. The choice of decontamination method for these patients must be individualized using both evidence-based medicine and clinical acumen. No patient should undergo any of the available procedures unless it is anticipated that decontamination will provide clinical benefits that outweigh the potential risks. Emesis, either by mechanical stimulation (i.e., placing a finger down the throat) or by use of syrup of ipecac, is contraindicated.

Gastric Lavage

The efficiency of gastric lavage to remove a marker significantly decreases with increasing time following ingestion. This is due to the fact that as time increases after ingestion, so too does the amount of marker that has been absorbed or left the stomach. It is rare that gastric lavage can be performed within the first hour after toxic ingestion. Not only does it take time for these patients to present to the emergency department, but initial evaluation and stabilization consume additional time before gastric lavage can take place. Based on the available literature, gastric lavage should not be routinely employed in the management of poisoned patients. Oral charcoal alone is considered superior to gastric lavage if the drug in question is adsorbed by charcoal.

The performance of gastric lavage is contraindicated in any person who demonstrates compromised airway protective reflexes, unless they are intubated. Gastric lavage is also contraindicated in persons who have ingested corrosive substances (i.e., acids or alkalis) or hydrocarbons (unless containing highly toxic substances, such as paraquat, pesticides, heavy metals, halogenated and aromatic compounds), in those with known esophageal strictures, and in those with a history of gastric bypass surgery. Caution should be exercised in performing gastric lavage in combative patients and in those who possess medical conditions that could be exacerbated by performing this procedure, such as patients with bleeding diatheses.

Numerous complications have been reported in association with gastric lavage. Depending on the route selected for tube insertion, damage to the nasal mucosa, turbinates, pharynx, esophagus, and stomach have all been reported. After tube insertion, it is imperative to confirm correct placement. Radiographic confirmation of tube placement should especially be considered in young children and intubated patients. Instillation of lavage fluid and charcoal into the lungs through tubes inadvertently placed endotracheally has been reported. Perforation of the esophagus is also a potential complication. The large amount of fluid administered during lavage has been reported to cause fluid and electrolyte disturbances. In the pediatric population, these disturbances have been seen with both hypertonic and hypotonic lavage fluids. Hypothermia is a possible complication if the lavage fluid is not pre-warmed. Pulmonary aspiration of gastric contents or lavage fluid is the primary risk during gastric lavage, especially in patients with compromised airway protective reflexes.

Activated Charcoal

Activated charcoal acts by adsorbing a wide range of toxins present in the gastrointestinal tract, as well as by enhancing toxin elimination if systemic absorption has already occurred. It accomplishes the latter by creating a concentration gradient between the contents of the bowel and the circulation. In addition, it has the potential to interrupt enterohepatic circulation if the particular toxin is secreted in the bile and enters the gastrointestinal tract prior to reabsorption. Oral activated charcoal is given as a single dose or in multiple doses.

Single-dose activated charcoal is indicated if the healthcare provider estimates that a clinically significant fraction of the ingested substance remains in the GI tract, that the toxin is adsorbed by charcoal, and that further systemic absorption may result in clinical deterioration. Multiple doses may be considered if the clinician anticipates that the charcoal will result in increased clearance of an already absorbed drug. Activated charcoal should not be routinely administered, but rather should be reserved for cases in which serious toxicity is anticipated. It is most effective within the first 60 minutes after oral overdose and decreases in effectiveness over time.

The administration of charcoal is contraindicated in any person who demonstrates compromised airway protective reflexes, unless they are intubated. Intubation will *reduce* the risk of aspiration pneumonia but will not totally eliminate it. Charcoal administration is contraindicated in persons who have ingested corrosive substances (i.e., acids or alkalis). Not only does charcoal provide no benefit in a corrosive ingestion, but its administration could precipitate vomiting, obscure endoscopic visualization, and lead to complications if a perforation developed and charcoal entered the mediastinum, peritoneum, or pleural space. Charcoal should also be avoided in cases of pure aliphatic petroleum distillate ingestion. Caution should be exercised in using charcoal in patients who possess medical conditions that could be further compromised by charcoal ingestion, such as those with gastrointestinal perforation or bleeding.

Whole Bowel Irrigation

Whole bowel irrigation (WBI) has emerged as the newest technique in gastrointestinal decontamination. It involves the enteral administration of an osmotically balanced polyethylene glycol–electrolyte solution (PEG-ES) in a sufficient amount and rate to physically flush ingested substances through the gastrointestinal tract, purging the toxin before absorption can occur. PEG-ES is isosmotic, is not systemically absorbed, and will not cause electrolyte or fluid shifts. Available data suggest that the large volumes of this solution needed to mechanically propel pills, drug packets, or other substances through the gastrointestinal tract are safe, even in pregnant women and in young children. WBI may be considered for ingestions of exceedingly large quantities of potentially toxic substances, ingestions of toxins that are poorly adsorbed to activated charcoal, ingestions of delayed-release formulations, late presentations after ingestion of toxins, pharmacobezoars, and in body stuffers or packers. Common indications for WBI in the emergency department include the treatment of toxic ingestions of sustained-release medications (e.g., calcium channel blockers, theophylline, lithium) and iron tablets. WBI is contraindicated in patients with gastrointestinal obstruction, perforation, ileus, or significant gastrointestinal hemorrhage. It should also be avoided in patients with hemodynamic instability, an unprotected airway, or when there is suspicion for a corrosive ingestion.

ANTIDOTES

The number of pharmacologic antagonists or *antidotes* is quite limited. There are few agents that will rapidly reverse toxic effects and restore a patient to a previously healthy baseline state. Administering some pharmacologic

Table 1-5. Antidotes

Agent or Clinical Finding	Antidote
Acetaminophen	N-acetylcysteine
Benzodiazepines	Flumazenil
Beta blockers	Glucagon
Cardiac glycosides	Digoxin immune Fab
Crotalid envenomation	Crotalidae polyvalent immune Fab
Cyanide	Hydroxocobalamin
Ethylene glycol	Fomepizole
Iron	Deferoxamine
Isoniazid	Pyridoxine
Methanol	Fomepizole
Methemoglobinemia	Methylene blue
Opioids	Naloxone
Organophosphates	Atropine & Pralidoxime
Sulfonylureas	Octreotide

antagonists may actually worsen patient outcome compared to optimization of basic supportive care. As a result, antidotes should be used cautiously and with clearly understood indications and contraindications. Table 1-5 provides a list of antidotes. Selected antidotes will be discussed in further detail later in this book.

CONCLUSION

Healthcare providers will often be required to care for poisoned patients. Many of these patients will do well with simple observation and never develop significant toxicity. However, for patients who present with serious toxic effects or after potentially fatal ingestions, prompt action must be taken. As many poisons have no true antidote and the poison involved may initially be unknown, the first step is competent supportive care. Attention to the latter, vital signs and the prevention of complications are the most important steps. Indeed, these considerations alone will often ensure recovery.

Identifying the poison, either through history, recognition of a toxidrome, or laboratory analysis may help direct patient care or disposition and should therefore be attempted. There are several antidotes available which can be life-saving, and prompt identification of patients who may benefit from these must be sought.

Chapter 2 — Medications

ACETAMINOPHEN

What is acetaminophen?

N-acetyl-*p*-aminophenol (APAP), an analgesic and antipyretic agent

Where is acetaminophen found?

Acetaminophen is found in a large number of products, both OTC and prescription. It is combined with opioids to make analgesics such as Percocet®, Vicodin®, and Darvocet®, with antihistamines to make sleep aids such as Tylenol PM®, and with antihistamines and decongestants to form products such as NyQuil® and the Tylenol Cold® preparations.

What is the potentially hepatotoxic single dose?

When there are no coexisting health problems, a single acute overdose of over 150 mg/kg in an adult or 200 mg/kg in children under age 12 is potentially hepatotoxic.

How is acetaminophen metabolized?

The majority is usually metabolized in the liver through sulfation and glucuronidation with 5% to 10% metabolized by the cytochrome P450 system.

What is the elimination half-life?

4 hrs

How does overdose result in toxicity?

Acetaminophen overdose overwhelms the sulfation and glucuronidation pathways, shunting metabolism to the cytochrome P450 system and producing the toxic metabolite.

What is the hepatotoxic metabolite of acetaminophen?

N-acetyl-*p*-benzoquinoneimine (NAPQI)

How is this metabolite normally metabolized by the liver?

In sub-toxic doses, NAPQI is quickly conjugated with glutathione in hepatocytes, then renally eliminated. In overdose, the quantity of NAPQI overwhelms glutathione stores which results in accumulation of the toxin.

What is the mechanism of toxicity of this metabolite?

NAPQI binds to hepatic proteins → hepatic centrilobular necrosis

What groups are at high risk for acetaminophen toxicity?

1. Chronic alcoholics who overdose (↑ risk of liver damage)
2. Pregnant patients who overdose (↑ risk of fetal death)
3. Patients taking inducers of CYP2E1 (e.g., isoniazid)
4. Patients suffering from malnutrition (lower glutathione stores)

What are the classic clinical stages of acetaminophen poisoning?

Stage 1 (time of ingestion to 24 hrs) – anorexia, nausea, vomiting
Stage 2 (24–72 hrs post-ingestion) – elevation of transaminases, bilirubin and PT; nausea and vomiting may resolve
Stage 3 (72–96 hrs post-ingestion) – worsening hepatic necrosis with corresponding elevation in AST and ALT; may progress to coagulopathy, jaundice, hepatic and renal failure, encephalopathy, and death, or may progress to stage 4
Stage 4 (>96 hrs post-ingestion) – healing of liver damage with eventual resolution of enzymatic and metabolic abnormalities

What laboratory tests should be performed?

Plasma acetaminophen level 4 hrs post-ingestion for nonextended release preparations. BUN, creatinine, AST, ALT, PT/INR, and glucose are also warranted.

What is the Rumack-Matthew nomogram?

A graph depicting the treatment line for probable hepatic toxicity

What is the 4-hr treatment level?	150 mcg/mL
Is this the same level as in Europe?	No, the original treatment line was 200 mcg/mL at 4 hrs. The level was lowered to 150 mcg/mL in the U.S. to provide an extra margin of safety.
What is the recommended treatment for overdose?	1. Activated charcoal – if presenting within 1 hr of ingestion 2. N-acetylcysteine (NAC) – most efficacious if given within 8 hrs of ingestion 3. Antiemetics – ondansetron is preferred; avoid antiemetics with sedative properties or that are metabolized by the liver
How does NAC work?	Acts primarily by repleting glutathione. It also may enhance the sulfation pathway, $\uparrow$ blood flow to the liver, bind NAPQI, and help to reduce NAPQI back to acetaminophen.
How is NAC supplied?	Both IV and PO formulations. IV form appears to be as efficacious as PO form and can be given over 20 hrs as opposed to the 72-hr PO dose.
What is the traditional PO dosing schedule as approved by the U.S. Food and Drug Administration (FDA)?	140 mg/kg $\times$ 1 dose, then 70 mg/kg q4 hrs for 17 more doses
How do you treat a patient who is an unreliable historian with a suspected acetaminophen overdose?	In patients with an unknown time of ingestion and a detectable acetaminophen level, treat with NAC until acetaminophen level is undetectable and transaminases are normal or declining.
Does acetaminophen cause an acidosis?	While not part of the traditional MUDILES, acetaminophen in very large doses appears to act as a metabolic poison and can cause an anion gap metabolic acidosis.

AMANTADINE

What are the indications for amantadine?

It is an antiviral agent that is also used in the treatment of parkinsonian symptoms and as an arousal agent in patients with traumatic brain injury.

What is the mechanism of action of amantadine?

Its antiviral properties are mediated by its interference with the M2 protein, which is necessary for viral "uncoating." Amantadine's anti-parkinsonian properties are mediated by the release of dopamine and the blockade of its reuptake. It also may act as an NMDA antagonist.

What are some common side effects of amantadine?

Nervousness, anxiety, agitation, insomnia, exacerbations of seizures, and suicidal ideation in some patients

What are the clinical signs of acute toxicity?

In high doses, amantadine has anti-cholinergic effects including dry mucous membranes, tachycardia, and delirium. It also may cause visual hallucinations, ataxia, tremor, myoclonus, and dysrhythmias. There have been rare reports of seizures.

What is the treatment for acute toxicity?

Only supportive care, no antidote available

What syndrome can abrupt withdrawal precipitate?

NMS

What is NMS?

Neuroleptic malignant syndrome results from the relative lack of dopaminergic activity, either from addition of a dopamine blocker (e.g., antipsychotic agent) or the withdrawal of a dopaminergic agent (e.g., amantadine, carbidopa/levodopa, bromocriptine). This produces the symptoms of altered mental status, muscle rigidity, hyperthermia, and autonomic instability.

What physical exam findings help to differentiate NMS from serotonin syndrome?

NMS classically lacks hyperreflexia and clonus.

What is the treatment for NMS?

1. Aggressive cooling for temperatures >39°C (102°F) secondary to NMS induced by amantadine withdrawal
2. Benzodiazepines for agitation
3. Reinstitution of amantadine or other dopamine agonists should be considered.

ANESTHETICS

CENTRAL

What is malignant hyperthermia?

A rare condition occurring in genetically-susceptible individuals. It is triggered by exposure to halogenated general anesthetic agents and/or succinylcholine.

What are the clinical signs of malignant hyperthermia?

Hypercarbia, tachypnea, tachycardia, hyperthermia, muscle rigidity, hyperthermia, metabolic acidosis, skin mottling, and rhabdomyolysis

What is the most valuable early sign of malignant hyperthermia?

A rise in end tidal CO_2. Masseter muscle spasm may also herald the onset of malignant hyperthermia.

What are the possible consequences of malignant hyperthermia?

Sustained hypermetabolism can cause rhabdomyolysis due to cellular hypoxia. This can lead to profound hyperkalemia, resulting in dysrhythmias or myoglobinuric renal failure. Other complications include compartment syndrome due to muscle swelling, mesenteric ischemia, CHF, and disseminated intravascular coagulation (DIC).

What is the treatment for malignant hyperthermia?

1. Discontinue offending drug
2. Hyperventilate patient
3. Administer dantrolene

4. Actively cool patient to a maximum of 38.5°C (101.3°F)
5. Treat hyperkalemia

How does dantrolene work?

It inhibits sarcoplasmic calcium release, thereby relaxing skeletal muscle by disassociating excitation-contraction coupling.

What screening tests can be used in susceptible patients?

Caffeine-halothane contracture test

What adverse effects can occur with chronic abuse of nitrous oxide?

Megaloblastic anemia and myeloneuropathy can occur due to a functional vitamin B_{12} deficiency.

How does the myeloneuropathy present?

Paresthesias in the feet and hands, impaired gait, loss of manual dexterity, and hypoactive reflexes

By which mechanism can nitrous oxide use or abuse cause death or brain injury?

It can displace oxygen and act as a simple asphyxiant. This can occur if pure nitrous oxide is delivered during anesthesia.

What are the indications for etomidate?

Induction of anesthesia

What is the mechanism of action of etomidate?

Depresses the reticular activating system and mimics the effects of GABA

What is a common reaction with etomidate?

Myoclonus, due to disinhibition of extrapyramidal activity in some patients

What is a possible consequence of long-term exposure to etomidate?

Adrenocortical suppression; this is of particular concern in critically ill patients.

Propofol is in what class of anesthetics?

Sedative-hypnotic agents

What is the mechanism of action of propofol?

1. Activation of the $GABA_A$ receptor chloride channel
2. Antagonism of the NMDA receptor

What are the indications for propofol?

1. Rapid induction for general anesthesia
2. Sedation

Prior to propofol administration, what drug may be given to decrease pain at the injection site?

Lidocaine

What are some common adverse effects of propofol?

Hypotension, bradycardia, and conduction disturbances; the risk of these adverse effects increases with rapid boluses in the elderly.

What is propofol infusion syndrome?

A syndrome of bradycardia leading to cardiovascular collapse, accompanied by at least one of the following: metabolic acidosis, rhabdomyolysis, hyperlipidemia, or fatty liver.

What are the risk factors for propofol infusion syndrome?

Prolonged high-dose infusion (>48 hrs), concurrent catecholamine administration, high-dose steroids, and acute neurological injury.

How is propofol infusion syndrome treated?

1. Stop propofol infusion
2. Hemodynamic support
3. Hemodialysis or hemofiltration to correct acidosis, clear lipemia, and remove propofol

LOCAL

How are local anesthetics administered?

SQ, topical (e.g., skin, mucous membranes), nerve blocks (e.g., epidural, spinal, regional)

What are the indications for local anesthesia?

Local anesthetics are sold OTC for such afflictions as dental and hemorrhoid pain and are used in procedures such as laceration repair and endoscopy.

What is the mechanism of action of local anesthetics?

They inhibit sodium influx through the neuronal sodium channels to prevent an action potential, thereby inhibiting signal conduction.

What are the main classes of local anesthetics? Name some common drugs in each.

1. Ester-linked (aminoesters) – benzocaine, cocaine, procaine, tetracaine

2. Amide-linked (aminoamides) – lidocaine, bupivacaine, mepivacaine, prilocaine

This class contains two "**I's**" in the name (i.e., bup "**I**"vaca "**I**"ne).

What are the clinically relevant differences between these classes?

1. Aminoesters are metabolized by plasma cholinesterases
2. Aminoamides are metabolized by the liver

What are the half-lives of some local anesthetics?

1. Bupivacaine – 120–300 min
2. Cocaine – 60–150 min
3. Lidocaine – 60–120 min
4. Procaine – 7–8 min
5. Tetracaine – 5–10 min

What are the signs and symptoms of toxicity?

1. Local effects – prolonged anesthesia
2. Systemic – acute toxicity during infusion or infiltration results in AMS, including confusion and disorientation which may progress to seizures.
3. CV – manifests as hypotension, dysrhythmias, AV block, and asystole

Which local anesthetics carry a risk of methemoglobinemia?

This is most commonly reported with topical benzocaine; however, there have also been reports with lidocaine, procaine, and tetracaine.

How common are allergies to local anesthetics?

1 in 10,000

Can local anesthetics be used if a patient has an established allergy to a specific agent?

Yes, with caution. Use the opposite class of anesthetic (ester or amide) if allergy is known. If the class of anesthetic to which the patient is allergic is unknown, diphenhydramine can be used as an acceptable alternative as a local anesthetic.

What drug is often given with local anesthetics and why?

Epinephrine, to provide local vasoconstriction and slow the systemic absorption of the local anesthetic

What are the implications of co-administration of this drug on the half-life and maximum adult SQ dose of lidocaine?	Longer half-life (120 min) and larger maximum adult SQ dose (7 mg/kg with epinephrine vs. 4 mg/kg without)
Which local anesthetic can be used as an antidysrhythmic?	Lidocaine (type Ib antidysrhythmic)
What specific antidote may be used in toxicity due to local anesthetics?	None. Treatment is primarily supportive care. Direct-acting vasopressors (e.g., norepinephrine) should be used for refractory hypotension and benzodiazepines for seizures. Lipid emulsions have been studied but cannot be recommended at this time.

ANGIOTENSIN-CONVERTING ENZYME INHIBITORS

What commercially available medications are found in this class?	Captopril, enalapril, ramipril, quinapril, perindopril, lisinopril, benazepril, fosinopril
What is the mechanism of action of ACE inhibitors?	ACE converts inactive angiotensin I to angiotensin II in the pulmonary vasculature. Angiotensin II stimulates both vasoconstriction and release of aldosterone and vasopressin, resulting in ↑ BP. ACE inhibitors ↓ production of angiotensin II → ↓ BP.
What clinical uses exist for ACE inhibitors?	1. Treatment of hypertension 2. Prevention of diabetic renal failure in patients suffering from diabetic nephropathy 3. Prevention of CHF and other cardiac events, even in the absence of hypertension
What are the adverse effects of this medication?	Dry persistent cough, angioedema, hypotension, hyperkalemia, headache, dizziness, fatigue, nausea, renal impairment

How does ACE inhibitor-related angioedema present?	Well-demarcated, nonpitting edema, most commonly of the tongue and mucous membranes of the upper airway, lips and eyes; usually painless and nonpruritic
When does ACE inhibitor-related angioedema occur?	At anytime during treatment, with reports of days to many years after initiation
What is the incidence of ACE inhibitor-related angioedema?	Commonly reported as 0.1% to 0.2%. Some report incidence approaching 0.7%.
What peptide is thought to cause both ACE inhibitor-related angioedema and cough?	Bradykinin, normally degraded by ACE
What is the treatment of angioedema?	Airway management should be of primary concern. IV diphenhydramine, corticosteroids, and SQ epinephrine should be considered in appropriate cases, but these agents may not significantly alter clinical progression.
What are the predominant signs and symptoms of ACE inhibitor overdose?	Acute ACE inhibitor overdose does not often result in significant toxicity. Hypotension and, occasionally, bradycardia may occur. Hyperkalemia may be seen, even in therapeutic doses.
What treatments are recommended for overdose of ACE inhibitors?	1. Activated charcoal, if given within 1 hr of overdose 2. Supportive care (e.g., IV fluids for hypotension) 3. Rarely, vasopressors may be indicated in refractory hypotension. 4. If hyperkalemia develops, treat with standard therapies.

ANGIOTENSIN RECEPTOR BLOCKERS

What commercially available medications are found in this class?	Valsartan, telmisartan, losartan, irbesartan, olmesartan, candesartan, eprosartan

What is the mechanism of action of angiotensin receptor blockers?

Angiotensin receptor blockers prevent activation of angiotensin II (AT_1) receptors, reducing BP. Angiotensin II normally stimulates vasoconstriction, aldosterone, and vasopressin release $\rightarrow \uparrow$ BP.

What clinical uses exist for angiotensin receptor blockers?

1. Treatment of hypertension in patients intolerant of ACE inhibitors
2. Some efficacy in treatment of CHF and prevention of diabetic renal failure in patients with diabetic nephropathy

What are the adverse effects of this class of drugs?

Dizziness, headache, hyperkalemia, first-dose orthostatic hypotension, and rare cases of angioedema

What are the signs and symptoms of angiotensin receptor blocker overdose?

Acute angiotensin receptor blocker overdose data is limited. Hypotension and bradycardia may occur in rare cases. Hyperkalemia may be seen, even in therapeutic doses.

What treatments are recommended for angiotensin receptor blocker overdose?

1. Activated charcoal, if given within 1 hr of overdose
2. Supportive care (e.g., IV fluids for hypotension)
3. Rarely, vasopressors may be indicated in refractory hypotension.
4. If hyperkalemia develops, treat with standard therapies.

ANTIBACTERIAL AGENTS

What mechanism causes most serious adverse reactions to antibacterial agents?

Allergic reactions

What symptoms are typically seen with oral overdose of antibacterial agents?

Primarily GI (i.e., nausea, vomiting, diarrhea)

What cardiovascular toxicity is typically associated with macrolides (e.g., erythromycin) and quinolones (e.g., ciprofloxacin)?

QT prolongation with subsequent torsade de pointes. This is especially relevant when given with other drugs known to prolong the QT interval (i.e., antipsychotics, cyclic antidepressants, antihistamines).

What neuromuscular condition may be exacerbated by administration of erythromycin or aminoglycosides?

Myasthenia gravis. These agents may also potentiate pharmacologic neuromuscular blockade.

Which class(es) of antibacterial agents are associated with ototoxicity?

Aminoglycosides (e.g., gentamicin, tobramycin), vancomycin, macrolides. Macrolide-induced ototoxicity typically reverses with cessation of drug.

Which class(es) of antibacterial agents are associated with nephrotoxicity?

Aminoglycosides, vancomycin, polymyxins, tetracyclines, first-generation cephalosporins (chronic use)

Which class(es) of antibacterial agents, in acute overdose, may present with seizures and by what mechanism?

High-dose IV penicillin (>50 million units) and imipenem. Both bind to picrotoxin site on neuronal chloride channels and indirectly antagonize nearby GABA binding site.

Which antibacterial agents are known to cause a disulfiram-like reaction when combined with ethanol?

Metronidazole is the classic example. However, chloramphenicol, nitrofurantoin, and certain cephalosporins have been implicated.

Which antibacterial agent(s) may cause nephrogenic diabetes insipidus?

Demeclocycline

Which antibacterial agent(s) is known to cause hemolysis in patients with G6PD deficiency?

Nitrofurantoin

Which antituberculosis agent is associated with red coloration of tears and urine?

Rifampin

What syndromic reactions can be seen with IM or IV administration of large doses of penicillin G?

1. *Hoigne syndrome* (minutes post-injection) – hallucinations (auditory and/or visual), fear of death, perceptions of changes in body shape, tachycardia, hypertension
2. *Jarisch-Herxheimer reaction* (hours post-injection for syphilis treatment) – myalgias, fever, chills, diaphoresis, rash, hypotension, rigors, headache. This self-limited reaction may also be seen with treatment of tick-borne diseases.

Overdose with which antibacterial agents may result in crystalluria?

Ampicillin, amoxicillin, sulfonamides (older, less-soluble forms), norfloxacin, ciprofloxacin

What classic syndrome is seen with vancomycin administration?

Red man syndrome. Anaphylactoid reaction named for the prominent skin flushing, but also includes hypotension, dyspnea, pruritis, urticaria. It is related to the rate of IV administration.

How may this complication of vancomycin use be avoided?

Administer slowly and pretreat with diphenhydramine.

How does acute and chronic chloramphenicol toxicity present?

1. Acute – nausea, vomiting, hypotension, hypothermia, metabolic acidosis, abdominal distention, cardiovascular collapse
2. Chronic – bone marrow suppression, "gray baby syndrome"

What is "gray baby syndrome"?

Associated with chloramphenicol use in neonates and toddlers and includes vomiting, abdominal distention, cyanosis, irregular respirations, metabolic acidosis, hypothermia, flaccidity, hypotension, cardiovascular collapse. Rarely seen prior to the second day of therapy.

Why are infants at greater risk for "gray baby syndrome"?	A limited ability to conjugate chloramphenicol (by glucuronyl transferase) leaves an abundance of the active form in the blood.
What specific treatment is indicated for isoniazid (INH) toxicity?	Pyridoxine (Vitamin B_6)
What specific treatment is indicated for trimethoprim toxicity?	Leucovorin (folinic acid)
What toxic effects can occur with dapsone poisoning?	Methemoglobinemia, sulfhemoglobinemia, and hemolysis
Which antibiotic is associated with serotonin syndrome?	Linezolid

ANTICHOLINERGICS

What common drug classes may have anticholinergic effects?	Antihistamines, antiparkinsonian drugs, antispasmodics (GI, urinary), skeletal muscle relaxants, tricyclic antidepressants, belladonna alkaloids, antipsychotics
What are some natural sources of anticholinergic alkaloids?	1. Jimson weed (*Datura stramonium*) 2. Black henbane (*Hyocyamus niger*) 3. Deadly nightshade (*Atropa belladonna*)
Name the classic drug that causes the anticholinergic toxidrome.	Atropine
What is the mechanism of toxicity of the anticholinergic agents?	Competitive antagonism of ACh at muscarinic cholinergic receptors; nicotinic cholinergic receptors (neuromuscular junction) remain unaffected.
What part(s) of the body is/are most affected by anticholinergic drugs?	Exocrine glands (e.g., sweat, salivary), muscle cells (smooth and cardiac), CNS

What is the typical clinical presentation of the anticholinergic toxidrome?

Warm, dry, and flushed skin; dry mucous membranes; hyperthermia; tachycardia; mydriasis; cycloplegia; delirium; ileus; urinary retention

What are the key aspects to differentiate this from the sympathomimetic toxidrome?

Dry skin and mucous membranes, hypoactive bowel sound, urinary retention

What is the mnemonic (and the classic findings) of the anticholinergic toxidrome?

"**Dry** as a bone (dry skin); **blind** as a bat (mydriasis); **red** as a beet (flushed skin); **hot** as a hare (hyperthermia); **mad** as a hatter (delirium); **full** as a flask (urinary retention)"

What is the classic antihistamine that causes anticholinergic toxicity?

Diphenhydramine

What are the other features of diphenhydramine poisoning?

Seizures and QRS widening, with subsequent risk of ventricular dysrhythmias

What is the mechanism of QRS widening?

Sodium channel blockade

How is sodium channel blockade treated?

IV sodium bicarbonate

What is the mechanism by which diphenhydramine causes seizures?

Antihistamine effect; pure anticholinergic agents rarely cause seizures

How does the chemical structure of the anticholinergic agent govern its effects?

Tertiary amines (e.g., atropine, scopolamine) exhibit more central effects owing to their penetration of the blood-brain barrier, whereas quaternary amines (e.g., glycopyrrolate) are not well-absorbed centrally.

How does anticholinergic overdose affect other ingestions?

Decreased GI motility may delay absorption and cause delayed or prolonged toxicity.

How is the diagnosis of anticholinergic toxicity made?	Principally based upon the history and features of the classic toxidrome
Is there an antidote?	Physostigmine may provide improvement or reversal of symptoms if used in the appropriate context. Physostigmine inhibits acetylcholinesterase and ↑ ACh available at the synaptic cleft.
What are the side effects of physostigmine?	Salivation, weakness, nausea, vomiting, diarrhea, and ↑ respiratory secretions. There have been reports of seizures and asystole when given to patients intoxicated with tricyclic antidepressants.

ANTICONVULSANTS

PLEASE NOTE THAT THE FOLLOWING COMPOUNDS ARE ADDRESSED IN THEIR OWN SECTIONS: BARBITURATES, BENZODIAZEPINES, CARBAMAZEPINE, PHENYTOIN, AND VALPROIC ACID.

What are the known mechanisms of anticonvulsants? Give an example for each mechanism.	1. Affect ion flux (especially sodium ion currents) across cell membranes (e.g., zonisamide, felbamate) 2. Enhance postsynaptic action of GABA (e.g., tiagabine, vigabatrin) 3. Inhibit release of excitatory neurotransmitters (e.g., lamotrigine) 4. Inhibit carbonic anhydrase (possibly topiramate and zonisamide)
What signs and symptoms are commonly seen with an anticonvulsant overdose?	1. AMS (including lethargy, anxiety, confusion, irritability, somnolence) 2. Ataxia 3. Nausea and vomiting 4. Coma, respiratory depression, and hypotension are typically seen only with large overdoses.
What are the common chronic adverse reactions to anticonvulsants?	Rash, dizziness, hangover, behavioral disturbances (e.g., emotional lability, depression, suicidality, impaired judgment, inattention to personal hygiene)

What forms of anticonvulsant toxicity necessitate immediate cessation of treatment?	Allergic reaction and hemotoxicity
What are the pertinent considerations of anticonvulsant therapy in special populations?	1. Pregnancy – almost all anticonvulsants are teratogenic 2. Children – anticonvulsants often induce hyperactivity
Which anticonvulsant carries a "black-box" warning?	Lamotrigine, due to its potential to induce life-threatening rashes (i.e., Stevens-Johnson syndrome, toxic epidermal necrolysis)
Which anticonvulsants have been associated with seizures in overdose?	Tiagabine, lamotrigine, topiramate, carbamazepine, and phenytoin in massive overdose
Which anticonvulsant is associated with non-anion gap metabolic acidosis and hyperkalemia?	Topiramate, due to carbonic anhydrase inhibition
Which anticonvulsants are associated with anticonvulsant hypersensitivity syndrome?	Phenytoin, carbamazepine, phenobarbital, primidone, lamotrigine

ANTIDEPRESSANTS

CYCLIC

What are cyclic antidepressants (CA)?	Ring-structured antidepressants used to treat disorders such as depression, chronic pain, migraines, and attention deficit hyperactivity disorder (ADHD)
What are some examples of commonly prescribed CAs?	Amitriptyline, amoxapine, clomipramine, dothiepin, doxepin, imiprimine, maprotiline, nortriptyline, protriptyline, trimipramine
What should the clinician anticipate in the CA overdose patient?	Be prepared for <u>rapid</u> deterioration, which includes CNS depression, seizures, dysrhythmias, and/or cardiovascular instability. Even an asymptomatic patient

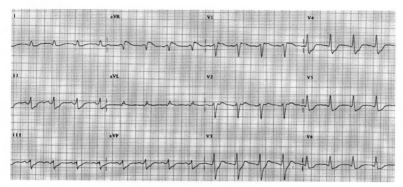

Figure 2-1. QRS prolongation.

can decompensate in <1 hr following overdose.

What are the reported ECG manifestations of CA toxicity?

1. Sinus tachycardia
2. QRS complex widening >100 msec (Fig. 2-1)
3. QTc prolongation that can result in torsade de pointes (Fig. 2-2)
4. A rightward axis often is present at the frontal plane terminal 40 msec (T 40-msec) of the QRS. This manifests as a negative S wave in lead I and a tall, positive R wave in lead aVR ("terminal R wave") (Fig. 2-3).
5. Right bundle branch block; this decreased conduction to the right fascicle is the presumed mechanism by which reentrant ventricular rhythms develop, causing VT in severe ingestions (Fig. 2-4).

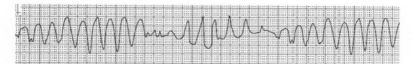

Figure 2-2. Torsade de pointes.

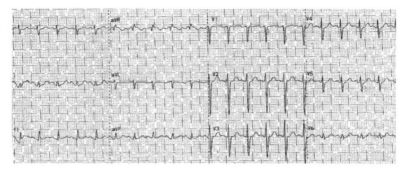

Figure 2-3. Right axis deviation and "terminal R wave."

Which ECG findings predict serious toxicity?

A QRS interval >100 msec and/or a terminal R wave in lead aVR measuring over 3 mm in height. One study showed that half the patients with a QRS interval >160 msec experienced dysrhythmias.

What are the 7 mechanisms of CA toxicity and the subsequent effects of each?

1. Fast cardiac Na^+ channel blockade – slows phase 0 depolarization, widening the QRS; decreased cardiac contractility and dromotropy lead to hypotension
2. Cardiac K^+ efflux channel blockade – slows phase 3 repolarization of the action potential, resulting in elongation of the QT interval
3. Alpha 1-adrenergic receptor blockade – peripheral vasodilation leads to hypotension

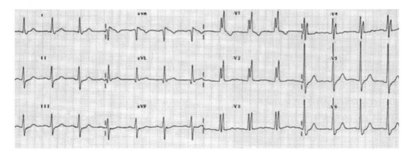

Figure 2-4. Right bundle branch block.

4. Cholinergic (muscarinic) receptor blockade – anticholinergic toxidrome
5. Histaminergic (H_1) receptor blockade – sedation and seizures
6. GABA receptor blockade – seizures
7. Presynaptic monoamine reuptake inhibition (serotonin, norepinephrine, dopamine) – tachycardia and hypertension seen during initial stages of toxicity, followed by hypotension due to depletion of norepinephrine

What are the hallmark signs of CA toxicity?

1. Cardiotoxicity – dysrhythmias and/or QRS duration $\geq$100 msec
2. CNS toxicity – seizures and/or AMS

Which CAs have been reported to cause isolated status epilepticus with no QRS widening or anticholinergic signs?

Amoxapine and maprotiline

What considerations should be made regarding the CA-toxic patient experiencing seizures?

1. Treat seizures with IV benzodiazepines.
2. Avoid phenytoin as it may exacerbate cardiac Na^+ channel blockade.
3. Monitor for acidosis and hyperthermia.
4. Avoid paralytic agents, as they can mask seizure activity.

How should the CA overdose be treated?

1. QRS prolongation – sodium bicarbonate
2. Hypotension unresponsive to IV fluids and sodium bicarbonate – direct vasopressors (e.g., phenylephrine; avoid dopamine)
3. Seizures – benzodiazepines
4. QT prolongation – magnesium sulfate

Does sodium bicarbonate treat seizures?

No, seizures are caused by other mechanisms. However, sodium bicarbonate can attenuate the acidosis caused by prolonged seizure activity that may predispose the patient to dysrhythmias.

Are there any other contraindicated treatments?	1. Physostigmine has been reported to induce seizure activity and asystole. 2. Flumazenil may induce seizure activity. 3. Type Ia and Ic antidysrhythmics may ↑ QRS interval and the likelihood of dysrhythmias.

MONOAMINE OXIDASE INHIBITORS

What is monoamine oxidase?	An enzyme that degrades biogenic amines. It, along with catechol-O-methyl transferase (COMT), prevents the build-up of biogenic amines in the neuronal synapse.
What are the indications for MAOIs?	1. Severe depression (especially atypical depression) 2. Phobias and anxiety disorders 3. Parkinson's disease (selegiline only)
What are the broad classes of MAOIs?	1. 1st generation – isocarboxazid, phenelzine, tranylcypromine 2. 2nd generation – selegiline, moclobemide
What are the subtypes of MAO, and where are they found?	1. MAO-A – found in neurons, the liver, and intestinal walls 2. MAO-B – found in neurons
Which neurotransmitters are preferentially degraded by MAO-A?	Biogenic amines – serotonin, tyramine, norepinephrine
Which neurotransmitters are preferentially degraded by MAO-B?	Dopamine
What are some common foods that interact with MAOIs?	Primarily tyramine-containing products, including beer, fava beans, aged cheese, aged meats, pickled foods, red wine, yeast extracts, and pepperoni
What is the mechanism by which foods cause MAOI toxicity?	MAOIs inhibit intestinal MAO-A, allowing dietary tyramine to be absorbed in the intestine. Tyramine indirectly

releases norepinephrine, causing a hyper-adrenergic response.

Which MAOIs are less likely to cause food interactions?

Selegiline is selective for MAO-B, and moclobemide binds reversibly to MAO. Both are unlikely to cause food interactions.

Name some common drugs that may precipitate a hyperadrenergic response in association with MAOIs.

Amphetamines, cocaine, phentermine, PCP

What is the mechanism?

These drugs cause release of norepinephrine from the presynaptic terminal, resulting in a sympathomimetic syndrome.

What hyperthermic syndrome can result from MAOI use?

Serotonin syndrome

Which medications increase this risk?

Concurrent use of any medication that ↑ serotonin levels, including SSRIs, LSD, dextromethorphan, meperidine, and tramadol

What are the clinical signs of serotonin syndrome?

AMS, hyperthermia, autonomic instability, hyperreflexia, and clonus

What is the primary treatment for serotonin syndrome?

Benzodiazepines for sedation, aggressive cooling for hyperthermia, and IV fluids

What 5-HT$_{2A}$ antagonist is considered an "antidote" for serotonin toxicity?

Cyproheptadine

Are there any drawbacks to using cyproheptadine?

It can only be administered PO, and it has anticholinergic properties.

What are the clinical signs of an acute MAOI overdose?

Severe hypertension, hyperthermia, delirium, seizures, cardiovascular collapse, and multi-system organ failure

What is the treatment of MAOI toxicity?

Supportive care. Short-acting IV agents should be used to control hypertension.

Beta-blockers are contraindicated secondary to the risk of worsening hypertension due to unopposed alpha-adrenergic activity. As vital signs may be labile, hypotension should be treated with a direct-acing agent like norepinephrine. First-line treatment for seizures is benzodiazepines; however, pyridoxine should be considered in refractory seizures, as some of the MAOIs are derived from hydrazine.

What other common drugs exhibit MAOI-like activity?

Procarbazine and linezolid

SELECTIVE SEROTONIN REUPTAKE INHIBITORS

What is the mechanism of action of selective serotonin reuptake inhibitors (SSRIs)?

Inhibition of serotonin reuptake into the presynaptic neuron, resulting in ↑ serotonin in the synaptic cleft

Why are SSRIs preferred over cyclic antidepressants (CAs)?

Safety profile; unlike CAs, SSRIs are lethal only in very high doses and essentially lack serious cardiovascular effects.

What are some common adverse effects of SSRIs?

Nausea, drowsiness, headache, vivid dreams, weight gain, anorgasmia

What is the clinical presentation of an SSRI overdose?

CNS effects – sedation, ataxia, tremor, lethargy, seizures, coma

Is there a specific treatment for SSRI overdose?

No

What is serotonin syndrome?

A constellation of varied symptoms that occurs secondary to a large dose of a serotonergic drug or combination of two or more serotonergic agents

Name some of the agents that induce serotonin syndrome.

1. Medications that inhibit serotonin reuptake (e.g., SSRIs, CAs, venlafaxine, meperidine, dextromethorphan, tramadol)
2. Medications that inhibit serotonin breakdown (e.g., MAOIs, linezolid)

3. Agents that ↑ serotonin release (e.g., amphetamines, cocaine, reserpine)
4. Agents that act as serotonin agonists (e.g., lithium, LSD, sumatriptan)
5. Agents that ↑ serotonin synthesis (e.g., L-tryptophan)

How does serotonin syndrome present?

It is classically described as a triad of AMS, autonomic instability, and neuromuscular hyperactivity. It presents as a continuum of symptoms, often starting with milder nonspecific symptoms, such as akathisia, agitation, diaphoresis, tachycardia, and hypertension. These progress to delirium, hyperthermia, clonus, and hyperreflexia. If not recognized and treated, it can lead to coma, rigidity, rhabdomyolysis, multisystem organ failure, and death.

How is serotonin syndrome treated?

1. Discontinue and avoid any serotonergic medicines.
2. Aggressive supportive care is the preferred treatment for this condition. Cyproheptadine is an antihistamine with $5HT_{1a}$ and $5HT_{2a}$ antagonist properties and has been proposed as an antidote for serotonin syndrome; however, it can only be administered orally, has potential side effects, and has little solid evidence of efficacy.
3. Benzodiazepines should be given and titrated to control agitation and neuromuscular hyperactivity.
4. Monitor temperature and treat hyperthermia with active cooling.
5. Monitor for rhabdomyolysis and administer IV fluids.

What is "discontinuation syndrome"?

A constellation of withdrawal symptoms seen within 24 hrs of stopping or rapidly decreasing the dose of SSRIs

What are the symptoms associated with the abrupt discontinuation of SSRIs?

Xerostomia, headache, insomnia, tremor, akathisia, "brain zap" or electric shock sensations

What population is at increased risk for suicide when starting SSRIs?

A black box warning exists for patients <18 years of age

OTHER

List the 4 categories of atypical antidepressants.

1. Serotonin and norepinephrine reuptake inhibitors (SNRIs)
2. Norepinephrine and dopamine reuptake inhibitors (NDRIs)
3. Serotonin antagonist and reuptake inhibitors (SARIs)
4. Norepinephrine and serotonin antagonists (NASAs)

List examples of each class.

1. SNRIs – venlafaxine, duloxetine, atomoxetine
2. NDRIs – bupropion
3. SARIs – nefazodone, trazodone
4. NASAs – mirtazapine

What are the toxic effects of SNRIs?

CNS depression, tachycardia, seizures, QTc prolongation (may be delayed), QRS prolongation has been reported, serotonin syndrome

What are the toxic effects of NDRIs?

CNS depression, seizures (bupropion lowers seizure threshold), sinus tachycardia, exacerbation of psychosis

What are the toxic effects of both SARIs and NASAs?

Peripheral alpha-adrenergic blockade, CNS depression, serotonin syndrome

How does atypical antidepressant toxicity typically present?

Acute mental status change, ataxia, nausea and vomiting, tachycardia with hypotension, seizures, and serotonin syndrome

Which atypical antidepressants can cause hypotension and priapism, and by what mechanism?

SARIs (e.g., trazodone) and NASAs (e.g., mirtazapine), due to alpha-adrenergic blockade

How can bupropion exacerbate psychosis?

Excessive dopaminergic effects at higher doses

Which atypical antidepressant may cause QT prolongation?

Venlafaxine

How is atypical antidepressant toxicity diagnosed?

Principally clinical. Should be suspected if there is a history of depression.

Are drug serum levels helpful?

Drug levels are not routinely available

List the basic principles of treatment for atypical antidepressant toxicity.

1. Supportive care and monitoring
2. Activated charcoal, if available shortly following ingestion
3. Benzodiazepines for seizures
4. QTc prolongation may be treated with IV magnesium sulfate
5. QRS prolongation may be treated with IV sodium bicarbonate
6. Direct-acting vasopressors are indicated for hypotension unresponsive to IV fluids

What syndrome may result from use of antidepressants?

Serotonin syndrome

Define serotonin syndrome.

An iatrogenic toxidrome due to excessive serotonergic activity in the CNS by overdose or combination of serotonergic medications

Name some of the agents that induce serotonin syndrome.

1. Medications that inhibit serotonin reuptake (i.e., SSRIs, CAs, venlafaxine, meperidine, dextromethorphan, and tramadol)
2. Medications that inhibit serotonin breakdown (i.e., MAOIs and linezolid)
3. Agents that ↑ serotonin release (i.e., amphetamines, cocaine, and reserpine)
4. Agents that act as serotonin agonists (i.e., lithium, LSD, and sumatriptan)
5. Agents that ↑ serotonin synthesis (L-tryptophan)

What is the triad of effects of serotonin syndrome?

1. CNS effects – mental status change, hypomania, agitation, coma
2. Autonomic effects – shivering, fever, flushing, hypertension, tachycardia, nausea, vomiting, diarrhea
3. Neuromuscular effects – myoclonus, tremor, hyperreflexia

How is serotonin syndrome diagnosed?

History consistent with exposure and the above toxidromic features. There is no specific diagnostic test.

How is serotonin syndrome treated?

1. Stop the offending agents
2. Supportive care (e.g., IV fluids)
3. Benzodiazepines for sedation
4. Cooling for hyperthermia

What 5-HT$_{2A}$ antagonist is considered an "antidote" for serotonin toxicity?

Cyproheptadine

Are there any drawbacks to using cyproheptadine?

It can only be administered PO and it has anticholinergic properties.

ANTIDIARRHEAL AGENTS

What are the three primary classes of antidiarrheal drugs, and which is most dangerous in overdose?

1. Antimotility agents (most dangerous)
2. Intraluminal agents
3. Antisecretory agents

The antimotility agent Lomotil® contains a combination of drugs from which two classes?

Opioids and anticholinergics (diphenoxylate and atropine, respectively)

Why should patients who overdose on Lomotil® be observed?

Both components contribute to slowed gut activity and result in delayed absorption

How long should a child suspected of ingesting any amount of Lomotil® be observed?

At least 18 hrs

In toxicity due to these combination agents, when do the anticholinergic effects typically present relative to the opioid effects?	Unpredictable; can be before, during, or after
Diphenoxylate is a structural analog of which opioid analgesic?	Meperidine
What metabolite of diphenoxylate is 5 times more potent as an opioid than its parent compound and has a longer elimination half-life?	Difenoxin
What is the antidote for severe diphenoxylate or loperamide overdose?	Naloxone. Repeat dosing may be necessary due to short duration of action relative to these opioids.

ANTIEMETIC AGENTS

What are the two primary mechanisms for antiemetic drugs?	1. Serotonin (5-HT$_3$) receptor antagonism (e.g., ondansetron, dolasetron, granisetron, palonosetron) 2. Dopamine antagonism, such as phenothiazines (e.g., prochlorperazine, promethazine), butyrophenones (e.g., droperidol), and benzamides (e.g., metoclopramide)
What is the most common adverse reaction with the antiemetic dopamine antagonists?	Extrapyramidal reactions (i.e., akathisia and dystonic reactions). These can be seen with any antiemetic which acts through central dopamine antagonism.
What drugs can you use to treat extrapyramidal reactions?	1. Dystonic reactions should be treated with either diphenhydramine or benztropine (i.e., anticholinergic agents). 2. Akathisia can be treated with diphenhydramine; propranolol and

benzodiazepines have also been successfully utilized.

Why does droperidol have a "black box" warning?

Concerns about QT prolongation, torsade de pointes, and unexplained deaths

What are the possible clinical effects of an overdose of the phenothiazine antiemetics?

1. CNS depression (common)
2. Extrapyramidal reactions due to dopamine blockade
3. Hypotension and/or reflex tachycardia due to alpha-adrenergic blockade
4. QT interval prolongation due to cardiac potassium channel blockade

Which antiemetics can cause NMS?

The dopamine antagonists

Which antiemetic has been associated with methemoglobinemia?

Metoclopramide

In which type of patient should metoclopramide be avoided?

In patients with suspected mechanical bowel obstruction; it causes accelerated GI motility via 5-HT$_4$ agonist activity and theoretically could worsen colic.

ANTIFUNGAL AGENTS

How is amphotericin B administered therapeutically?

IV

What is the mechanism of action of amphotericin B?

Binds to ergosterol on cell membranes of fungi → ↑ permeability and cell death

How is amphotericin B eliminated?

Renal

What is the elimination half-life of amphotericin B?

15 days

What are the acute adverse effects of therapeutic amphotericin B administration?

Fever, chills, nausea, vomiting, diarrhea, chest discomfort, tachycardia, dyspnea

How can these effects be minimized?	1. Slow infusion rate 2. Pre-treat with antihistamines, acetaminophen, NSAIDs, and steroids
What adverse effect is commonly seen during treatment with amphotericin B?	Renal dysfunction
What is the maximum therapeutic dose of amphotericin B?	1.5 mg/kg/day
What may be seen with an acute overdose of amphotericin B?	Fatal cardiac dysrhythmias
How is flucytosine administered?	PO
What is the mechanism of action of flucytosine?	Converted to fluorouracil in fungal cells, which inhibits DNA synthesis by interfering with thymidylate synthetase
How is flucytosine eliminated?	Renal
What is the elimination half-life of flucytosine?	2.5 to 6 hrs
What is the principal mechanism of toxicity of flucytosine?	Bone marrow suppression
Are enhanced elimination methods effective for flucytosine?	Hemodialysis has been shown to enhance elimination of the drug (minimally protein-bound)
What specific treatments are available for flucytosine overdoses?	Generally supportive. Colony stimulating factor has been used for neutropenia.
What is the mechanism of action of fluconazole?	Inhibits sterol synthesis in fungi

How is fluconazole eliminated?	Renal
What is the elimination half-life of fluconazole?	30 hrs
What are the untoward effects of fluconazole?	Elevated liver enzymes, nausea, vomiting, headache, rash, pruritus
By which mechanism do some azole antifungals (e.g., fluconazole and miconazole) cause drug interactions?	Inhibition of CYP3A4

ANTIHISTAMINES

What are the indications for the use of antihistamines?	1. Allergy-related symptoms 2. Common cold symptoms, including cough 3. Motion sickness 4. Mild insomnia
What differentiates first- and second-generation antihistamines?	Second-generation antihistamines are less lipid-soluble and are thus unable to cross the blood-brain barrier, rendering them nonsedating. Second-generation agents are generally less toxic.
What are examples of first-generation antihistamines?	Diphenhydramine, promethazine, meclizine, chlorpheniramine
What are examples of second-generation antihistamines?	Loratadine, desloratadine, cetirizine, fexofenadine
What is the mechanism of toxicity of first-generation antihistamines?	Blockade at H_1 receptors and antimuscarinic (anticholinergic) effects
What antihistamines were taken off the market for reports of cardiac toxicity (QT prolongation and torsade de pointes)?	Terfenadine and astemizole

What is the clinical presentation of first-generation antihistamine overdose?

Flushed skin, anhydrosis, tachycardia, dry mucous membranes, mydriasis, ileus, urinary retention, fever, and delirium. In severe cases, this can progress to seizures, coma, and rhabdomyolysis. QRS and QT prolongation, as well as wide complex dysrhythmias have been reported with specific antihistamines (e.g., diphenhydramine) in overdose.

What is the toxidrome this constellation of symptoms represents?

Anticholinergic

What is the mnemonic for the anticholinergic toxidrome?

"**Dry** as a bone (dry skin); **blind** as a bat (mydriasis); **red** as a beet (flushed skin); **hot** as a hare (hyperthermia); **mad** as a hatter (delirium); **full** as a flask (urinary retention)"

How does diphenhydramine produce QRS widening?

Na^+ channel blockade

What is the treatment for QRS prolongation?

IV sodium bicarbonate

How is the diagnosis of antihistamine overdose made?

Primarily based on history and anticholinergic toxidrome. In addition, labs including electrolytes, glucose, CPK, and ECG should be obtained.

What specific antidotes exist for treating antihistamine toxicity?

Physostigmine can be used to reverse anticholinergic symptoms, but should be used with extreme care.

Which medicines are contraindicated for antihistamine-induced dysrhythmias?

Class Ia, Ic, and III antidysrhythmics (may further prolong QRS or QT interval)

How long should patients with antihistamine overdose be monitored?

Signs or symptoms are expected to develop within 4 hrs of overdose.

What is the recommended treatment for antihistamine overdose?

1. Benzodiazepines for agitation, seizures, hyperthermia (if related to ↑ muscle activity)
2. Assess for co-ingestions (e.g., acetaminophen-containing products)
3. Aggressive cooling for severe hyperthermia >40°C (104°F)
4. Sodium bicarbonate (1–2 mEq/kg) for QRS prolongation
5. Consider physostigmine for delirium or diagnostic purposes
6. Activated charcoal may be of benefit, even if the patient's presentation is delayed (slowed gut motility due to anticholinergic effects)

Are H$_2$ antagonists as toxic as H$_1$ antagonists?

H$_2$ antagonists have a high toxic-to-therapeutic index; these agents rarely cause significant toxicity, and treatment consists of supportive care.

ANTIHYPERLIPIDEMIA AGENTS

What is another name for HMG-CoA reductase inhibitors?

"Statins"

What is the mechanism of action of these agents?

Competitive inhibition of 3-hydroxy-3-methylglutaryl-coenzyme A (HMG-CoA) reductase, blocking the enzymatic conversion of HMG-CoA to mevalonate, an early step in hepatic cholesterol synthesis

What adverse effect on muscle may occur with the therapeutic use of HMG-CoA reductase inhibitors?

Myopathy with subsequent rhabdomyolysis and hyperkalemia

What are the effects of acute HMG-CoA reductase inhibitor toxicity?

Overall, HMG-CoA reductase inhibitors have limited toxicity in acute overdose.

Is there a specific treatment for HMG-CoA reductase inhibitor toxicity?

Supportive care only

What are some common bile acid sequestrants?	Cholestyramine, colesevelam, colestipol
What is the mechanism of action of the bile acid sequestrants?	Bind bile acids in the GI tract, forming an insoluble complex that undergoes fecal elimination
Are bile acid sequestrants absorbed in the GI tract?	No
What are the potential toxic effects of bile acid sequestrants?	Bloating, constipation, impaired GI absorption of other xenobiotics
What is the mechanism of action of niacin?	Several mechanisms have been proposed. Among these are that niacin inhibits release of free fatty acids from adipose tissue, ↓ hepatic lipoprotein synthesis, ↑ fecal sterol elimination, and ↑ activity of lipoprotein lipase.
Extended-release niacin has been associated with what organ system dysfunction?	Severe hepatotoxicity
What untoward effect of therapeutic niacin therapy on the skin may occur?	Flushing ("niacin flush")
What medication can reduce the side effect of niacin flush?	ASA
What untoward ocular effect of therapeutic niacin therapy may occur?	Amblyopia
What substance adds to the hepatotoxic effects of niacin?	Ethanol
What is the only approved drug in the cholesterol absorption inhibitor class?	Ezetimibe

What is the mechanism of action of ezetimibe?	Inhibits the absorption of cholesterol in the small intestine
What drugs are included in the fibrates category?	Gemfibrozil, fenofibrate, clofibrate
What is the mechanism of action of fibrates?	Generally, they decrease hepatic triglyceride production and inhibit peripheral lipolysis.
What adverse effect on the gallbladder is associated with fibrates?	Cholelithiasis
Increased anticoagulant effects are seen when fibrates are used with which other drug?	Warfarin

ANTIMALARIAL AGENTS

Which medications are used for malaria prophylaxis and treatment?	Doxycycline, chloroquine, quinine, tetracycline, clindamycin, atovaquone-proguanil, mefloquine, hydroxychloroquine, dapsone
What are the common side effects of all antimalarial medications?	Abdominal pain, nausea, vomiting, diarrhea
Which medications can cause methemoglobinemia and hemolysis in patients with G6PD deficiency?	Primaquine, dapsone, quinine, chloroquine
Which medication causes photosensitivity?	Doxycycline
What complication of quinine, chloroquine, and hydroxychloroquine can lead to death in overdose?	Cardiovascular complications; these agents act both as cardiac fast sodium channel blockers and potassium efflux blockers, causing QRS prolongation and QTc prolongation, respectively. Poisoning can lead to AV block and dysrhythmias.

Which aminoquinones are also used for rheumatoid arthritis?

Chloroquine and hydroxychloroquine

What is the classic "syndrome" caused by quinine?

"Cinchonism," a constellation of nausea, vomiting, diarrhea, tinnitus, hearing loss, vertigo, headache, and syncope, all associated with therapeutic dosing.

What medication is a type Ia antidysrhythmic, which has been used for leg cramps and may cause retinal ischemia?

Quinine

Which medication may cause prominent neuropsychiatric symptoms?

Mefloquine; it has been associated with sleep disturbance, anxiety, depression, and hallucinations.

What specific treatment steps are implemented in cases of acute toxicity of most antimalarial medications?

1. QRS prolongation – IV sodium bicarbonate
2. QTc prolongation – IV magnesium sulfate
3. Methemoglobinemia – IV methylene blue

ANTIPSYCHOTIC AGENTS

What are the names of commonly used antipsychotics?

1. Phenothiazines – chlorpromazine, thioridazine
2. Butyrophenones – haloperidol, droperidol
3. Atypical antipsychotics – risperidone, chlorpromazine, quetiapine, olanzapine, ziprasidone

What classification system is typically used to describe the older versus newer antipsychotics?

Typical vs. atypical

How do they differ?

Typical antipsychotics exert most of their affects on the dopamine receptor, while atypical antipsychotics also inhibit serotonin action and treat both the "positive" and "negative" symptoms of schizophrenia.

What are the primary and secondary mechanisms of action of antipsychotics?

Dopamine receptor antagonism is the primary action; however, atypicals also block serotonin activity, and many antipsychotics have some degree of antimuscarinic activity.

What neurotransmitter receptor is associated with movement disorders?

Dopamine (D2) receptor

What are the clinical components to an acute dystonic reaction?

Involuntary muscle contractions that typically affect the neck (torticollis), jaw (trismus), trunk (opisthotonus), or eye (oculogyric crisis)

What other class of medications can cause an acute dystonic reaction?

Antiemetics (e.g., metoclopramide, promethazine)

What is akathisia?

Uncontrollable restlessness, an adverse effect of antipsychotics

How do you treat akathisia or acute dystonic reaction?

Diphenhydramine or benztropine (anticholinergic agents)

What is the rare, life-threatening adverse effect of antipsychotics, and how does it present?

NMS, which is associated with muscular rigidity, hyperthermia, autonomic instability, and AMS.

What is the mortality rate of NMS?

~5% to 10%

How do you treat this disorder?

Supportive care. Benzodiazepines are appropriate for sedation. Aggressive cooling is warranted for hyperthermia. Dopamine agonists (e.g., bromocriptine, levodopa, amantadine) may be beneficial, but their efficacy is unproven.

What are the typical exam findings in an atypical antipsychotic overdose?

CNS depression, hypotension, tachycardia, and miotic pupils

What is the antipsychotic mechanism of miosis and hypotension?	Alpha 1-adrenergic blockade
What ECG change may be associated with an antipsychotic overdose?	QT prolongation due to myocardial potassium efflux channel blockade
What ventricular dysrhythmia may be associated with this ECG change, and how is it treated?	Torsade de pointes. Treat with magnesium and/or overdrive pacing
The atypical antipsychotic clozapine causes what life-threatening adverse effect?	Agranulocytosis

ANTIVIRAL AND ANTIRETROVIRAL AGENTS

What are the clinical uses of antiviral and antiretroviral agents?

Treatment of viral infections

What are typical mechanisms of toxicity for each category of this class of drugs?

1. Antiherpes drugs – renal crystal deposition causing obstructive acute renal failure
2. Nucleoside reverse transcriptase inhibitors (NRTI) – disturbs neuronal mitochondrial function leading to neurotoxicity, lactic acidosis, and hepatic steatosis thought to be caused by impairment of ability to replicate mitochondrial DNA. This may occur in acute overdose or with therapeutic use.
3. Nonnucleoside reverse transcriptase inhibitors (NNRTI) – little information is known about acute overdose; however, they generally appear to be safe.
4. Protease inhibitors – in chronic use, peripheral lipodystrophy due to impaired fat storage and some

hepatotoxicity may occur. In acute
overdose, GI symptoms predominate,
and rash may occur.

5. Fusion inhibitors – unknown

**What antiherpes agent has
been associated with
seizures?**

Foscarnet

**What is the common clinical
presentation of antiviral and
antiretroviral agent
overdose?**

Primarily GI, although lactic acidosis
(usually with NRTIs) can occur

**What treatments should be
performed in the event of
antiviral and antiretroviral
agent overdose?**

Supportive care is the primary treatment. GI symptoms may be treated with
antiemetics and IV fluids. When ingestion of an NRTI occurs, evaluation for
lactic acidosis is warranted. Benzodiazepines should be the first-line therapy
for seizures. Renal failure should
warrant admission with standard
supportive therapy.

BARBITURATES

What are barbiturates?

Medications of the sedative-hypnotic
class that have been used for anesthesia
induction, seizure management, and
pain control. Secondary to their sedative
properties, barbiturates also have a high
abuse potential.

**Which drugs are in the
barbiturate class?**

1. Ultra short-acting – thiopental,
   methohexital
2. Short-acting – pentobarbital,
   secobarbital
3. Intermediate-acting – amobarbital,
   aprobarbital, butabarbital, butalbital
4. Long-acting – mephobarbital,
   phenobarbital

**What are some common
street names for
barbiturates?**

Downers, yellow jackets, purple hearts,
double trouble

Describe the mechanism of action of barbiturates.

They bind to GABA-mediated chloride channels, increasing the *duration* of opening, which results in synaptic inhibition.

What are the signs of barbiturate intoxication?

Signs of CNS depression, including slurred speech, somnolence, and ataxia. If severe, hypotension, coma, and respiratory arrest can occur.

What are physical exam findings characteristic of barbiturate intoxication?

Patients typically have somnolence and respiratory depression. They may have nystagmus and in severe cases, mid-fixed pupils. Deep barbiturate comas may result in loss of primitive reflexes causing the patient to appear brain-dead.

What are "barbiturate burns"?

Cutaneous bullae that may appear following overdose, seen not only on regions where the body has pressure points, but also on nondependent areas of the body

Can barbiturates be detected in either the serum or the urine?

Yes, both. Barbiturates are detected on most standard urine drug screens.

What treatments are possible for barbiturate intoxication?

1. Supportive care is considered standard therapy.
2. Activated charcoal may be helpful if given within 1 hr after ingestion.
3. Alkalinization of the urine may help ↑ phenobarbital excretion.
4. Hemodialysis can ↑ elimination of the longer-acting agents but is rarely indicated.
5. Because barbiturate-induced coma can resemble brain death, patients should not be pulled from life support without documenting that the levels are nontoxic.

BENZODIAZEPINES

How are benzodiazepines used?

Benzodiazepines are sedative-hypnotics. They are used primarily for sedation, anxiolysis, and seizure management.

What is the mechanism of action of benzodiazepines?

Benzodiazepines induce a conformational change in the GABA receptor to enhance binding of endogenous GABA, resulting in ↑ *frequency* of chloride channel opening and subsequent neuronal hyperpolarization.

What is the result of overdose?

CNS depression, but typically mild in isolated overdose. Coma and respiratory arrest are more common if used in combination with other CNS/respiratory depressants (e.g., barbiturates, ethanol).

What other signs and symptoms may be seen in overdose?

Ataxia, slurred speech, lethargy, hypotension, hypothermia, memory impairment (short-term)

What physical exam findings are characteristic of benzodiazepines?

Other than CNS depression, the exam may be unremarkable. Pupillary exam is variable.

Which benzodiazepines have active metabolites that prolong their effects during overdose?

Chlordiazepoxide, clorazepate, diazepam, flunitrazepam, flurazepam, midazolam, quazepam

Which benzodiazepine is known as the date rape drug "roofies"?

Flunitrazepam

Why is flunitrazepam used for nefarious purposes?

It is a potent sedative that induces amnesia, has a rapid onset, and is easily dissolved in liquids. It is often not detected on routine urine benzodiazepine drug screens.

What laboratory methods are used to evaluate exposure to benzodiazepines?

Urine screening and serum drug levels

What is the specific antidote for benzodiazepine toxicity?

Flumazenil. Its effect is limited, so resedation may occur.

Are there any pitfalls in using flumazenil?

Yes. Flumazenil may precipitate seizures in chronic benzodiazepine users and in patients with multi-drug ingestions. Use can be considered in the "benzo-naïve," following iatrogenic overdose, or possibly to avoid painful or difficult procedures (e.g., an anticipated difficult intubation).

BETA 2-ADRENERGIC AGONISTS

What are some examples of beta 2-adrenergic agonists?
Albuterol, metaproterenol, ritodrine, terbutaline

What is the mechanism of beta 2-adrenergic activity?
These agents stimulate the beta 2-adrenergic receptor → ↑ intracellular cAMP. This stimulation causes smooth muscle relaxation (vascular, bronchial, uterine).

How do beta 2-adrenergic agonists cause tachycardia?
Reflex tachycardia, secondary to vasodilation and to nonspecific activation of beta 1-adrenergic receptors (all adrenergic agents tend to lose specificity in high doses)

What are the signs and symptoms of beta 2-adrenergic agonist toxicity?
Tachycardia, hypotension with widened pulse pressure, tremor, agitation, headache, vomiting, seizures, dysrhythmias. Ischemic events may occur in those with heart disease.

What laboratory abnormalities may be seen in cases of toxicity?
Hypokalemia and hyperglycemia are two common findings. Elevation of CPK can occur, as can lactic acidosis.

Describe the mechanism of hypokalemia.
Beta-adrenergic stimulation causes potassium influx.

What are some clues to diagnosis?
Tachycardia and hypotension with hypokalemia and hyperglycemia are suggestive of toxicity.

What specific treatments are indicated?
1. Hypotension is commonly ameliorated simply with IV fluids
2. Hypotension refractory to IV fluids should be treated with peripheral alpha-adrenergic agonists (e.g., phenylephrine)

3. Nonselective beta-adrenergic blockers (e.g., propranolol) may, theoretically, block the hypotension (beta 2-adrenergic) and tachycardia (beta 1-adrenergic); however, extreme care should be taken when administering them secondary to potential worsening of hypotension. Avoid beta-adrenergic blockers in asthma/severe COPD.
4. Hypokalemia rarely warrants treatment, as total body stores are not usually depleted.

BOTULIN (BOTULISM)

What is botulism?	A syndrome of symmetric, descending, flaccid paralysis caused by a bacterial exotoxin
Which bacterium causes botulism?	*Clostridium botulinum*, a gram-positive, spore-forming obligate anaerobe
How does botulinum toxin cause paralysis?	Inhibits ACh release at peripheral voluntary motor and autonomic synapses
How many different botulinum exotoxins exist?	7, named A, B, C, D, E, F, G
Which exotoxins are most frequently involved in human toxicity?	A, B, and E
What is the major cause of death from botulism?	Respiratory failure due to respiratory muscle weakness
Name the most potent toxin known.	Botulinum toxin (inhalation LD_{50} is 0.01 $\mu g/kg$)
Name the major forms of botulism.	Food-borne, infant, wound, inhalational
What are the symptoms of adult type (food-borne) botulism?	Nausea and vomiting may initially be present, followed by dysphonia; blurred vision; dysphagia; diplopia; and descending, bilaterally symmetric motor paralysis.

Which form of botulinum toxin is used as a medical treatment?

Botulinum toxin subtype A, administered as a local injection

What are approved FDA uses for botulinum toxin type A?

1. Strabismus
2. Blepharospasm
3. Cervical dystonias
4. Cosmesis – for glabellar facial lines
5. Axillary hyperhydrosis

What factor primarily determines side effects to botulinum toxin type A treatment?

Location of injection site, as the toxin produces local side effects

Is there an antidote for botulinum toxin?

Yes, equine bivalent (A, B) and trivalent (A, B, and E) are the classic antitoxins; however, a heptavalent form has recently been approved for use in humans.

Does the antidote reverse symptoms?

No, the SNARE (docking) proteins at the nerve terminal are destroyed by the toxin and must be regenerated for symptoms to improve.

What are the symptoms of infant botulism?

Constipation, feeble cry, diffusely ↓ muscle tone, and difficulty feeding and sucking

What is the preferred treatment for infant botulism?

Human IV botulism immune globulin

Can botulism be used as an agent of terrorism?

Yes, the toxin is small, easily aerosolized, and readily absorbed in the lungs. Identification of types C, D, F, or G in humans should raise suspicion.

CAFFEINE

Where is caffeine found?

It is found naturally in plants such as *Coffea arabica* (coffee), *Theobroma cacao* (cocoa), and *Thea sinesis* (tea) and is ubiquitous in our society, as it is found in coffee, tea, energy drinks, energy tabs, and chocolate.

What is caffeine used for?

Caffeine is a stimulant, diuretic, appetite suppressant, and analgesic agent.

In what structural class is caffeine found?

Methylxanthines

What are two metabolites of caffeine?

Theophylline and theobromine

What is the mechanism of toxicity of caffeine?

It inhibits the adenosine receptor; it causes release of endogenous catecholamines; it also acts as a phosphodiesterase inhibitor.

What is the significance of adenosine blockade?

Activation of adenosine receptors causes cerebral vasodilatation and helps to attenuate seizure activity. Blocking these receptors can cause prolonged, refractory seizure activity with a relative lack of blood flow to the brain.

How is caffeine metabolized?

In the liver by the cytochrome P450 enzymes

What is the half-life of caffeine in overdose?

Up to 15 hrs

What drugs can interact with caffeine metabolism?

Metabolism by CYP1A2 is inhibited by oral contraceptives, cimetidine, norfloxacin, ethanol

What other habits affect caffeine metabolism?

Smoking (tobacco or marijuana) increases the metabolism

What are commonly reported caffeine contents in foods and supplements?

1. Brewed coffee – 100–200 mg
2. Espresso – 30–90 mg
3. Energy drinks – 70–140 mg
4. Energy tabs – 100–200 mg
5. Soda – 30–40 mg
6. Tea – 40–120 mg

What is the lethal PO dose of caffeine?

150–200 mg/kg or about 10 g in adults

What are the signs and symptoms of caffeine toxicity?	Tremor and restlessness, which may progress to nausea, vomiting, tachycardia, tachydysrhythmias, and seizures
What are two commonly seen metabolic abnormalities in caffeine toxicity?	1. Hypokalemia (beta-adrenergic stimulated influx into the cell) 2. Hyperglycemia
By what mechanism does caffeine overdose cause hypotension?	Beta 2-adrenergic stimulation, also resulting in bronchodilation
What are the effects of chronic caffeine ingestion?	Chronic ingestion can lead to insomnia, tremulousness, irritability, anxiety, and palpitations.
How is caffeine toxicity diagnosed?	Clinically. A history of caffeine exposure helps, but tremor, tachycardia, vomiting, and seizures (especially refractory) with hypokalemia are strongly suggestive.
Is there a diagnostic test for caffeine?	Yes, but caffeine levels are only available at large institutions. A theophylline level, since it is a metabolite, may be more readily available and may clue the provider in to the presence of caffeine.
What intervention has been utilized in severe caffeine toxicity?	Hemodialysis

CAMPHOR AND OTHER ESSENTIAL (VOLATILE) OILS

What is camphor?	A volatile, aromatic compound initially isolated from the *Cinnamomum camphora* tree
What are the major uses of camphor?	Liniments, plasticizers, preservatives in pharmaceuticals and cosmetics, moth repellants, decongestants

What are the signs and symptoms of camphor intoxication, and how long is the onset of action?

Nausea, vomiting, tachycardia, confusion, agitation, sedation; seizures often develop within 30 min of ingestion. Camphor odor may be evident on the breath.

What oral doses of camphor may be toxic in adults and children?

Adults – as little as 2 g
Children – as little as 1 g

What is the treatment for a camphor ingestion?

Supportive care is the primary treatment, including benzodiazepines for seizures. There is no role for activated charcoal in the management of camphor oil ingestion due to its rapid absorption.

What are essential oils?

Volatile, polyaromatic hydrocarbons that are used in liniments, cold preparations, and herbal remedies. There are more than 100 of these oils.

What is the general sign of intoxication with essential oils?

Primarily sedation; pneumonitis may develop if aspiration occurs

What is the active ingredient in oil of wintergreen?

Methyl salicylate

What products contain oil of wintergreen?

Topical analgesics

Why is this oil so dangerous?

Each teaspoon of oil of pure oil of wintergreen is equivalent to 7 g (or about 21 tablets) of ASA. It is rapidly absorbed and is a potentially lethal dose to a child.

Which essential oils have caused fulminant hepatic failure?

Clove oil and pennyroyal oil

Which essential oil causes coma following less than a 5 mL ingestion?

Eucalyptus oil

Which essential oil is used as an illicit abortifacient?	Pennyroyal oil
Which oil has been abused for its hallucinogenic properties?	Nutmeg
What is the hallucinogenic ingredient in nutmeg?	Myristicin
Which oils may cause gynecomastia and photosensitivity?	Lavender and tea tree oils
What is the treatment for an essential oil ingestion?	Supportive care including benzodiazepines for seizure activity; N-acetylcysteine may be effective for hepatonecrosis in pennyroyal and clove oil ingestions.

CARBAMAZEPINE

What is carbamazepine?	An anticonvulsant used for the treatment of epilepsy, trigeminal neuralgia, psychiatric illnesses, restless leg syndrome, and alcohol withdrawal
To which class of drugs is carbamazepine structurally similar?	Tricyclic antidepressants; therefore, urine drugs screens may be positive for cyclic antidepressants in patients taking carbamazepine.
What is the mechanism of action?	In therapeutic doses, carbamazepine blocks neuronal sodium channels and is an adenosine receptor agonist. In overdose, it becomes an adenosine receptor antagonist.
What is the rate of absorption?	Absorption is typically slow and erratic. Peak levels can be delayed 6–24 hrs following overdose.
Where is carbamazepine metabolized?	Liver, by P450 oxidation
What is considered a therapeutic level of carbamazepine?	4–12 mg/L

What neurotransmitter receptors are blocked in toxicity?

Adenosine receptors

What are the clinical effects of carbamazepine toxicity?

CNS symptoms predominate with altered consciousness, dizziness, ataxia, headache, and nystagmus. GI symptoms may be present. Severe toxicity can result in cardiac dysrhythmias and seizures.

What cardiac effects have been reported with carbamazepine toxicity?

QRS and QTc prolongation → ventricular dysrhythmias

Name the standard treatments for QRS and QTc prolongation.

IV sodium bicarbonate and IV magnesium sulfate, respectively

What endocrine abnormality can result from toxicity?

Syndrome of inappropriate anti-diuretic hormone (SIADH)

Are there any specific antidotes for carbamazepine toxicity?

No

CHEMOTHERAPEUTIC AGENTS

What are the clinical uses and major classes of chemotherapeutic agents?

Inhibit tumor growth and progression. Major classes include alkylating agents, antibiotics, antimetabolites, hormones (prevent synthesis of, or competitively antagonize hormones), mitotic inhibitors, monoclonal antibodies, platinum complexes, topoisomerase inhibitors, and miscellaneous.

What are typical therapeutic mechanisms of action of this class of drugs?

1. Interference with DNA synthesis and replication
2. Interference with growth signaling pathways
3. Generation of free radicals which damage/destroy rapidly dividing cells
4. Interference with RNA synthesis
5. Inhibition of cell division

6. Inhibition of specific enzymes or receptors over-expressed in cancerous cells
7. Inhibition of protein synthesis

What are typical mechanisms of toxicity for this class of drugs?

Most are cytotoxic by nature, thus toxic effects resemble extremes of pharmacologic effects. Those that target DNA replication and cell division exert toxic effects most readily on the GI and hematopoietic systems (i.e., those systems with rapid turnover). Free radical generation can be a major side effect, particularly with antibiotics. Local tissue damage may be caused by extravasation.

What are possible clinical manifestations of chemotherapeutic agent overdose?

1. Heme – leukopenia (with subsequent infection), thrombocytopenia (with subsequent hemorrhage), anemia
2. GI – nausea, vomiting, and diarrhea (with resultant dehydration), stomatitis, peptic ulcer formation, GI bleeding
3. Skin necrosis at injection sites due to extravasation injury

What is the standard rescue therapy for methotrexate overdose?

Leucovorin (folinic acid)

Which agents commonly cause cardiotoxicity?

Anthracyclines (dactinomycin, doxorubicin)

Name two agents known to cause hemorrhagic cystitis.

Cyclophosphamide and ifosfamide

Overdose of what agents can result in seizures?

Nitrogen mustards

What treatments may be considered in specific chemotherapeutic agent extravasation?

1. Actinomycin, daunorubicin, doxorubicin, idarubicin, and mitoxantrone – ice to injection site (15 min, QID × 3d), consider topical dimethyl sulfoxide (DMSO) to alleviate symptoms

2. Mitomycin – moderate heat to injection site, consider topical DMSO
3. Mechlorethamine, dacarbazine, and cisplatin – flush injection site with 10 mL sterile 2.5% sodium thiosulfate solution
4. Etoposide, paclitaxel, vincristine, and vinblastine – heating pad to injection site (intermittently × 24 hrs), elevate limb, consider local injection of hyaluronidase

CHLOROQUINE AND OTHER AMINOQUINOLINES

Name the commonly used aminoquinolines.	Chloroquine, hydroxychloroquine, primaquine, mefloquine
What are these drugs used for?	Malaria, systemic lupus erythematosus, rheumatoid arthritis
How does chloroquine work?	Inhibits DNA and RNA synthesis
What are some of the adverse effects of aminoquinolines?	GI upset, anxiety, depression, pruritus, headache, visual disturbance
How do the aminoquinolines produce cardiotoxic effects in humans?	Chloroquine and hydroxychloroquine possess quinidine-like cardiotoxicity, resulting in QRS prolongation. QT prolongation may also occur through potassium channel blockade.
What are the effects of acute chloroquine/ hydroxy-chloroquine overdose?	CNS and respiratory depression, hypokalemia, hypotension, cardiac dysrhythmias, possibly seizures
Which aminoquinoline is highly associated with neuropsychiatric disturbance?	Mefloquine
What hematological abnormality is associated with primaquine and quinacrine?	Methemoglobinemia and subsequent hemolysis

What electrolyte abnormality is associated with chloroquine toxicity?	Hypokalemia, from direct intracellular shifts
Describe the management of acute overdose.	Secondary to severe toxicity, aggressive decontamination should be considered in the airway-protected patient. Early mechanical ventilation may be required. Seizures should be treated with benzodiazepines. Vasopressors may be needed for hypotension.
How should cardiotoxicity be treated?	For QRS widening, sodium bicarbonate boluses are the standard treatment. QTc prolongation may be treated with IV magnesium sulfate.

CLONIDINE AND RELATED AGENTS

What are some common uses for clonidine?	Hypertension and attenuation of opioid withdrawal symptoms
What are the pharmacologic mechanisms of action of clonidine?	1. Stimulation of presynaptic alpha 2-adrenergic (inhibitory) receptors centrally, thereby reducing sympathetic outflow 2. Stimulation of alpha 2-adrenergic receptors peripherally → transient, paradoxical ↑ HR and ↑ BP 3. Stimulation of imidazoline receptors
What other medicines act as centrally-acting adrenergic antagonists?	Oxymetazoline (e.g., nasal spray), tetrahydrozoline (e.g., eye drops), tizanidine, guanfacine, methyldopa, guanabenz
What are the routes of administration of clonidine?	PO, transdermal patches
When is the usual time to onset of effect of oral clonidine?	30–60 min
What type of overdose can a clonidine overdose mimic?	Opioid overdose (triad of miosis, CNS, and respiratory depression)

**What are the primary
cardiovascular effects of a
clonidine overdose?**

Hypotension and bradycardia

**Should paradoxical
hypertension from an acute
clonidine overdose be
treated?**

No, it is self-limited.

**What is characteristic about
the pupils of a patient who
has overdosed on clonidine?**

Pinpoint

**Is there an antidote for
clonidine overdose?**

1. Naloxone has been reported to reverse
   CNS depression.
2. Yohimbine and tolazoline have been
   reported to reverse hypotension and
   bradycardia, but their use is
   controversial.

COLCHICINE

**For what condition is
colchicine most commonly
prescribed?**

Gout

**What is the mechanism of
action of colchicine?**

It primarily acts to disrupt cellular microtubule formation, which halts chemotaxis,
phagocytosis, and mitosis. Therapeutically, this results in anti-inflammatory
properties.

**What is the maximum
therapeutic dose?**

8–10 mg daily

**What plants contain
colchicine?**

1. Autumn crocus (*Colchicum
   autumnale*)
2. Glory lily (*Gloriosa superba*)

**What are the effects of an
acute overdose of
colchicine?**

Symptoms are delayed in onset, usually
from 2–12 hrs depending on the dose.
Initial symptoms are GI in nature and
include nausea, vomiting, and bloody
diarrhea. Severe volume loss may result,
followed by multisystem organ failure.

Are there cardiovascular complications of colchicine overdose?	Colchicine is directly toxic to both cardiac and skeletal muscle. This may lead to dysrhythmias and cardiovascular collapse, as well as rhabdomyolysis.
What are late complications of a colchicine overdose?	The arrest of cellular division results in bone marrow suppression with leukopenia and thrombocytopenia. Hair loss may also occur.
What are some side effects of chronic colchicine therapy?	Myopathy and polyneuropathy
Is there a test for colchicine intoxication?	No blood or urine test exists; however, bone marrow biopsies may reveal "pseudo-Pelger-Huet" cells, which are cells in metaphase arrest.
How is a colchicine overdose treated?	1. Aggressive supportive care with fluid and electrolyte monitoring 2. Orogastric lavage can be considered if the patient presents within 1 hr of ingestion, as colchicine possesses extreme toxicity with little available treatment. 3. Neutropenia precautions should be followed for those with bone marrow suppression. 4. Case reports of granulocyte colony-stimulating factor (G-CSF) improving neutropenia have been reported.
Is hemodialysis effective?	No, due to extensive volume of distribution and tissue-binding
What other natural toxin has colchicine-like properties?	Podophyllin, from the American man-drake (*Podophyllum peltatum*)

DAPSONE

What is dapsone?	Dapsone is an antibiotic agent that can be administered for leprosy, toxoplasmosis,

malarial prophylaxis, and *Pneumocystis* pneumonia prophylaxis in immunocompromised individuals. It is used topically for acne vulgaris.

What is the approximate half-life of dapsone?

30 hrs for therapeutic dosing, up to 77 hrs in overdose

What is the mechanism of action of dapsone?

It prevents the formation of folate by inhibiting dihydropteroate synthase.

How is dapsone metabolized?

Acetylation and cytochrome P450 oxidation

What is the mechanism of acute toxicity of dapsone?

Dapsone is an oxidizing agent. Oxidation of iron in heme produces methemoglobinemia. Oxidative stress on red blood cells may result in hemolysis. Sulfhemoglobinemia may result from sulfation of heme groups.

Are certain patients more affected by dapsone exposure?

Yes, patients with congenital hemoglobin abnormalities and G6PD deficiency are more likely to experience toxicity.

What are acute effects of dapsone toxicity?

Nausea, vomiting, abdominal pain, hemolytic anemia, methemoglobinemia, sulfhemoglobinemia, tachycardia, dyspnea, headache, and CNS stimulation (including hallucinations and agitation)

What is the clinical presentation of dapsone-induced methemoglobinemia?

Fatigue, cyanosis, and dyspnea may be present. Cyanosis is refractory to O_2 therapy, as hemoglobin is unable to become saturated. If significant methemoglobin is present ($\geq15\%$–20%), blood may appear brown in color.

What is the diagnostic test for methemoglobinemia?

An arterial blood gas with co-oximetry

What is the antidote for methemoglobinemia?

Methylene blue

How does methylene blue work?	It induces the reduction of ferric iron (Fe^{3+} = methemoglobin) back to ferrous iron (Fe^{2+} = hemoglobin).
What clinical and laboratory findings indicate sulfhemoglobinemia?	Primarily indicated by cyanosis that fails to respond to methylene blue in the appropriate clinical setting
What finding is seen on a peripheral blood smear in patients with dapsone-induced hemolytic anemia?	Heinz bodies (evidence of precipitated Hgb). Hemolytic anemia may be delayed up to 1 week.
What is the toxic dose of dapsone?	Toxic dose varies by individual, but generally 3–15 g for severe toxicity in adults. Deaths reported at doses as low as 1.4 g.

DECONGESTANTS

Which general class of medications is primarily utilized as decongestants?	Sympathomimetics
Which peripheral neuroreceptors mediate vasoconstriction?	Alpha-adrenergic receptors
Which sympathomimetics are used in decongestant preparations?	Pseudoephedrine and phenylephrine
What other medications are used as decongestants?	Imidazoline and propylhexedrine
Why was phenyl-propanolamine removed from the market?	Due to ↑ risk of hypertensive crisis and hemorrhagic stroke associated with its use
What are the most common classes of medications used in combination with decongestants in OTC "cold" medications?	Antihistamines, acetaminophen, salicylates, dextromethorphan
Name some specific imidazoline preparations.	Oxymetazoline, naphazoline, tetrahydrozoline, xylometazoline

How are imidazolines generally used?	As topical vasoconstrictors—ophthalmic or nasal preparations
What is the therapeutic mechanism of action for the imidazoline class of medications?	Topical use produces vasoconstriction by activating alpha-adrenergic receptors.
What is the toxic affect of imidazolines?	Toxic effects are similar to a clonidine ingestion and include miosis, lethargy, hypotension, bradycardia, respiratory depression, and coma. This is due to a central alpha 2-adrenergic agonist effect when absorbed systemically.
Which ophthalmic solution that is known to "get the red out" produces diarrhea?	None. This is an urban legend and, in fact, the CNS depression produced by imidazolines, combined with their liquid formulation, makes them popular for drug-facilitated sexual assault or robbery.
What is the mechanism of action of propylhexedrine, and what are its toxic effects?	Alpha-adrenergic agonist, similar to amphetamine; toxic effects include hypertension, pulmonary edema, ophthalmoplegia, nystagmus, CNS stimulation, injection site necrosis.
What are the signs and symptoms of pseudoephedrine, phenylpropanolamine, and phenylephrine toxicity?	Tachycardia, mydriasis, hypertension (especially with phenylpropanolamine), agitation, tremor, visual and auditory hallucinations, seizures
What ephedrine-containing herbal supplement used to be used as a decongestant and is now banned in the United States?	Ma Huang

DIGOXIN

In what class of drugs is digoxin found?	Cardiac glycosides
Where may cardiac glycosides be found in nature?	*Digitalis purpurea* (foxglove), *Nerium oleander* (oleander), *Thevetia peruviana* (yellow oleander), *Convallaria majalis*

(lily of the valley), *Urginea maritima* (red squill), secretions of *Bufo alvarius* (Colorado River toad)

What are the typical indications for digoxin?

Digoxin is used as an inotropic agent in CHF and as an AV nodal blocker in atrial tachydysrhythmias.

What is the mechanism of action of digoxin?

Digoxin binds to the extracellular surface of the Na-K-ATPase, blocking its activity and increasing residual sodium inside the cell. This decreased gradient drives the sodium-calcium antiporter to extrude sodium from the cell, driving calcium into the cell. The increased calcium inside the cell during systole increases the force of contraction. Digoxin-induced increase in vagal tone decreases SA and AV nodal dromotropy.

What are the adverse effects of sodium-potassium pump blockade?

Increasing calcium inside the cell elevates the membrane potential, allowing for easier depolarization and predisposition to dysrhythmias. At the same time, increased vagal tone leads to AV nodal blockade, which results in the classic atrial tachycardia with AV block seen in digoxin toxicity.

What ECG abnormalities are associated with *therapeutic* dosing?

Scooped ST segments and T wave inversions in the lateral leads

Describe the distribution of digoxin.

It follows the two-compartment model.

How is digoxin eliminated?

Primarily by the kidneys

What is the therapeutic level of digoxin?

0.5–2.0 ng/mL

What are the signs and symptoms of acute overdose?

GI distress (e.g., nausea, vomiting, abdominal pain), lethargy, confusion, atrial and ventricular ectopy (including progression to VT or VF), sinus bradycardia, sinus arrest, high-degree AV block

What laboratory abnormality is classically associated with acute digoxin toxicity?

Hyperkalemia

What is the most common dysrhythmia associated with digoxin toxicity?

PVCs

What dysrhythmia is pathognomic of digoxin toxicity?

Biventricular tachycardia

What are the signs and symptoms of chronic toxicity?

GI distress (e.g., nausea, vomiting, abdominal pain); anorexia with weight loss; delirium; headaches; seizures; visual disturbances; weakness; sinus bradycardia; ventricular dysrhythmias (more common than in acute toxicity)

What laboratory testing should be done?

Digoxin levels, but these may not accurately indicate severity of ingestion for the initial 6 hours due to distribution kinetics. Serum potassium levels reflect the amount of sodium-potassium pump poisoning in acute overdose.

What is the role of calcium in digoxin toxicity?

While normally an integral part of treatment in hyperkalemia, there have been case reports of cardiac standstill when giving calcium for hyperkalemia in digoxin toxicity.

What is the treatment of digoxin overdose?

1. In acute overdose, digoxin-specific antibody (Fab) fragments are indicated for patients with potassium levels greater than 5.0 mEq/L for high degree heart blocks, and for dysrhythmias.
2. Standard therapy is indicated for hyperkalemia.
3. Use caution in cardioversion of atrial dysrhythmias (use lowest energy possible), as the irritable myocardium is prone to ventricular dysrhythmias.

4. Atropine can be used for bradycardia. Use caution with temporary cardiac pacemakers.
5. Phenytoin may be used for ventricular irritability if Fab fragments are not available.

Does hemodialysis have a role in cardiac glycoside poisoning?

No, as digoxin has a large volume of distribution

For a known steady state digoxin blood level, what is the dose calculation for Fab fragments?

[Drug level (ng/mL) × patient weight in kg]/100 = number of vials (round up)

DISULFIRAM

What is the chemical name of disulfiram, and how is it used?

Tetraethylthiuram disulfide—a chemical used in the treatment of alcoholism to produce an unpleasant effect following ingestion of ethanol

By what route is disulfiram administered?

Primarily PO, although SQ implants are available outside the U.S.

What are the modes of toxicity of disulfiram?

Acute overdose, disulfiram-ethanol interaction, and chronic toxicity

What are the primary mechanisms of toxicity of disulfiram?

1. Inhibition of aldehyde dehydrogenase, causing systemic accumulation of acetaldehyde, an intermediate product in the metabolism of ethanol
2. Blockade of dopamine beta-hydroxylase, a crucial enzyme in norepinephrine synthesis, causing depletion of presynaptic norepinephrine, resulting in vasodilation and orthostatic hypotension

What industrial solvent and toxin is produced during the metabolism of disulfiram?

Carbon disulfide

When is the peak efficacy of disulfiram reached?	8–12 hrs
Where is disulfiram metabolized?	Liver
What is the elimination half-life of disulfiram?	7–8 hrs, with the potential for clinical effects to persist for several days
What is the toxic dose of ethanol when on disulfiram therapy?	Patients on maintenance therapy of 200 mg/day have had severe reactions to as little as 7 mL of ethanol.
What are the signs and symptoms of an acute disulfiram overdose (without ethanol)?	Vomiting, confusion, lethargy, ataxia, coma
What are the signs and symptoms of ethanol ingestion in patients on chronic disulfiram therapy?	Flushing, headache, vomiting, dyspnea, vertigo, confusion, and orthostatic hypotension with peripheral vasodilation
What anti-protozoal medicine commonly causes a disulfiram-like reaction?	Metronidazole

DIURETICS

What is the primary medical use of diuretics?	As antihypertensives
What type of OTC medications may contain diuretics?	Weight-loss drugs
What groups of people are likely to abuse diuretics?	Athletes, dieters, people with eating disorders
What organ do diuretics primarily act upon?	Kidney
Describe the mechanism of the four major classes of diuretics.	1. Thiazide and thiazide-like diuretics— inhibit sodium-chloride transporter in distal convoluted tubule, increasing Na^+/Cl^- excretion

2. Loop diuretics—inhibit $Na^+/K^+/2Cl^-$ transporter in thick ascending limb, blocking reuptake of these electrolytes, as well as calcium and magnesium
3. Potassium-sparing diuretics—act at a variety of sites (depending upon the drug) including distal tubule and collecting duct to prevent the reabsorption of sodium while inhibiting potassium excretion
4. Carbonic anhydrase inhibitors— inhibit renal carbonic anhydrase, preventing the reabsorption of $NaHCO_3$ from the tubular lumen

What is the most common, reversible side effect of loop diuretics?

Hearing loss

What is the effect of diuretics in acute overdose?

In general, diuretics have low toxicity in acute overdose. Nausea, vomiting, and diarrhea may occur, as may dehydration.

What is the effect of chronic use/abuse?

Electrolyte and acid-base abnormalities

How do you treat a diuretic overdose?

Fluid resuscitation and electrolyte repletion as needed

ERGOT DERIVATIVES

What are ergot alkaloids?

Derivatives of methylergoline that possess central serotonergic activity and peripheral vasoconstrictive properties

From which fungus is ergot derived?

Claviceps purpurea

Name the common medicinal preparations included in each of the three groups of ergot alkaloid derivatives.

1. Amine alkaloids—ergonovine, methylergonovine, methysergide, pergolide
2. Amino acid alkaloids—ergotamine, bromocriptine
3. Dihydrogenated amino acid alkaloids—dihydroergotamine

Classically, ergotism is divided into what two syndromes?

1. Convulsive—the symptoms include headache, muscle spasms, miosis, paresthesias, mania, psychosis, lethargy, and seizures. GI effects (i.e., nausea, vomiting, and diarrhea) precede CNS effects. Hallucinations may occur, resembling those produced by LSD.
2. Gangrenous—the dry gangrene is ultimately a result of profound tissue hypoxia and subsequent peripheral ischemic injury. Symptoms include cool/mottled extremities, loss of peripheral sensation and/or an irritating "burning" sensation, edema, severe distal pain, diminished peripheral pulses, and possible loss of affected tissues or digits.

How do people develop ergotism?

1. Ingesting grain contaminated with ergot fungus
2. Ergotamine treatment for diseases such as migraines
3. Drug–drug interactions between any ergot therapy and drugs that inhibit the cytochrome CYP3A4 enzymes (e.g., macrolide antibiotics)

Ergot is theorized to have contributed to what 1692 Massachusetts event?

The Salem witch trials

Gangrenous ergotism during the Middle Ages was also known by what other name?

St. Anthony's fire (*ignis sacer*)

In 1951, a case of mass-poisoning occurred following the consumption of bread in the French village of Pont-Saint-Esprit. Although misidentified as ergotism, what fungicidal compound has been implicated as the cause of the toxic event?

Mercury

What is the treatment for ergot poisoning?	1. Withdraw drug 2. Benzodiazepines for seizures 3. Sodium nitroprusside or phentolamine for treatment of vasoconstriction 4. Nitroglycerin for myocardial ischemia 5. Vascular surgery consultation for irreversible ischemia

HEPARIN

What are the different types of heparin?	Unfractionated and low molecular weight (LMWH) forms
What are the different routes of administration?	1. IV (intermittent or continuous) 2. SQ
What is the mechanism of action of heparin?	Heparin acts as a catalyst for antithrombin III, increasing its activity by approximately a thousand times. Antithrombin III is a plasma enzyme that inactivates certain activated serine proteases of the coagulation cascade, most importantly activated factors II (thrombin) and X. The larger heparin species (found in unfractionated heparin) catalyzes the inactivation of activated factor II and X. In contrast, LMWH chiefly inactivates activated factor X.
What is the half-life of heparin?	1–2 hrs in healthy adults, which increases with long-term IV administration
What is the half-life of LMWH?	4–7 hrs
Where is heparin metabolized?	Primarily hepatic, with some metabolism in the reticuloendothelial system
How are LMWHs eliminated?	Renal
What lab test is used to monitor patients on heparin?	aPTT

What two forms of thrombocytopenia are induced by heparin?

Two forms of heparin-induced thrombocytopenia (HIT) have been observed. The first (HIT I) is a transient, mild, and benign thrombocytopenia seen soon after initiation of heparin therapy (usually within 2 days) and is thought to be due to inherent platelet-aggregating properties of heparin. A second, more severe form of HIT (HIT II) is typically seen later and is immune-mediated. The incidence of HIT II is estimated at 3% to 5%. The onset is generally 3–14 days after initiation of heparin therapy but may occur sooner with repeat exposure. HIT II may occur with any dose and type of heparin, but the frequency is highest with continuous IV infusions of unfractionated heparin. HIT with subsequent thrombosis is a feared complication. These thrombi can form in the venous or arterial circulation. Thrombotic complications include necrotic skin lesions, myocardial infarction, stroke, and gangrene.

What type of electrolyte disorder may occur with heparin therapy?

Hyperkalemia may be seen with heparin therapy due to inhibition of aldosterone synthesis.

Is heparin safe in pregnancy?

Pregnancy category C. It does not cross the placenta and is not expressed in breast milk.

What is the antidote to heparin?

Protamine sulfate

What is protamine?

A protein found in fish sperm that binds and inactivates heparin

HYPOGLYCEMIC AGENTS

INSULIN

What are the pharmacokinetics of insulin?

IV insulin has a circulating half-life of 5–10 min. SQ insulin has a bioavailability of 55% to 77% and a half-life that differs based on the type of insulin. It is excreted unchanged by the kidneys and metabolized by the kidneys and liver. Insulin does not cross the placenta.

What does insulin do?

1. Stimulates cellular uptake and metabolism of glucose
2. Stimulates entry of proteins into the cell
3. Shifts potassium and magnesium intracellularly
4. Promotes formation of glycogen, fatty acids, and proteins

What is the duration of action of the 7 common insulins when administered SQ?

1. Regular—5–8 hrs
2. Lispro—3–8 hrs
3. Aspart—3–5 hrs
4. NPH—16–24 hrs
5. Lente—16–24 hrs
6. Ultralente—28–36 hrs
7. Glargine—22–24 hrs

What patients are at an increased risk for hypoglycemia?

Renal failure, hypopituitarism, adrenal failure, autonomic neuropathy, those on beta-blocker therapy

How does hypoglycemia present?

Confusion, tachycardia, diaphoresis, coma, seizures, and stroke-mimicking symptoms. The sympathetic response may be blunted in patients taking beta-blockers.

What are diagnostic clues in the evaluation of hypoglycemia?

1. History of insulin or sulfonylurea use
2. Physical exam findings that include injection sites
3. Finger-stick blood sugar should be used to rapidly assess glucose status.
4. Potassium may be low after insulin injection.
5. ↑ BUN and creatinine may explain ↓ renal excretion.
6. ↑ LFTs may reveal ↓ liver function.

How can hyperinsulinemia from exogenous insulin administration be differentiated from that due to oversecretion of endogenous insulin (e.g., in patients with an insulinoma)?

C-peptide will be present in the blood of patients with endogenous insulin secretion.

How can sulfonylurea poisoning be differentiated from an insulinoma?

The two can be differentiated only by obtaining a sulfonylurea panel. Both an insulinoma and sulfonylurea poisoning will have elevated insulin and C-peptide levels.

How should insulin-induced hypoglycemia be treated?

1. Oral glucose therapy if the patient is awake and alert
2. IV dextrose if the patient is obtunded
3. The patient must be observed past the peak of the type of insulin used.
4. Check for renal insufficiency that may have contributed to ↓ insulin metabolism.

What is the disposition for patients with accidental insulin overdose?

With short- to medium-acting agents, patients may be discharged with a responsible party if their blood glucose remains elevated 3–4 hrs following a standard carbohydrate meal. Admission is recommended after accidental over-dose of a long-acting insulin, especially in those patients who develop hypoglycemia.

What is the usual bolus dose of IV glucose in hypoglycemic patients with AMS?

Adults—1–2 mL/kg D50W
Children—2–4 mL/kg D25W
Infants—2 mL/kg D10W

Is there a role for activated charcoal or gastric lavage in patients who have ingested insulin?

No. Enteral administration of insulin is harmless, as no insulin is absorbed from the GI tract.

METFORMIN

In what class of antidiabetic agents is metformin found?	Biguanides
What biguanide was taken off the U.S. market in 1976 due to its association with lactic acidosis?	Phenformin
What is the mechanism of action of metformin?	1. ↓ hepatic glucose production 2. ↓ intestinal glucose absorption 3. ↓ fatty acid oxidation 4. ↑ insulin sensitivity
What is the mechanism of elimination of metformin?	Almost no hepatic metabolism, 90% to 100% excreted unchanged by the kidneys
Does an acute overdose of metformin induce hypoglycemia?	No, metformin does not cause insulin release; therefore, hypoglycemia with an isolated metformin overdose does not occur.
What is the most serious adverse effect of metformin?	Lactic acidosis, which can present with nonspecific symptoms such as fatigue, nausea, vomiting, myalgias, and abdominal pain.
What are risk factors for lactic acidosis with metformin use?	Renal insufficiency, cardiovascular disease, severe infection, alcoholism, advanced age
What is a potential treatment option following a metformin overdose that induces a marked lactic acidosis?	Hemodialysis or continuous venovenous hemodiafiltration can speed the elimination of metformin and may be used to correct life-threatening lactic acidosis.

SULFONYLUREAS

What are sulfonylureas?	PO hypoglycemic agents that ↑ insulin secretion
Name some common sulfonylureas.	Chlorpropamide, glipizide, glyburide, glimepiride, tolbutamide
What is the mechanism of action?	1. Inhibits an ATP-dependent potassium channel on pancreatic

beta-islet cells, resulting in cell membrane depolarization. This causes calcium influx and subsequent release of stored insulin from secretory granules.

2. ↓ hepatic insulin clearance → ↑ serum insulin
3. ↑ peripheral insulin receptor sensitivity
4. ↓ glycogenolysis

What is the average duration of action of the second- and third-generation agents?

16–24 hrs

What is the principal effect of toxicity associated with sulfonylureas?

Hypoglycemia

What factors contribute to an increased risk of hypoglycemia?

Young or advanced age, poor nutrition, alcohol consumption, renal and hepatic insufficiency, polypharmacy

By what mechanism does octreotide help in sulfonylurea-induced hypoglycemia?

Suppresses the secretion of insulin and glucagon by coupling to G proteins on beta-islet cells

What is the mechanism by which diazoxide treats sulfonylurea-induced hypoglycemia?

Although not the preferred method of treatment, diazoxide enhances the release of glucose from the liver, inhibits endogenous insulin release, and decreases peripheral glucose utilization. Although diazoxide may be used for this indication, octreotide is preferred.

How long should asymptomatic patients with sulfonylurea overdose be observed?

All sulfonylureas show a time-to-peak effect of less than 8 hrs, except for extended-release glipizide. A patient who is receiving no supplemental glucose parenterally and who has normal blood glucose checks during an 8-hr observation period can be safely discharged. Any significant drop in blood glucose after initial stabilization warrants admission to the hospital.

With what other toxicity/side effect is chlorpropamide associated?	Hyponatremia, due its induction of inappropriate antidiuretic hormone secretion (SIADH)
Which sulfonylureas have active metabolites eliminated by the kidney and should not be used in patients with renal insufficiency?	Chlorpropamide, glyburide, glimepiride

OTHER

What are some examples of thiazolidinediones (TZDs)?	Rosiglitazone and pioglitazone
What TZD was taken off the market in 2000 after cases of acute liver failure?	Troglitazone
What is the mechanism of action of TZDs?	TZDs bind to peroxisomal proliferator-activated receptors and change insulin-dependent gene expression to enhance the effect of insulin in skeletal muscle and in adipose and hepatic tissues.
How are TZDs eliminated?	Extensive hepatic metabolism with products excreted in urine and feces
What adverse effects are seen with TZDs?	No hypoglycemia is expected to occur in overdose; only fluid retention, peripheral edema, and the potential for hepatotoxicity
What TZD has recently been associated with serious adverse cardiac events?	Rosiglitazone
What are the names of the meglitinides on the market?	Nateglinide and repaglinide
What is the mechanism of action of meglitinides?	Binds to ATP-sensitive potassium channels on pancreatic beta-islet cells to stimulate insulin secretion
How is this drug eliminated?	Predominately metabolized by the liver, then excreted in the bile, with 6% excreted by the kidneys

What are the clinical effects of overdose?

Meglitinides cause the release of insulin from the pancreas and, therefore, have the potential to cause hypoglycemia. Overdose data is limited, but hypoglycemia seems to be brief and easily treated with dextrose solutions.

What is the treatment of meglitinide-induced hypoglycemia?

PO or IV glucose

What are the common alpha-glucosidase inhibitors?

Acarbose and miglitol

What is the mechanism of action of the alpha-glucosidase inhibitors?

Inhibit alpha-glucosidase, an intestinal brush border enzyme that aids in carbohydrate absorption

What are the side effects of alpha-glucosidase inhibitors?

Primarily GI—bloating, flatulence, diarrhea, abdominal pain

What is the mechanism of elimination of the alpha-glucosidase inhibitors?

1. Acarbose is poorly absorbed and eliminated predominantly in the feces.
2. Miglitol is fully absorbed with unknown implications for its systemic absorption. It is cleared by the kidney and may thus exhibit toxicity in the presence of renal impairment.

What are the contraindications for alpha-glucosidase inhibitor use?

Cirrhosis, inflammatory bowel disease, predisposition for bowel obstruction, malabsorption syndromes

What is the presentation of an alpha-glucosidase inhibitor overdose?

Limited data exists, but patients would likely present with GI symptoms and electrolyte abnormalities. No hypoglycemia is expected to occur.

What are the dipeptidyl peptidase-4 (DPP-4) inhibitors?

A new class of drugs for glycemic control in type 2 diabetes.

What are the names of the DPP-4 inhibitors?

Vildagliptin, sitagliptin, saxagliptin

What is the mechanism of action of the DPP-4 inhibitors?

Inhibits the degradation of incretin hormones, causing:
1. ↑ insulin synthesis and release
2. ↓ glucagon release
3. ↓ hepatic glucose production
4. Delayed gastric emptying
5. ↑ satiety

What are the adverse effects of the DPP-4 inhibitors?

They appear to be relatively benign in overdose. While overdose data is sparse, hypoglycemia seems to be limited.

IMMUNOSUPPRESSANTS

What are some of the indications for immunosuppressant drugs?

1. Prevent rejection of transplanted organs
2. Management of autoimmune diseases (e.g., Crohn's disease, systemic lupus erythematosus, myasthenia gravis)
3. Management of chronic nonautoimmune disease (e.g., asthma)

What are the types of immunosuppressants?

Monoclonal and polyclonal antibodies, interferons, methotrexate, cyclosporine, sirolimus, glucocorticoids

What are some of the major adverse effects of these drugs?

1. Action can be nonselective.
2. Can impair ability to fight infection
3. Hypertension
4. Specific organ toxicity (especially liver, lung, and kidney)
5. Dyslipidemia

How do patients with acute immunosuppressant overdose present?

Nausea and vomiting may be followed by diarrhea, myelosuppression, and signs of immunosuppression (e.g., infection).

What about individual drugs and their toxicities?

1. Mono/polyclonal antibodies – fever, rigors, anaphylaxis, serum sickness
2. Methotrexate – nausea, vomiting, myelosuppression, anemia, aphthous ulcers, neutropenia

3. Cyclosporine – gingivitis, burning paresthesias, hepatotoxicity, nephrotoxicity, neurotoxicity
4. Sirolimus – interstitial lung disease
5. Glucocorticoids – adrenal suppression, hyperglycemia, osteoporosis

Name the rescue therapy for methotrexate poisoning.

Leucovorin (folinic acid)

What herbal product used for depression may enhance cyclosporine elimination and result in transplant rejection?

St. John's wort – it induces CYP3A4. Both are metabolized via CYP3A4.

Name the number one cause of secondary adrenal insufficiency.

Chronic glucocorticoid use

How should a patient poisoned with an immunosuppressant agent be managed?

1. CBC, electrolytes, and renal function studies can evaluate for myelosuppresion and nephrotoxicity.
2. Hyponatremia and hyperkalemia may indicate adrenal insufficiency in patients that have been on long-term glucocorticoids.
3. While data is limited, treatment is primarily supportive. Granulocyte colony-stimulating factor (G-CSF) has been used to treat myelosuppression.

IPECAC SYRUP

What is ipecac syrup?

An alkaloid oral suspension that induces vomiting

Where is this found in nature?

It is derived from the plant *Psychotria ipecacuanha*, which belongs to the family *Rubiaceae*.

Name the two key components.

1. Emetine
2. Cephaeline

How is ipecac used?

Historically, ipecac was used as an emetic in the case of a potentially poisonous ingestion or intentional overdose. Ipecac is no longer recommended for GI decontamination.

What is the mechanism of action of ipecac?

Emetine produces irritation of the gastric mucosa, while cephaeline causes stimulation of the chemoreceptor trigger zone in the medulla.

What two groups of patients are reported to have chronic ipecac toxicity?

1. Bulimics who regularly use ipecac syrup to induce vomiting
2. Victims of Munchausen's syndrome by proxy

How long is the onset of action of ipecac?

15–30 min

What are the symptoms of an acute ingestion?

Nausea, vomiting, and diarrhea

What are the cellular effects of chronic use?

Emetine-mediated inhibition of protein synthesis in skeletal muscle

How do acutely toxic patients present?

Nausea, vomiting, lethargy, and electrolyte abnormalities; gastritis. Gastritis, gastric rupture, Mallory-Weiss tears, and pneumomediastinum all have been reported. Airway compromise may occur secondary to aspiration.

How do chronic ipecac-toxic patients present?

Dehydration and electrolyte abnormalities secondary to vomiting and diarrhea, muscle weakness and tenderness, and ↓ reflexes. Elevated serum CPK indicates skeletal muscle myopathy. Cardiomyopathy with resultant dysrhythmias and CHF have been reported.

How is ipecac toxicity diagnosed?

Primarily by patient history. Suspect chronic exposure in patients with eating disorders. Urine emetine levels (present for several weeks following ingestion) can confirm the diagnosis.

ISONIAZID (INH)

What is the indication for isoniazid (INH) therapy?	Tuberculosis
What is the mechanism of action of INH?	Isoniazid is a prodrug and must be activated by bacterial catalase; it inhibits the synthesis of mycolic acid in the mycobacterial cell wall.
How is INH metabolized?	Hepatic
What is the half-life of INH?	0.5–1.6 hrs in fast acetylators, 2–5 hrs in slow acetylators
What is the mechanism of toxicity of INH?	INH metabolites inhibit pyridoxine kinase and bind pyridoxal-5-phosphate, a cofactor for glutamic acid decarboxylase, thereby decreasing levels of the inhibitory neurotransmitter GABA.
What are the signs of acute overdose?	Nausea, vomiting, slurred speech, ataxia, CNS depression, and seizures
What are the metabolic effects of acute overdose?	A marked lactic acidosis may develop in patients who present with seizures. INH inhibits lactate dehydrogenase that converts lactate to pyruvate, thereby prolonging the metabolic acidosis.
How is the diagnosis made?	Generally by history; however, INH toxicity should be in the differential diagnosis for all refractory seizures, especially in high risk patients (history of HIV, tuberculosis, homelessness, or incarceration).
What are the adverse effects of chronic overdose?	Peripheral neuritis, optic neuritis, hepatitis, pancreatitis, drug-induced systemic lupus erythematosus, and pyridoxine deficiency
What drugs are used to treat INH overdose?	Pyridoxine (vitamin B_6) – 1 g IV for each g of INH ingested or 5 g IV for an unknown amount ingested. Standard seizure treatments also apply (i.e., benzodiazepines).

KETAMINE

What is ketamine?	A psychoactive, dissociative agent similar to phencyclidine (PCP), which is often used as a sedative agent in medical and veterinary practice, but has a high abuse potential secondary to its ability to cause an "out-of-body" experience.
Which demographic group is most likely to abuse ketamine?	Teenagers and young adults who frequent "rave" or "techno" parties popular in large urban cities
What are some common street names for ketamine?	Bump, Cat Valium, Green, Honey Oil, Jet, K, Purple, Special K, Special LA Coke, Super Acid, Super C, Vitamin K
What are street sources of ketamine?	Veterinary offices. Mexico is a major country of origin.
What is the reported street price of ketamine?	$20–$40 per dosage unit, $65–$100 per 10 mL vial containing 1 g of ketamine
What desirable effects of ketamine support its illicit use?	Distorts perceptions of sight and sound, makes the user feel disconnected and not in control. Sensations ranging from a pleasant feeling of floating to being separated from one's body have been reported.
What undesirable effects of ketamine are reported by illicit users?	Terrifying feeling of almost complete sensory detachment, likened to a near-death experience
What are recreational doses of ketamine?	10–250 mg intranasally, 40–450 mg PO/PR, 10–100 mg IM
How is ketamine prepared and administered for illicit uses?	Generally evaporated to form a powder. It is often adulterated with caffeine, ephedrine, heroin, cocaine, or other illicit drugs. The powder is usually snorted, mixed in drinks, compressed into pills, or smoked. Liquid ketamine is injected,

applied on a smokeable material, or consumed in drinks.

What are the clinical effects of ketamine, and by what route(s) is it administered?

Short-acting dissociative anesthesia with little or no depression of airway reflexes or ventilation. Clinically, it is administered IM or IV.

With which CNS receptors does ketamine interact, and what is the effect of each?

Blocks N-methyl-D-aspartate (NMDA) receptor (dose-dependent), which inhibits catecholamine and dopamine reuptake, resulting in elevated BP and heart rate. In significant overdoses, it stimulates the sigma (σ) opioid receptor, resulting in coma.

What is the NMDA receptor?

A voltage-gated ligand-dependent calcium channel to which glutamate (the main excitatory CNS neurotransmitter) naturally binds. Activation allows for inward calcium and sodium currents (and some potassium efflux), resulting in neuronal depolarization and action potential initiation.

What is the clinical presentation of ketamine abuse?

Similar to PCP (lethargy, euphoria, hallucinations, occasional bizarre or violent behavior), but much milder and of shorter duration. Also, hypersalivation and lacrimation; vertical and horizontal nystagmus may be prominent with intoxication.

What other effects are seen clinically (and how is each managed)?

1. Stimulation of salivary and tracheobronchial secretions (treated with atropine and glycopyrrolate)
2. Laryngospasm during oral procedures (treated with positive-pressure ventilation, rarely endotracheal intubation)
3. Slight increase in muscle tone and myoclonic movements

What is the behavioral effect of ketamine intoxication?

Patients may be oblivious to pain and surroundings due to dissociative anesthetic effects; therefore, self-inflicted injuries and injuries due to resisting physical restraints are frequent. A low index of suspicion for rhabdomyolysis should be maintained.

What is an "emergence reaction"?

Bizarre behavior characterized by a confused state, vivid dreaming, and hallucinations observed during the recovery phase of use

How are emergence reactions treated?

Sedation with benzodiazepines or haloperidol

Can anything be done to decrease the risk of an emergence reaction?

1. Avoid rapid IV administration of the drug
2. Avoid excessive stimulation during recovery

What are therapeutic anesthetic doses of ketamine?

1–4 mg/kg IV or 2–4 mg/kg IM

What is the duration of effect of ketamine?

Route-dependent – 15 min for IV, 45–90 min after snorting, 30–120 min for IM, 4–8 hrs after PO/PR

What are illicit uses of ketamine, and what "advantages" does it have over PCP?

Hallucinogen. A "Special K" trip is touted as better than that of LSD or PCP because its hallucinatory effects are of relatively short duration, lasting ~30–60 min vs. several hours.

For what other illicit purpose is ketamine used, and what properties allow this use?

Date-rape drug. It is odorless and tasteless, so it can be added to beverages without detection; it also induces amnesia.

Is there a readily available diagnostic test for detection of ketamine in hospitals?

No. Diagnosis is suggested by rapidly fluctuating behavior, vertical nystagmus, and sympathomimetic signs. Ketamine can cross-react with a urine PCP immunoassay.

What OTC drug is abused for its dissociative effects that are similar to ketamine?	Dextromethorphan, a widely available cough suppressant analog of codeine. In high doses, dextromethorphan and its first-pass metabolite, dextrorphan, produce PCP/ketamine-like effects due to interaction with the PCP binding site of NMDA receptors.

LITHIUM

What are the indications for lithium administration?	As a mood stabilizer, most often in patients with bipolar disorder
How is lithium metabolized?	Excreted unchanged by the kidney
What is the etiology of lithium toxicity?	Acute toxicity occurs when a patient takes a single large dose. Chronic toxicity usually occurs in those taking their regularly prescribed dose. The levels become toxic through any mechanism which alters renal function, including dehydration, diabetes insipidus, and the use of diuretics, ACE inhibitors, or NSAIDs.
What renal side effect is associated with lithium therapy?	Nephrogenic diabetes insipidus
What are the signs and symptoms of acute toxicity?	Nausea and vomiting predominate. With a large enough ingestion, lithium can cause delayed neurological effects after redistribution to the tissues.
What signs and symptoms are seen with chronic toxicity or in patients in later stages of acute toxicity?	Tremor, confusion, ataxia, slurred speech, myoclonus, and hyperreflexia are common. Severe poisoning can cause agitated delirium, coma, hyperthermia, and convulsions.
What does the ECG show in lithium toxicity?	T-wave flattening or inversions. Prolongation of the QT interval has also been reported

What important considerations must be observed when ordering lithium levels?

1. Peak levels may be delayed, so serial levels should be obtained.
2. Avoid lithium heparin tubes as they can cause false positive results.
3. A patient with chronic toxicity can have significant clinical findings even with a mildly elevated serum level.

How is lithium toxicity treated?

1. Whole bowel irrigation can be considered after significant acute ingestions.
2. Activated charcoal is not effective.
3. Administer IV normal saline (use care to avoid hypernatremia).
4. Hemodialysis or continuous venovenous hemodialysis can be considered in those with severe intoxication (i.e., seizures, AMS).

What must be considered if hemodialysis is employed?

Lithium commonly redistributes from the tissues into the serum, and serum lithium levels will rebound.

What drug interaction can be seen?

Combining lithium with serotonergic drugs (e.g., SSRIs) can precipitate serotonin syndrome.

MAGNESIUM

What are the medical preparations of magnesium?

1. Magnesium citrate (i.e., oral cathartic)
2. Magnesium hydroxide (i.e., milk of magnesia as an antacid)
3. Magnesium sulfate (i.e., Epsom salt)
4. Magnesium IV preparations

What is the major source of magnesium in occupational exposures?

Inhalation of magnesium oxide dust

What is the major source of exposure to magnesium in healthcare settings?

Oral and parenteral administration in medicinal preparations

What percent of an oral dose of magnesium is absorbed?

15% to 30% in the small bowel, negligible amount exchanged across the large bowel mucosa

How is magnesium filtered and excreted in the body?

1. Filtered at the glomerulus with 95% reabsorbed at the proximal tubule by active transport
2. Excess magnesium is excreted in the urine.

Can hypermagnesemia occur in individuals with normal renal function?

Rarely, as the renal elimination rate can exceed the maximum rate of GI absorption.

Can a person overdose on oral cathartics/antacids?

Most patients with a single acute overdose will have only mild symptoms (nausea, vomiting, diarrhea); however, after a very large ingestion or with multiple repeat overdoses, more severe symptoms may occur.

What are the signs and symptoms of magnesium poisoning?

Nausea, vomiting, weakness, flushing, loss of reflexes, sedation, paralysis, dysrhythmias

What neurological signs are seen with acute magnesium toxicity?

1. CNS depression progressing to lethargy and coma
2. Hyporeflexia and muscular paralysis
3. Hypotonicity

What ECG findings are indicative of hypermagnesemia?

Bradycardia, PR interval prolongation, QRS widening

For what ECG abnormality is magnesium considered the "antidote"?

QTc prolongation

What can increase the renal excretion of magnesium?

Hypercalcemic and hypernatremic states, loop diuretics

How should I decontaminate a patient from a magnesium exposure and/or hazardous materials scene?

Remove the patient from the scene, and gently brush any magnesium off of the patient prior to the use of water for decontamination, as magnesium will readily react with water.

What laboratory tests should I get for suspected magnesium exposure/toxicity?

Electrolytes with serum magnesium, CBC, BUN, serum creatinine

Does the serum magnesium level correspond to the severity of symptoms?

Generally yes, but intracellular concentration is more predictive than plasma concentration.

What symptoms correspond with a given serum magnesium concentration?

1. 3–9 mEq/L – erythema (cutaneous vasodilation), vomiting, hypotension, hyporeflexia, bradycardia, sedation
2. 10–14 mEq/L – muscle paralysis (including respiratory), hypoventilation, cardiac conduction abnormalities, stupor
3. >14 mEq/L – asystolic cardiac arrest

Can the inhalation of magnesium dust cause lung injury?

Yes, it may incite local injury leading to pulmonary edema. Also, this may lead to systemic toxicity, as magnesium is readily absorbed across alveolar-capillary membranes.

What is the treatment of acute magnesium toxicity?

1. Gastric emptying with an NG tube may be attempted within 1 hr of ingestion.
2. Calcium for cardiac conduction abnormalities or respiratory symptoms
3. IV fluids and dopamine for hypotension
4. Hemodialysis for severe cases
5. Activated charcoal does not bind magnesium and is ineffective.

How does calcium work?

Direct antagonism of magnesium at neuromuscular and cardiovascular sites

What dose of calcium should I give?

1 g of IV calcium gluconate slowly (over 3–5 min)

Which magnesium-toxic patients should be treated with calcium?

Symptomatic patients with serum magnesium >5 mEq/L

NEUROMUSCULAR BLOCKERS

What are the two kinds of neuromuscular blockers (NMB)?

1. Depolarizing neuromuscular blockers (DNMB)

2. Nondepolarizing neuromuscular
   blockers (NDNMB)

What is the effect common to both therapeutic and nontherapeutic uses of all NMBs?

Paralysis and subsequent respiratory arrest

What is the mechanism of action of a DNMB?

Agonist at the neuromuscular nicotinic ACh post-junctional receptor, causing prolonged depolarization of the muscle fiber with subsequent paralysis

What is the only DNMB currently in use?

Succinylcholine

What is the mechanism of action of a NDNMB?

Competitive antagonist of ACh at the neuromuscular nicotinic post-junctional receptor, causing paralysis by preventing depolarization of the muscle

Name some side effects of succinylcholine administration.

↑ potassium and ↑ intracranial, intraocular, and intraabdominal pressures

The normal initial dose of succinylcholine is ~1–1.5 mg/kg. By what amount does this raise the serum potassium in most patients?

0.5 mEq/L

What patient conditions can be adversely affected by this rise in serum potassium?

Recent burns, multi-system trauma/crush injuries; recent (days to months) CNS injuries (e.g., paraplegia) or denervation processes; stroke; neuropathy; myopathy; renal failure; malignant hyperthermia; or prolonged NDNMB use

What are the signs and symptoms of potentially fatal malignant hyperthermia (rarely) associated with succinylcholine?

Fever, hypercapnia, metabolic acidosis, mottled skin, muscle rigidity, tachydysrhythmias

What factors prolong the effects of succinylcholine?

A decrease in pseudocholinesterase levels in the plasma, the presence of a genetically atypical pseudocholinesterase, or the presence of a competitive pseudo-cholinesterase substrate (e.g., cocaine)

Laudanosine is a metabolite of certain NDNMBs that causes seizures by inhibiting GABA. Since all NMBs are polar, why does this metabolite affect the CNS?

Laudanosine is nonpolar and readily crosses the blood-brain barrier.

What class of drugs can reverse the effects of NDNMBs?

Cholinesterase inhibitors

Can cholinesterase inhibitors be used to reverse succinylcholine?

No, they will prolong neuromuscular blockade in this setting.

NITRATES

What are the major therapeutic uses of nitrates?

Angina pectoris, AMI, CHF

What are some other uses of nitrates?

1. Industrial uses – explosives (e.g., nitroglycerine in dynamite), food preservation
2. Therapeutic uses – antidiarrheals and topical cautery devices (e.g., silver nitrate)

What is the mechanism of action?

Within smooth muscle cells, nitrates re-lease nitric oxide with the downstream effect of increasing cGMP, resulting in smooth muscle relaxation.

What are the effects on the cardiovascular system?

Peripheral vasodilation $\rightarrow \downarrow$ preload and $\downarrow$ afterload (with higher doses)

What are the most common toxic effects of nitrate ingestion?

Related to vasodilation, most notably hypotension

What are the clinical signs and symptoms of nitrate toxicity?	Tachycardia, headache due to meningeal artery dilatation, orthostatic hypotension
What adverse effect to hemoglobin may occur following exposure to nitrates?	Methemoglobin
What drug class should be used with caution with nitrates?	Phosphodiesterase inhibitors (e.g., sildenafil)
When nitrates and these agents are used together, what adverse effects occur?	Both ↑ cGMP → synergistic vasodilatation and hypotension with potential hypoperfusion

NITRITES

What are examples of nitrites?	Sodium nitrite, amyl nitrite, butyl nitrite, methyl nitrite
What are the clinical uses of nitrites?	Sodium nitrite (injectable) and amyl nitrite (inhalant) are components of the cyanide antidote package. They oxidize hemoglobin to methemoglobin, which binds cyanide.
How are nitrites abused?	Amyl nitrite ampules are called "Amy," "poppers," "rush," or "snappers" and are inhaled.
What is the "high" achieved by abusing "poppers"?	A "rush" characterized by warm sensations and feelings of dizziness. May also delay and prolong orgasm.
What is the mechanism of action of nitrites?	Oxidizes hemoglobin to methemoglobin and also functions as a vasodilator.
What are signs of acute toxicity?	Headache, skin flushing, orthostatic hypotension with reflex tachycardia, acidosis, cyanosis, seizures, coma, dysrhythmias, "chocolate brown blood" if methemoglobinemia is present

What labs are helpful in the diagnosis of nitrite toxicity?

Direct measurement of methemoglobin level through co-oximetry

How should nitrite toxicity be treated?

High-flow oxygen and methylene blue (if methemoglobin level >30% or the patient is symptomatic)

NITROPRUSSIDE

What two active metabolites are released when nitroprusside is hydrolyzed, and what are their effects?

1. Nitric oxide (NO) – causes vasodilation
2. Cyanide (CN) – cellular toxin

What are the indications for nitroprusside use?

Treatment of severe hypertension and for inducing hypotension in certain surgical procedures

What is the normal fate of cyanide in patients treated with nitroprusside?

Cyanide is rapidly converted to thiocyanate by the enzyme rhodanese. Thiocyanate is then cleared by the kidneys.

What infusion rate of nitroprusside may cause cyanide toxicity?

Infusion rates >10 μg/kg/min for >1 hr put patients at risk for cyanide toxicity.

A patient with renal insufficiency becomes nauseated, confused, and progressively hypertensive after being treated with nitroprusside for 3 days. What toxin is implicated?

Thiocyanate, produced from the metabolism of cyanide, may accumulate to toxic levels in patients treated with nitroprusside. Symptoms include nausea, vomiting, somnolence, delirium, tremors, hyperreflexia, hypertension, and seizures.

What factors can cause thiocyanate accumulation?

Renal insufficiency and prolonged infusion. Nitroprusside infusion should not be run for >72 hrs.

Does hemodialysis help eliminate nitroprusside or cyanide?

No. Nitroprusside and cyanide are both metabolized rapidly; however, hemodialysis may be useful in clearing thiocyanate, particularly in patients with impaired renal function.

NITROUS OXIDE

How is nitrous oxide (N_2O) used clinically?	As a weak anesthetic, mostly in outpatient dentistry mixed with oxygen at a concentration of 25% to 50% for analgesia and sedation; principal adjunct to inhalation and IV general anesthetic
What are the street names for nitrous oxide?	Laughing gas, hippie crack
How is it commonly obtained by abusers?	1. "Crackers" are nitrite-containing metal or plastic canisters. "Poppers" are nitrite-containing ampules that are broken or "popped" to release vapors. 2. "Whipits" are small cartridges of N_2O used for dispensing whipped cream.
What is the onset of action and method of delivery?	2–5 min by inhalation
By what mechanism is anesthesia achieved?	It may act by inhibition of NMDA-activated currents and stabilize axonal membranes to partially inhibit action potentials, leading to sedation.
What are signs and symptoms of acute toxicity?	Acute inhalation may lead to euphoria; however, acute toxicity is related to asphyxia, causing headache, dizziness, confusion, syncope, seizures, and cardiac dysrhythmias.
What are the results of chronic abuse?	Megaloblastic anemia, thrombocytopenia, leukopenia, peripheral neuropathy (especially posterior column findings), myelopathy, birth defects, and spontaneous abortion
Name the vitamin depleted by chronic inhalation.	Vitamin B_{12} (cyanocobalamin)
What is the effect of nitrous oxide on the cardiovascular system?	Hypotension has been reported, as has methemoglobinemia, which may result from contaminants (nitrates/nitrites).

How is it eliminated?	Almost completely by the lungs, with some minimal diffusion through the skin
What lab tests could aid in diagnosis?	CBC with differential, vitamin B_{12}, and folic acid levels
Is there a treatment for chronic toxicity?	Folinic acid may help with bone marrow suppression

NONSTEROIDAL ANTI-INFLAMMATORY DRUGS

What are the common specific drugs that fall into the five major categories of NSAIDs?	1. Propionic acids – ibuprofen, fenoprofen, ketoprofen, naproxen, oxaprozin 2. Acetic acids – diclofenac, etodolac, indomethacin, ketorolac, sulindac 3. Fenamic acids – mefenamic acid, meclofenamic acid 4. Oxicams – piroxicam 5. Pyrazolones – phenylbutazone
Which NSAID is most commonly taken in an overdose?	Ibuprofen
What is the general mechanism of action for NSAIDs?	Inhibition of cyclooxygenase enzymes (COX) I and II with subsequent blockade of prostaglandins
Are there NSAIDs with selective COX inhibition properties?	Yes. Celecoxib, rofecoxib, and meloxicam are more COX II selective.
How are NSAIDs metabolized and eliminated?	Absorbed primarily in the small intestine and undergo hepatic oxidation and glucuronidation. Metabolites are mainly excreted in the urine, but most have some enterohepatic excretion and reabsorption.
At what dose may symptoms emerge in children following ibuprofen overdose?	100 mg/kg
Which two NSAID classes require more aggressive management?	Pyrazolones and fenamic acids

Which drug has the highest incidence of seizures?

Mefenamic acid, usually 2–7 hrs post-ingestion

What are the most common side effects with ibuprofen?

Mild GI symptoms (e.g., nausea, vomiting, abdominal pain), which can be followed by mild CNS disturbances (e.g., drowsiness, headaches). Seizures, hypotension, metabolic acidosis, and renal and hepatic dysfunction may develop after massive overdoses.

What is the mechanism of acidosis?

Anion gap metabolic acidosis may be related to acidic metabolites and hypotension. This tends to occur only in large overdoses.

Are there toxicities associated with chronic ingestion?

Yes. GI bleeding and renal dysfunction

Are hemodialysis and urine alkalinization indicated in NSAID overdoses?

Mild renal dysfunction can be seen with acute overdoses; however, the renal failure usually resolves with fluid administration. NSAIDs are highly protein-bound, and the metabolites are excreted in the urine, thus hemodialysis and alkalization of urine have not been proven to enhance elimination.

Do serum NSAID levels predict toxicity?

No

OPIOIDS

What are the three opiate receptors?

Delta, kappa, mu

What are some slang terms for various opiates?

China white, brown, superbuick, black tar, hot shot, bird's eye, homicide

How are opioids abused?

Depending on the specific substance, opioids can be insufflated, injected, smoked, or taken orally.

What is the opioid toxidrome?

CNS and respiratory depression with miotic pupils

How do opiates differ from opioids?

Opiates are specific substances derived from the opium poppy. Opioids include all substances (both natural and synthetic) that are capable of producing opium-like effects.

With opioid urine drug screens, what three opioids are reliably detected?

These screens detect morphine metabolites; therefore, only morphine, as well as heroin and codeine (both of which are metabolized to morphine), are detected by such screens. Other opioids (i.e., fentanyl, oxycodone, hydrocodone, meperidine, propoxyphene, hydromorphone, tramadol) may not be detected.

Which synthetic opioid should be avoided in patients taking MAOIs and why?

Meperidine. MAOIs block the reuptake of serotonin, and the interaction between meperidine and the serotonin receptors could induce serotonin syndrome.

Which by-product of illicit opioid production causes parkinsonian symptoms?

Illicit synthesis of the meperidine analogue MPPP (1-methyl-4-phenyl-4-propionoxypiperidine) has been shown to accidentally produce MPTP (1-methyl-4-phenyl-1,2,3,6-tetrahydropyridine) as a by-product. When MPTP is used intravenously, it is subsequently metabolized into MPP^+ (by MAO-B), which interferes with mitochondrial oxidative phosphorylation at complex I and causes free radical-mediated cell destruction within the substantia nigra.

How are opioids metabolized and excreted?

Hepatic metabolism with renal excretion

What percentage of the population lacks the ability to metabolize codeine to morphine?

Approximately 7% of the Caucasian population lacks the appropriate enzyme (CYP2D6).

Is there an antidote for opiate overdose?

Naloxone. It should be given slowly (0.4 mg over a few min) and titrated with the return of spontaneous respiratory effort. As the half-life of naloxone is shorter than that of most opioids, the patient should be monitored for re-sedation or development of opioid-induced non-cardiogenic pulmonary edema, typically manifesting within 4 hrs in people with normal renal function.

What is the general treatment of opioid poisoning?

Primarily supportive care. Respiratory depression will be the main concern. Naloxone may be used as a diagnostic tool or to avoid intubation.

Other than respiratory depression, what acute pulmonary complication is associated with opioid use?

Noncardiogenic pulmonary edema

What are the signs of withdrawal?

CNS excitation (e.g., restlessness, agitation, anxiety, dysphoria), nausea, vomiting, abdominal cramps, diarrhea, piloerection, lacrimation, rhinorrhea, diaphoresis. AMS and fever are not associated with opioid withdrawal and those signs should prompt further diagnostic testing.

Which medications have been used to alleviate opioid withdrawal symptoms?

Methadone, clonidine, buspirone

Name three opioids that do not cause miosis.

Meperidine, propoxyphene, tramadol

PHENYTOIN

What electrolyte channel is primarily affected by phenytoin?

Neuronal sodium channels are blocked

Why does rapid IV administration of phenytoin cause myocardial depression and cardiac arrest?

While originally thought to come solely from the propylene glycol diluent, phenytoin also seems to have a direct cardio-depressant effect.

How should IV phenytoin be administered?

Slowly (maximum 50 mg/min) and with ECG monitoring

Is oral phenytoin cardiotoxic?

No

Why is it important that phenytoin not be administered IM or through an infiltrated IV?

It causes tissue necrosis.

What is fosphenytoin?

A disodium phosphate ester of phenytoin that does not contain propylene glycol, is better tolerated IV and can be administered IM

What happens to the half-life of phenytoin as the levels rise?

First-order elimination switches to zero-order elimination, and the half-life increases.

How is phenytoin metabolized?

Cytochrome P450 pathway, resulting in multiple drug interactions

What are the symptoms of mild to moderate intoxication?

Nystagmus, dysarthria, ataxia, nausea, vomiting, diplopia

What are the symptoms of a severe intoxication?

Stupor, coma, respiratory arrest

What are some potential side effects of phenytoin?

Fever, rash, blood dyscrasia, hepatitis, Stevens-Johnson syndrome, gingival hyperplasia

Can a serum phenytoin level be obtained?

Yes, the therapeutic range is 10–20 mg/L.

What is the correlation between phenytoin levels and symptoms?

1. >20 mg/L – nystagmus
2. >30 mg/L – ataxia, slurred speech, nausea, vomiting
3. >40 mg/L – lethargy, confusion, stupor
4. >50 mg/L – coma, seizures

Is there a specific antidote for phenytoin toxicity?

No, treatment is supportive.

RAUWOLFIA ALKALOIDS

In what general class of medications are rauwolfia alkaloids found?

Antihypertensives

From where are rauwolfia alkaloids derived?

The roots of *Rauwolfia serpentina*, a plant native to India

What was once a commonly used rauwolfia alkaloid?

Reserpine

What is the significance of reserpine?

First drug used in the modern era of hypertension management

Describe the mechanism of action of reserpine.

It depletes stores of serotonin, dopamine, and norepinephrine by initially preventing their reuptake, then binds to catecholamine storage vesicles in the presynaptic adrenergic neuron terminals. This is effectively a pharmacological sympathectomy, which leads to decreased vascular tone and bradycardia with subsequent hypotension.

Why was reserpine used as a treatment for schizophrenia?

Depletion of catecholamines in the brain can produce a sedative effect.

Why is reserpine not used commonly in the United States?

CNS side effects and newer drugs that are as effective

List some of the common side effects of reserpine.

Sedation and inability to concentrate are most common. Also, psychotic depression, parkinsonism, headache, nightmares, dysrhythmias, bradycardia, hypotension. Concomitant use of MAOIs can lead to adrenergic storm.

What is the clinical presentation of acute reserpine toxicity?

Symptoms are typically seen within 3–7 hrs post-ingestion and may last 2–4 days. Signs and symptoms are related to initial catecholamine excess, then subsequent depletion with unbalanced parasympathetic activity.

1. CNS – ataxia, AMS, stupor, coma
2. CV – tachycardia followed by bradycardia, hypertension followed by hypotension
3. Parasympathetic effects – miosis, facial flushing, excessive salivation, hypothermia, diarrhea, excessive gastric acid secretion

What neurologic disorders may be induced with chronic reserpine use?

Parkinson's disease and depression

Why is reserpine starting to be used more in the United States?

Reserpine at low doses, used in combination with diuretics, has proven effective in the treatment of hypertension, specifically in the elderly.

Why is reserpine use still prevalent in developing nations?

The cost is cheaper than that of other antihypertensives.

How long does it take to synthesize vesicles once reserpine is stopped?

2–3 wks

How long after the first dose of reserpine does it take for hypotensive effects to be seen?

2–3 wks

What is the treatment of acute reserpine overdose?

Supportive care. Short-acting, titratable cardiovascular agents should be used, as initial hypertension may progress to hypotension.

SALICYLATES

What are the clinical uses of salicylates?

Analgesia, anti-inflammatory, anti-pyretic

What are common forms of salicylates?

1. Aspirin (acetylsalicylic acid)
2. Oil of wintergreen (methyl salicylate)
3. Bismuth salicylate

How many grams of aspirin are equal to 5 mL of oil of wintergreen?

About 7 g or 21 regular strength aspirin tablets

What factors can dramatically delay absorption in salicylate overdoses?

1. Large tablet masses (bezoars) in the GI tract
2. Enteric-coated products
3. Pylorospasm
4. ↓ gastric motility

What are the metabolic effects of a salicylate overdose?

1. Respiratory alkalosis – stimulation of the central respiratory center causes hyperpnea and tachypnea. Also occurs to compensate for metabolic acidosis in more severe cases.
2. Metabolic acidosis – uncoupling of oxidative phosphorylation and interruption of Krebs cycle dehydrogenases → ↑ CO_2 production
3. Metabolic alkalosis – may occur secondary to vomiting

How are salicylates eliminated?

Hepatic metabolism predominates at therapeutic doses, but due to saturation of hepatic metabolism, renal excretion is also important in overdoses.

What is the toxic dose in acute ingestions?

1. <150 mg/kg – no toxicity to mild toxicity
2. 150–300 mg/kg – mild to moderate toxicity
3. 300–500 mg/kg – severe toxicity

What is the clinical presentation of an acute overdose of salicylates?

Initial symptoms include GI upset, tinnitus, and tachypnea/hyperpnea, followed in severe cases by coma, seizures, hyperthermia, hypotension, pulmonary and cerebral edema, and death.

What is the clinical presentation of chronic toxicity?

Hearing loss/tinnitus, confusion, dehydration, metabolic acidosis, seizures, lethargy, pulmonary and cerebral edema, coma

Which has higher morbidity and mortality, acute or chronic overdose?

Chronic

What acid-base abnormality is seen on ABG analysis with salicylate overdoses?

Mixed respiratory alkalosis and metabolic acidosis

What is considered a toxic salicylate level?

Above 30 mg/dL (300 mg/L). Note the units, as some laboratories report in mg/dL and others in mg/L. Failure to pay attention to this detail can lead to unnecessary transfers and treatment.

How often should salicylate levels be drawn following acute overdose?

Initially, consider drawing levels every 2 hrs until the salicylate level begins declining, then every 4 hrs until they return to the therapeutic range.

How should a salicylate overdose be treated?

GI decontamination with activated charcoal. Sodium bicarbonate should be given to alkalinize the urine and serum in order to prevent salicylate from crossing the blood-brain barrier and to promote excretion. Dialysis should be considered in severe overdoses.

Why is charcoal important in treatment?

Due to the possibility of delayed absorption, even if administered late, charcoal has the potential to bind a significant amount of the drug.

How should sodium bicarbonate be administered?

Boluses of 1–2 mEq/kg, followed by an infusion of 5% dextrose in water with 150 mEq of sodium bicarbonate to maintain the urine pH at 7.5 to 8. After assuring urine output, add potassium to each liter of fluid to avoid hypokalemia.

If a salicylate toxic patient is intubated, how should they be ventilated?

Hyperventilate to compensate for the metabolic acidosis. Placing an acute salicylate overdose on typical ventilator settings may kill the patient.

What are the indications for urgent hemodialysis?

1. Salicylate level >100 mg/dL after acute overdose
2. Salicylate level >60 mg/dL after chronic overdose with AMS or acidosis
3. Severe manifestations – coma, seizures, cerebral edema, acute respiratory distress syndrome (ARDS), renal failure, severe / refractory acidosis or electrolyte abnormality
4. Inability to tolerate sodium bicarbonate alkalinization (due to renal failure, pulmonary edema, etc.)

SEDATIVE-HYPNOTIC AGENTS

What are the common uses of sedative-hypnotic agents?

Anxiety, insomnia, sedation, alcohol withdrawal, seizure management

Name some common sedative-hypnotic agents.

Barbiturates, benzodiazepines, buspirone, zolpidem, chloral hydrate, carisoprodol

What is the sedative-hypnotic toxidrome?

CNS depression with variable respiratory depression. The remainder of the physical exam may be otherwise unremarkable.

What subversive acts are these drugs often used for?

Drug-facilitated sexual assault ("date-rape") or robbery

What benzodiazepine used in drug-facilitated assault is not detected on many routine drug assays?

Flunitrazepam (Rohypnol), also known as "Roofies"

What properties make it popular for this use?

It is a potent sedative-hypnotic that is tasteless, easily dissolved in liquids, and is not detectable on most routine urine drug screens. It is still legally manufactured in European countries but is Schedule I in the U.S. The manufacturer has recently added a blue dye to the formulation in an attempt to make it more detectable in beverages.

Which agent has been associated with ventricular dysrhythmias in children?

Chloral hydrate

What is the term used for the combination of chloral hydrate and ethanol?

"Mickey Finn"

What is the treatment of sedative-hypnotic overdose?

The mainstay of treatment of all sedative-hypnotics is supportive care. Respiratory support should be provided as needed, and evaluation for co-ingestions is important.

Is there an antidote for benzodiazepine overdose?

Yes. Flumazenil is a competitive benzodiazepine antagonist.

Do sedative-hypnotics have a withdrawal syndrome?

Yes. Withdrawal from these agents can have severe and life-threatening complications. CNS and autonomic excitation occur, resulting in tremor, tachycardia, hypertension, hyperthermia, and seizures.

SKELETAL MUSCLE RELAXANTS

What are some examples of common skeletal muscle relaxants?

Baclofen, carisoprodol, chlorzoxazone, cyclobenzaprine, metaxolone, methocarbamol, orphenadrine, tizanidine

Under what class do most of these medicines fall?

Sedative-hypnotic agents

Which three skeletal muscle relaxants are the most abused as recreational drugs?

Cyclobenzaprine, carisoprodol, baclofen

Does the clinical presentation of all skeletal muscle relaxants in overdose look the same?

No, as this is a broad class of drugs with varying effects on specific receptors.

What skeletal muscle relaxant has GABA-B agonist activity?

Baclofen. Overdose is consequently associated with coma, respiratory depression, seizures, and bradycardia.

What two skeletal muscle relaxants induce an anticholinergic syndrome in overdose?	Cyclobenzaprine and orphenadrine
What skeletal muscle relaxant has been associated with SVT and lidocaine-refractory VT in overdose?	Orphenadrine
Which skeletal muscle relaxant has alpha 2-adrenergic effects and acts like clonidine following overdose?	Tizanidine (CNS depression, miosis, bradycardia, and hypotension following overdose)
Is there a specific antidote for skeletal muscle relaxant overdoses?	No, management is supportive.

THEOPHYLLINE

What are the clinical uses for oral theophylline?	COPD and asthma
What is aminophylline, and how does it differ from theophylline?	Theophylline ethylenediamine, a salt of theophylline. It is less potent and may be given IV.
What are the clinical uses for aminophylline?	1. Refractory asthma 2. CHF 3. Nonasthmatic bronchospasm 4. Neonatal apnea, as a respiratory stimulant
By what mechanisms does theophylline exert its therapeutic and toxic effects?	1. Stimulation of beta 1- and beta 2-adrenergic receptors 2. Inhibition of phosphodiesterase 3. Inhibition of adenosine receptors
What is the significance of adenosine blockade?	Adenosine-1 receptors cause feedback inhibition of neuronal firing. Adenosine-2 receptors cause cerebral vasodilation. Theophylline toxicity may, therefore, result in refractory seizures with a relative lack of cerebral blood flow.

What is the toxic dose for theophylline?

>20 μg/kg, although toxicity may be seen with lower doses

What serum level signifies a severe theophylline acute overdose?

>80–100 mg/L

How does acute theophylline overdose present?

1. Mild or moderate toxicity – GI upset, tachycardia, anxiety, tremor, mild metabolic acidosis, and electrolyte abnormalities
2. Severe toxicity – refractory vomiting, hypotension, metabolic acidosis, dysrhythmias, seizures

What electrolyte and glucose abnormalities may be seen with acute theophylline overdose?

Hypokalemia, hypophosphatemia, hypomagnesemia, hypercalcemia, hyperglycemia

How does chronic theophylline toxicity differ from acute overdose?

In chronic toxicity, GI upset, hypokalemia, and hyperglycemia are less common, but severe symptoms (e.g., seizures, dysrhythmias) are more frequently seen than in acute overdose and may occur at lower serum concentrations (even at 40 mg/L).

What criteria may be used to positively diagnose theophylline overdose?

Serum theophylline levels. The diagnosis is suggested by a history of refractory vomiting, tachycardia, hypokalemia, tremors, hyperreflexia, and hyperglycemia.

What treatments should be performed in the event of theophylline overdose?

1. Primarily supportive
2. Nonselective beta blockers have been reported to improve hypotension and tachycardia in case reports but should be used cautiously, as no clinical trials have been conducted to determine efficacy.
3. Hypokalemia is usually transient and resolves without intervention.
4. Multiple-dose activated charcoal may be beneficial, as theophylline undergoes enteroenteric recirculation.
5. Hemodialysis should be considered for those with severe toxicity.

THYROID HORMONES

What forms of thyroid hormone are available for clinical use?	1. Synthetic triiodothyronine (T_3, or liothyronine) 2. Synthetic thyroxine (T_4, or levothyroxine) 3. Synthetic combination of T_3 and T_4 in 1:4 ratio (liotrix) 4. Natural desiccated animal thyroid (both T_3 and T_4), derived from porcine thyroid glands
For what medical condition are thyroid hormones administered?	Both T_3 and T_4 are used for hypothyroidism.
What form of thyroid hormone is considered to be most potent?	T_3 has $3\times$ more activity than T_4. T_4 undergoes peripheral conversion to T_3 by a $5'$-deiodinase, primarily in the liver and kidney.
How is thyroid hormone administered?	Oral (well-absorbed enterally)
What is the mechanism of action of thyroid hormones?	Bind to intracellular receptors that regulate transcription and translation of proteins that $\uparrow$ oxygen consumption by promoting Na-K-ATPase activity
In which compartments are thyroid hormones metabolized?	Liver and kidneys
What is a toxic dose of thyroid hormone?	A dose $>3–5$ mg T_4 or 750 µg T_3 acutely. The threshold is lower in those with baseline cardiac disease or chronic overexposure.
How is the diagnosis of acute thyroid hormone overdose made?	History consistent with ingestion and clinical presentation consistent with sympathetic adrenergic excess. Serum thyroid hormone levels are of little use clinically.
What is the mechanism of toxicity of thyroid hormone overdose?	Sympathetic adrenergic overstimulation (targets CV, GI, neuro)

How soon after acute ingestion of thyroid hormones will symptoms of overdose appear?

T_3 overdose may be evident as soon as 6 hrs post-ingestion. T_4 toxicity may not be clinically apparent until as long as 11 days post-ingestion (while being deiodinated to T_3).

What are the acute effects of thyroid hormone overdose?

Anxiety, agitation, tremor, GI symptoms, tachycardia, and hypertension on presentation may be followed by SVT, hypotension, hyperthermia, and seizures in severe overdose.

What is the treatment of thyroid hormone overdose?

Similar to hyperthyroidism – adrenergic symptoms can be treated with propranolol or esmolol. In cases of T_4 overdose, peripheral conversion to T_3 may be inhibited by propylthiouracil. Benzodiazepines also are appropriate for agitation.

TYPE I ANTIDYSRHYTHMIC AGENTS

What is the basic mechanism of action of the type I antidysrhythmics?

They reduce excitability of cardiac tissue by preventing fast acting sodium channels from converting from an inactivated state to a resting or "ready" state, thereby decreasing the number of active sodium channels available to generate an action potential.

What is the physiology behind this mechanism?

By inhibiting the fast acting sodium channels that are normally active during the upstroke (phase 0) of the action potential in cardiac tissue, they slow the rate of depolarization and propagation of conduction through the myocardium.

How are type I antidysrhythmics further subdivided?

Based on their effects on the duration of the action potential (AP)

What are the effects of type Ia, Ib, and Ic agents on the AP?

Ia – prolong
Ib – shorten
Ic – no effect on the AP

Which class binds primarily to inactivated sodium channels?

Ib

Which class also acts at myocardial potassium channels responsible for repolarization?

Ia and Ic

How does this potassium efflux blockade affect the ECG?

Prolongs the QTc

What rhythm can result from QTc prolongation?

Torsade de pointes

What are some type Ia agents?

Procainamide (prototypical type Ia agent), quinidine, disopyramide

What are the physiologic effects of type Ia agents at high concentrations?

1. Prolonged AV conduction
2. Depressed ventricular conduction velocity, resulting in prolonged QRS duration
3. Delayed repolarization, resulting in prolonged QT interval and progression to torsade de pointes
4. ↓ cardiac contractility and excitability

What organ systems are affected by type Ia toxicity?

Mostly CNS and cardiovascular effects

What are the clinical signs and symptoms of type Ia agent toxicity?

1. CNS – anticholinergic toxidrome with AMS (quinidine and disopyramide), seizures, respiratory depression, coma
2. CV – wide QRS-complex tachycardia (sodium channel blockade), anticholinergic-induced tachycardia, depressed contractility, and subsequent hypotension when confounded by alpha-adrenergic blockade or ganglionic blockade
3. GI – nausea, vomiting, diarrhea, hypoglycemia

Which agent is associated with a drug-induced lupus syndrome when used chronically?	Procainamide
What is cinchonism?	Syndrome of headache, tinnitus, vertigo, deafness, and visual disturbances
What agent is associated with cinchonism after chronic use?	Quinidine
What is the management of type Ia cardiac toxicity?	Sodium bicarbonate for ventricular tachy-dysrhythmias and undifferentiated wide complex tachycardias. Other agents, such as lidocaine, phenytoin, or pacing can be used. Never use type Ia or type Ic agents, as they may exacerbate toxic effects on the heart.
What is the prototypical type Ib agent?	Lidocaine
Name some other type Ib agents.	Tocainamide, mexiletine, phenytoin
Do type Ib agents cause QRS widening?	No, these agent have binding properties that are fast-on, fast-off and they prefer-entially bind to the sodium channel in the inactive state. In contrast, both type Ia and Ic agents may cause QRS widening.
What are the CNS effects with type Ib overdose?	CNS stimulation, confusion, seizures, res-piratory arrest
What the effects of toxic exposure to type Ib agents?	Asystole, sinus arrest, AV block, cardiac arrest
Can type Ib agents be associated with torsade de pointes?	No. They have no effect on potassium channels, do not prolong repolarization, and do not prolong the QTc.

Which of these agents is associated with agranulocytosis?

Tocainide

What are some examples of type Ic agents?

Flecainide, encainide, propafenone, moricizine

What the effects of toxic exposure to type Ic agents?

Ventricular dysrhythmias, bradycardia, SA and AV block, asystole

According to the Cardiac Arrhythmia Suppression Trial (CAST), which of these agents have been shown to increase overall mortality?

Flecainide, encainide, moricizine

What electrolyte disturbance increases the cardiac toxicity of all type I agents?

Hyperkalemia

Which type I agents (Ia, Ib, or Ic) are most associated with proarrhythmic effects?

Type Ic; thus, these agents are typically used only for dysrhythmias that are refractory to other drugs

TYPE II ANTIDYSRHYTHMIC AGENTS

What is the mechanism of action of type II agents?

Beta-adrenergic receptor blockade → ↓ cAMP → inhibition of sodium and calcium currents

What cardiac tissues are most sensitive to the antidysrhythmic actions of type II agents?

AV node

What are the effects of excessive beta-adrenergic blockade in patients requiring antidysrhythmics?

Same as those for patients taking beta blockers for other medical problems, including bronchospasm, bradycardia, hypotension, and first-degree heart block, but these patients are more prone to the depressive effects on cardiac output

Which type II agent is associated with coma, respiratory depression, and convulsions?	Propranolol. Because it is lipophilic, it has more severe CNS toxicity. It also has myocardial sodium channel blocking activity and can therefore lead to prolongation of the QRS complex.
What metabolic disturbances can occur with type II agent toxicity?	Hyperkalemia and hypoglycemia
Hypotension induced by overdose of beta-blockers can be reversed with which drug?	npc8a
What other therapy has been utilized to treat persistent hypotension and bradycardia induced by beta-blockers?	Hyperinsulinemia/euglycemia therapy

TYPE III ANTIDYSRHYTHMIC AGENTS

What is the basic mechanism of action of type III antidysrhythmics?	Delays repolarization, prolonging the action potential and increasing the effective refractory period by blocking the potassium current
At therapeutic levels, what ECG changes can be seen?	PR and QTc prolongation
Upon which cardiac tissues do these agents act?	Atrial and ventricular
Name examples of type III agents.	Amiodarone, sotalol, bretylium, dofetilide, ibutilide
What dysrhythmia may be induced by these agents?	Torsade de pointes
Can these agents cause toxic effects at therapeutic doses?	Yes. Because they have a narrow therapeutic index, these agents can be highly toxic with even small ingestions.
What other actions does sotalol have?	Type II effects (beta-adrenergic blockade) at low doses and mixed type II and type III effects at high doses

What other cardiovascular disturbances can this drug precipitate?	Bradydysrhythmias and hypotension
Which agent initially releases and later inhibits catecholamine release?	Bretylium
What can this cause?	Transient hypertension followed by hypotension that may last for hours after administration
Although amiodarone primarily acts as a type III agent, what other properties does it possess?	Types I, II, and IV (all of them)
Because amiodarone has type II (beta-adrenergic blocking) and type IV (calcium channel blocking) effects, what can amiodarone do to the heart rate?	Slows heart rate → bradycardia
How does this affect the arrhythmogenicity of this type III agent?	Reduces the propensity to cause new dysrhythmias
What extracardiac side effects are associated with chronic amiodarone use?	Pulmonary fibrosis, hypo- and hyperthyroidism, corneal deposits → vision loss, grayish discoloration of the skin

TYPE IV ANTIDYSRHYTHMIC AGENTS

What is the mechanism of action of type IV agents?	Calcium channel blockade that slows calcium entry into the myocardial cells → ↓ cardiac contractility and ↓ AV nodal conduction
What changes are typically seen on ECG at therapeutic levels?	PR interval prolongation
Which calcium channel blockers (CCB) are antidysrhythmic agents?	Verapamil and diltiazem

What are the toxic effects of calcium channel blockade?

AV block, bradycardia, hypotension, CNS depression

What drug interactions might exacerbate these effects?

Concomitant use with beta blockers, especially when given parenterally

Verapamil in overdose has been associated with what adverse effect on the heart (besides calcium channel blockade)?

Cardiac sodium channel blockade

CCBs in overdose are associated with what adverse insulin effects?

1. Prevention of insulin release from pancreatic beta cells
2. Peripheral insulin blockade

In severe CCB overdose, what is more commonly seen, hyperglycemia or hypoglycemia?

Hyperglycemia

What specific drugs can be used in type IV agent toxicity?

Calcium chloride or calcium gluconate can initially be used to augment calcium flow. Glucagon, adrenergic agents (e.g., epinephrine), and amrinone may ↑ intracellular cAMP to overcome calcium channel blockade. Hyperinsulinemia-euglycemia therapy has been shown to improve contractility.

Are CCBs dialyzable?

No, CCBs are highly protein bound and, therefore, not dialyzable.

VALPROIC ACID

For which indications is valproic acid prescribed?

1. Seizure disorders (prophylaxis or to abort status epilepticus)
2. Affective disorders
3. Chronic pain (not an approved use)
4. Migraine headache prophylaxis

Where is valproic acid metabolized?

Liver

What is the toxic dose?

Although highly variable, 200–400 mg/kg may cause coma. >400 mg/kg has an increased risk for an adverse outcome.

What organ system is most affected by an acute overdose?

CNS – causes depression

With chronic therapy, what organ may be adversely affected?

The liver – hepatic failure can occur.

What metabolic complications can be seen with valproic acid ingestion?

Primary hyperammonemia (without coexisting hepatic failure) may be seen with therapeutic use or following overdose. Anion gap metabolic acidosis may be seen in acute overdose with very large ingestions.

What is considered a toxic valproate level?

Levels >150 mg/L are considered toxic.

How should the overdose be treated?

Multi-dose activated charcoal has been used to ↑ elimination. Valproate-induced hyperammonemic encephalopathy may be treated with carnitine and lactulose. Hemodialysis may be used for patients with marked acidosis or very high serum concentrations.

What hematologic abnormality may be seen in overdose?

Bone marrow suppression can occur after massive overdose. This presents within 3 to 5 days and resolves spontaneously a few days later.

VASODILATORS

What medications are vasodilators?

This class includes a broad spectrum of medications that dilate peripheral arteries and veins, producing ↓ BP. Many medications fit this description, but only alpha-adrenergic blockers and direct-acting agents will be discussed here.

What are the names and mechanisms of the three direct-acting arterial vasodilators?

1. Hydralazine – acts via cGMP in the smooth muscle
2. Minoxidil sulfate – hyperpolarizes arteriolar smooth muscle cells by activating ATPase-sensitive potassium channels
3. Diazoxide – hyperpolarizes arteriolar smooth muscle cells by activating ATPase-sensitive potassium channels

How is the alpha-adrenergic receptor involved in vasodilation?

Peripheral alpha-1 receptors cause vasoconstriction when activated. Blockade of these receptors, therefore, causes vasodilation.

How does the typical vasodilator overdose patient present?

Hypotension with reflex tachycardia

How do vasodilators cause tachycardia?

Likely through a baroreceptor-mediated reflex causing sympathetic stimulation, increasing myocardial chronotropy, and inotropy

What treatment for male-pattern baldness is also used as a vasodilator?

Minoxidil

What types of immunologic reactions are associated with hydralazine?

Lupus-like syndrome, serum sickness, vasculitis, glomerulonephritis, hemolytic anemia

What test should every patient with suspected vasodilator toxicity undergo?

An ECG, as myocardial ischemia, tachycardia, and ECG changes all have been reported with vasodilator toxicity, particularly minoxidil

What is the primary treatment for overdose?

Fluid resuscitation followed by alpha-1 agonists (e.g., phenylephrine) as necessary

VITAMINS

Which vitamins are most likely to cause acute or chronic toxicities?

Fat-soluble vitamins (A, D, E, K)

Are the toxic levels of vitamins well-defined?	No. A wide variance in potential toxicity exists for both acute and chronic exposures.
What are the acute and chronic toxic doses of vitamin A?	1. Acute – 12,000 IU/kg 2. Chronic – 25,000 IU/day for 2–3 wks or 4,000 IU/day for 6–15 months
Name the food associated with vitamin A toxicity in Eskimos.	Polar bear liver
What are the clinical findings of acute vitamin A toxicity?	Nausea, vomiting, headache, drowsiness, desquamation
What are the clinical findings of chronic vitamin A toxicity?	↑ ICP (causing headache, papilledema, seizures, blurred vision); dry skin (may also see eczema, erythema, alopecia, or angular cheilitis); bone pain; hepatitis
The measurement of specific levels of which vitamins may assist in diagnosing an overdose?	Vitamins A and D
How are vitamin E and vitamin K toxicities monitored if not measuring their specific levels?	PT, aPTT, and bleeding times
What are the clinical findings of chronic vitamin D toxicity?	Hypercalcemia (may see metastatic calcifications and renal calculi); weakness; AMS; constipation; polyuria; polydipsia; backache; cardiac dysrhythmias (late sign associated with hypertension)
What is the mechanism by which vitamin E exerts its anticoagulant effects?	It antagonizes the effects of vitamin K and may act synergistically with warfarin, affecting factors II, VII, IX, and X.
Acute vitamin E toxicity may present with which signs and symptoms?	Nausea, vomiting, and weakness are most likely to be reported; however, in a malnourished patient or in those on warfarin, coagulopathy may be reported.

If a mother receives excess vitamin K during pregnancy, what symptoms may result in the newborn?

Hemolytic anemia, jaundice, and hyperbilirubinemia (particularly if comorbid G6PD deficiency)

Which vitamin is highly teratogenic in pregnancy?

Isotretinoin, a form of vitamin A used in the treatment of acne. Embryonic sensitivity is greatest during the first eight weeks of pregnancy.

How can chronic beta-carotene ingestion be differentiated from true jaundice?

In beta-carotene ingestion no scleral icterus is present, while in true jaundice scleral icterus may be one of the first signs.

Toxic amounts of vitamin K result in the inactivation of what drug class?

Oral anticoagulants

Which vitamin is also known as niacin?

Vitamin B$_3$

Toxic levels of niacin increase the release of which prostaglandin?

Prostaglandin D2

What signs and symptoms does prostaglandin D2 produce?

Cutaneous flushing, pruritus, headache, bronchoconstriction, vasodilation

What medication can be used to prevent this side effect of niacin?

Aspirin, 81 mg ingested 30 min before niacin

What is the acute toxic dose of niacin?

Ingestion of >1000 mg/day

Name the organ most likely affected in chronic niacin toxicity.

The liver. Elevated transaminases can occur with both acute and chronic overdose. Abnormalities usually improve after discontinuation of niacin.

Which vitamin is also known as pyridoxine?

Vitamin B$_6$

What are the symptoms of chronic pyridoxine overdose?	Ataxia, hyporeflexia, and sensory neuropathies, primarily affecting proprioception and vibratory sense
What is the chronic toxic dose of pyridoxine?	2–5 g/day for several months has resulted in peripheral neuropathy
Large doses of B vitamins may result in which benign clinical sign?	Intensification of the yellow color of urine. Riboflavin may cause yellow perspiration.

WARFARIN

How was warfarin discovered?	Researchers at the **W**isconsin **A**lumni **R**esearch **F**oundation found that cattle eating spoiled clover were developing coagulopathies. This also gave the name WARFarin.
How is warfarin used?	1. Therapeutic anticoagulant 2. Rodenticide, although longer-acting "superwarfarins" are now used
What is the mechanism of warfarin?	Blocks hepatic synthesis of vitamin K-dependent coagulation factors by inhibiting the enzyme vitamin $K_{(1)}$ 2, 3-epoxide reductase
Which coagulation factors are dependent on vitamin K for synthesis?	II, VII, IX, X
What is a "superwarfarin"?	A fat-soluble warfarin derivative that is used as a rodenticide because of its long-acting effects
How long does it take for anticoagulation effects to emerge?	Warfarin inhibits synthesis of new factors. While factor VII begins to degrade within 5 hrs, peak effects are not seen until 2–3 days.
What is the toxic dose of warfarin?	In patients who are not on chronic warfarin therapy, single acute ingestions of warfarin do not cause clinically significant

anticoagulation; however, small amounts (2–5 mg) repeated over multiple days can lead to significant anticoagulation.

What is the duration of anticoagulant effect after a single dose of warfarin?

2–7 days

What is the duration of anticoagulant effect after a single dose of a superwarfarin?

Weeks to months

How is warfarin metabolized?

Cytochrome P450 liver enzymes, resulting in numerous potential drug interactions

What drugs interfere with the anticoagulant effect of warfarin?

1. ↑ anticoagulation – allopurinol, amiodarone, cimetidine, disulfiram, ginkgo biloba, NSAIDS, salicylates, sulfa
2. ↓ anticoagulation – barbiturates, carbamazepine, nafcillin, PO contraceptives, phenytoin, rifampin

What is the primary adverse effect of warfarin?

Bleeding

Name two nonhemorrhagic complications of warfarin use.

Warfarin skin necrosis and purple toe syndrome

Is checking a warfarin level helpful for management of an overdose?

No, warfarin levels are not clinically useful in the acute management of a known warfarin overdose. The PT/INR should be checked; a normal PT/INR at 48 hrs post-ingestion rules out significant poisoning. Warfarin and superwarfarin (i.e., brodifacoum) levels can be measured if surreptitious poisoning is suspected.

Are there any specific antidotes for warfarin overdose?

Vitamin K_1 (phytonadione) restores production of clotting factors by bypassing the inhibitory effects of warfarin.

Is prophylactic vitamin K therapy warranted in treatment?

No. Prophylactic vitamin K therapy will make the 48-hr PT/INR inaccurate as a measure of toxicity.

How do monitoring parameters change after antidote administration?

Monitoring must continue at least 5 days following the last vitamin K_1 dose.

How is acute bleeding treated in the setting of a warfarin overdose?

Transfusions with fresh whole blood or fresh frozen plasma to replete coagulation factors rapidly

How is vitamin K administered?

PO, SQ, and IV

Chapter 3   Drugs of Abuse

AMPHETAMINES

What are amphetamines?

Chemicals with structures similar to phenylethylamine. Added side chains promote different levels of catecholamine and serotonin activity.

What is the mechanism of action of amphetamines?

Amphetamines bind to the monoamine transporters and ↑ extracellular levels of the biogenic amines dopamine, norepinephrine, and serotonin.

Which amphetamines are used in the treatment of narcolepsy and attention-deficit hyperactivity disorder (ADHD)?

1. Dextroamphetamine
2. Methylphenidate

Which amphetamines were used for weight loss but later recalled due to cardiopulmonary toxicity when used in combination with phentermine?

1. Fenfluramine
2. Dexfenfluramine

What amphetamine began to be used therapeutically in the mid-1970s after the chemist Alexander Shulgin introduced it to psychotherapist Leo Zeff?

3,4-methylenedioxy-N-methylamphetamine (MDMA, "ecstasy")

What illicit amphetamine is referred to as "ice"?

Methamphetamine in a smokable form

What is the bioavailability of amphetamines?

Good oral absorption with predominant hepatic metabolism. Urinary excretion is favored by an acidic environment.

What are the clinical signs of acute amphetamine intoxication?

Agitation, anxiety, AMS, mydriasis, hypertension, tachycardia, diaphoresis, tremor, muscle rigidity (sometimes with rhabdomyolysis), hyperthermia, seizures

What is the toxidrome for this constellation of symptoms?

The sympathomimetic toxidrome

What are adverse effects of chronic amphetamine intoxication?

Anorexia, paranoia, cardiomyopathy, pulmonary hypertension, vasculitis, aortic regurgitation, mitral regurgitation

What is an important class of drugs for counteracting the sympathomimetic effects of amphetamines?

Benzodiazepines. Large doses may be needed.

Amphetamine became a schedule II drug with the passage of what act in 1970?

The Controlled Substances Act

COCAINE

How is cocaine administered as a drug of abuse?

Intranasal (snorting), inhalation (smoking), IV injection, ingestion

By which method is the onset of action most rapid?

Inhalation (3–5 sec)

Which method provides the longest duration of action?

Intranasal or other mucosal administration (60–90 min)

What is a "speedball"?

IV injection of a combination of cocaine and heroin

What is a common alternative form of the hydrochloride salt?

Free base, including "crack"

Why is "free base" preferred over the HCl salt for smoking?

1. Lower temperature of volatilization
2. More heat-stable

Which form of cocaine is considered to be most addictive?

Crack

What is the approximate half-life of cocaine?

60 min

In which compartment(s) is cocaine metabolized?

1. Plasma
2. Liver

What is the mechanism of action of cocaine?

1. Blockade of presynaptic norepinephrine, dopamine, and serotonin reuptake centrally and peripherally
2. Na^+ channel blockade (neuronal and cardiac)

What are the desired effects of illicit cocaine use?

Euphoria and ↑ vigilance

What are the acute untoward effects of cocaine use?

Cerebral ischemia/infarction, intracranial hemorrhage, myocardial ischemia/infarction, cardiac arrhythmias, hyperthermia, seizures, anxiety, agitation, muscle rigidity, hypertension

What is the incidence of myocardial infarction associated with cocaine-induced chest pain?

5%

What active compound is enzymatically formed when cocaine and ethanol are co-administered?

Cocaethylene

What is the significance of this compound relative to cocaine?

1. Longer half-life
2. Significantly ↑ risk of sudden death
3. Less reinforcing
4. Less euphoria
5. Smaller increase in heart rate

By what methods can recent cocaine use be detected?

1. Direct blood or urine detection (several hrs after use)

    2. Detection of metabolites in blood or urine (24–36 hrs after use)

    3. Hair analysis (weeks to months after use)

What drug class is contraindicated for use in the cocaine intoxicated patient?

Beta blockers

In the agitated, cocaine intoxicated patient who is manifesting sympathomimetic overdrive, what drug class should initially be used in management?

Benzodiazepines

DESIGNER DRUGS

What is the definition of a designer drug?

A chemical substance intended for recreational use that results from the modification of a legitimate pharmaceutical agent

List some of the different classes of designer drugs.

1. Narcotic derivatives
2. Phenylethylamine/amphetamine derivatives
3. Tryptamine-based substances
4. Phencyclidine (PCP) analogs
5. Piperazine-based substances
6. Gamma-hydroxybutyrate (GHB) analogs

What are some common narcotic designer drugs and their street names?

1. Fentanyl analogs – 3-methylfentanyl and alpha-methylfentanyl ("China White" and "Tango and Cash," respectively)
2. Meperidine analog – 1-methyl-4-phenyl-4-propionoxy-pyridine (MPPP)

What is the typical triad of symptoms in opioid overdose?

AMS, miosis, respiratory depression

What are the side effects of the fentanyl-based designer drugs?

Usual potency is greater than that of heroin, resulting in excessive sedation and death. Higher than usual doses of naloxone may be needed to reverse effects.

What unique and serious presentation can occur after a single use of the meperidine analog MPPP?

This drug is often contaminated with the chemical 1-methyl-4-phenyl-1,2,3,6-tetrahydropyridine (MPTP), which is metabolized to 1-methyl-4-phenyl-1,2,5,6-tetrahydropyridine (MPP^+) by monoamine oxidase-B (MAO-B). The latter causes the destruction of the dopamine-containing cells in the substantia nigra. A parkinsonian-like syndrome can result after even a single use. Effects are often permanent, hence the name "frozen addicts."

Name some of the common amphetamine-based designer drugs.

1. Methamphetamine
2. 4-Methylaminorex
3. MDMA
4. 2,4-dimethoxy-4-propylthiophenylethylamine (2C-T7)

What is "ice"?

The translucent crystals of methamphetamine in a very pure form.

In what ways can methamphetamine be administered?

Injected, inhaled/smoked, ingested

How long can the effects of methamphetamine last?

2–24 hrs

What are some of the undesired and dangerous effects of methamphetamine use?

Delusions, paranoia, tics, compulsive behavior, GI distress, anorexia, weight loss, coronary ischemia/infarction, stroke, acute pulmonary edema, death

Mixing "ice" with what other commonly used drug results in increased cardiac and cerebrovascular toxicity?

Ethanol

What are the desired effects of MDMA?	Euphoria, verbosity, intimacy
How long do the desired effects last?	4–6 hrs
What is the usual route of administration of MDMA?	Orally ingested in tablet or capsule form
What is the mechanism of action of MDMA?	Induces the release and blocks the reuptake of serotonin, dopamine, and norepinephrine
What are the undesirable and dangerous effects of MDMA?	Hyperthermia, diaphoresis, muscle rigidity (including trismus), rhabdomyolysis, disseminated intravascular coagulation (DIC), cardiac dysrhythmias, anorexia, hyponatremia, metabolic acidosis

How should the drug-induced hyperthermia caused by MDMA be treated?

1. Active cooling – cold IV fluids, misting fans
2. Benzodiazepines
3. If resistant to active cooling and benzodiazepines, intubation with paralysis may be needed to ↓ muscle rigidity and prevent further hyperthermia and rhabdomyolysis (continuous EEG may be needed to monitor for seizure activity).

What is the long-term effect of MDMA use?	Destruction of serotonergic neurons → chronic dysphoria
The tryptamine analogs (e.g., alpha-methyltryptamine, dimethyltryptamine) are recreationally used as psychedelics and produce what desirable effects?	Euphoria, hallucinations, disinhibition
What are some of the undesirable effects of the tryptamine analogs?	Anxiety, insomnia, GI discomfort, muscle rigidity (including trismus)

The piperazine-based designer drugs have similar effects to what other drug?	MDMA
What designer drug is similar to the drug found in leaves of the khat bush (*Catha edulis*)?	Methcathinone

DEXTROMETHORPHAN

For what condition is dextromethorphan used?	OTC antitussive
What is the mechanism of action of dextromethorphan?	1. Serotonin reuptake inhibition 2. NMDA receptor antagonism
How is dextromethorphan abused?	By the oral route. Available in liquid, pill, and caplet form. Products containing dextromethorphan are often combined with other agents (e.g., acetaminophen, chlorpheniramine). Common slang terms include "Triple C's," "Dex," and "DXM."
Why is dextromethorphan abused?	While dextromethorphan is often classified as an opioid, the popularity of abuse comes from the "out-of-body" experience produced from blocking the NMDA receptor.
To what dissociative agent is dextromethorphan structurally similar?	PCP
Name the substance assay that cross-reacts with dextromethorphan on many urine drug screens.	PCP
Name two hyperthermic syndromes associated with dextromethorphan abuse.	1. Serotonin syndrome. The risks are especially great when the person abusing the drug is taking other pro-serotonergic agents (e.g., SSRIs).

2. Anticholinergic toxidrome, as dextromethorphan is often combined with anticholinergic agents

What electrolyte abnormality may be a clue to dextromethorphan abuse?

Dextromethorphan bromide may cause a falsely elevated chloride level, as bromide and chloride have the same valence on the periodic table.

Where is dextromethorphan absorbed?

GI tract, then crosses blood-brain barrier after absorption into vascular compartment

What is the half-life of dextromethorphan?

3–6 hrs

When is the onset of therapeutic effect?

15–30 min post-ingestion

What are the signs and symptoms of dextromethorphan toxicity?

Dizziness; ataxia; hallucinations (visual and auditory); dystonias; miosis; nystagmus; seizures; respiratory depression; stupor; coma; serotonin syndrome

How should dextromethorphan toxicity be treated?

Supportive care. Naloxone may be helpful for CNS and respiratory depression.

ETHANOL

Should ethanol be classified as a toxic alcohol or an antidote?

Both. It competitively inhibits alcohol dehydrogenase and may be used as an antidote for methanol and ethylene glycol poisonings when fomepizole is not available.

Action at what receptor is responsible for the major CNS effects of ethanol?

$GABA_A$ receptor binding and activation

Is the rate of absorption higher from a "straight shot" of ethanol or from a mixed drink?

Mixed drink. The fastest absorption comes from drinks containing 20% ethanol. High concentrations of ethanol cause pylorospasm and delay systemic absorption.

Alcohol dehydrogenase activity is higher in what groups of people?

Males and Pacific Rim Asians. High levels of acetaldehyde (from rapid ethanol conversion) are responsible for the skin flushing seen in some people after ethanol consumption. Pacific Rim Asians also tend to be slow metabolizers of acetaldehyde, leading to further accumulation.

What are the metabolites of ethanol in the major pathway (i.e., alcohol and aldehyde dehydrogenases)?

Acetaldehyde and acetate, respectively

What are the main symptoms of alcohol intoxication?

Slurred speech, ataxia, nystagmus, CNS depression

Name three commonly prescribed antibiotics which react with ethanol metabolism similarly to disulfiram.

Some cephalosporins, metronidazole, nitrofurantoin

What mechanism is responsible for ethanol-induced hypoglycemia?

The presence of ethanol favors conversion of pyruvate to lactate, leaving less pyruvate available for gluconeogenesis. Children, chronically malnourished alcoholics, and binge drinkers who do not eat are at particular risk.

Does ethanol intoxication alone produce an anion gap acidosis?

No; however, in alcoholic ketoacidosis (AKA), the high anion gap is caused by acetoacetate, beta-hydroxybutyrate, and lactate. Serum ethanol levels are usually not elevated in this setting.

What antidote cures ethanol intoxication?

None. Caffeine and cold showers are of no benefit. Hemodialysis can clear serum ethanol in life-threatening ingestions but is seldom necessary with airway protection and supportive care.

An intoxicated patient in the emergency department has a measured blood alcohol

While the average serum ethanol clearance is 15 mg/dL/hr, there is considerable individual variation. Discharge criteria

level of 140 mg/dL. When can this patient be safely discharged?

should be based on the clinical scenario and serial assessments of the patient.

Describe the ethanol withdrawal syndrome.

Tachycardia, tremor, hypertension, agitation. This may be followed by hallucinations (usually tactile or visual) or seizures. Seizures may be one of the first signs of ethanol withdrawal.

What is the treatment for ethanol withdrawal?

Benzodiazepines. High doses often are needed.

GAMMA-HYDROXYBUTYRATE (GHB)

What was the original intended indication for GHB?

Anesthesia

Why was GHB withdrawn for this indication?

Insufficient anesthesia, emergence delirium, myoclonus, bradycardia

Is GHB prescribed for any legitimate purpose?

Yes. It has been FDA-approved as the schedule III drug Xyrem®, or sodium oxybate, for narcolepsy since 2002; however, due to both the narrow scope and the extreme abuse potential it carries, GHB is concurrently listed as a schedule I drug.

What is the "street" purpose and delivery method of GHB?

GHB is abused as a "club drug" for its euphoric properties. It also may be used for drug-facilitated sexual assault ("date rape") secondary to its quick action and amnestic properties. For this purpose, GHB often is mixed with ethanol.

What other chemicals are converted to GHB?

1. Gamma-butyrolactone (GBL) is hydrolyzed to GHB either spontaneously or in the blood.
2. 1,4-butanediol (1,4-BD) is oxidized by alcohol dehydrogenase to gamma-hydroxybutyraldehyde, which is then metabolized to GHB by aldehyde dehydrogenase.

GHB is the structural analog of which endogenous neurotransmitter?

GABA; however, GHB also appears to be an endogenous neurotransmitter, possessing its own receptors in the brain.

What is the mechanism of toxicity of GHB?

It easily crosses the blood-brain barrier and exerts GABA-like CNS depressant effects.

What are the signs and symptoms of GHB toxicity?

CNS and respiratory depression, apnea, amnesia, hypotonia, euphoria, coma, bradycardia. Symptoms have a rapid onset and are followed by a rapid arousal in 6–8 hrs when the drug has cleared.

What is the antidote?

None available

What is the recommended hospital treatment for suspected GHB toxicity?

Supportive care

Does GHB have a withdrawal syndrome?

Yes. In heavy users, manifestations can occur within hours after the last dose and include anxiety, tremor, nausea, vomiting, possibly delirium, hallucinations, and mild autonomic instability. Treatment of GHB withdrawal syndrome can be difficult and requires large doses of benzodiazepines or barbiturates to control.

What are some common street names for GHB?

Easy Lay, Everclear, Fantasy, G, Grievous Bodily Harm, Georgia Home Boy, Great Hormones at Bedtime, G-riffick, Jolt, Liquid Ecstasy, Salty Water, Scoop, Soap, Vita G, Zonked

HALLUCINOGENS

Name some commonly abused hallucinogens.

1. Lysergic acid diethylamide (LSD)
2. MDMA ("ecstasy," "X")
3. Alpha-methyltryptamine (AMT)
4. Dimethyltryptamine (DMT)
5. Mescaline (Peyote)
6. Psilocybin ("Magic Shrooms")

What are the desired effects?

"Tripping," an altered state of perception usually associated with auditory and visual hallucinations. Senses are often distorted and can be merged, a phenomenon known as synesthesia.

How are hallucinogens abused?

Primarily ingested, although some may be smoked or injected:
1. LSD is taken on sugar cubes, blotter paper, and microdots.
2. Psilocybin mushrooms and peyote cactus are dried and eaten or brewed in tea.
3. Dimethyltryptamine may be smoked, snorted, or injected.

What is the mechanism for these drugs?

Pure hallucinogens bind serotonin, primarily 5-HT$_{2A}$, activating these receptors. Other drugs, such as anticholinergics and sympathomimetics, may cause hallucinations but are not considered primary hallucinogens.

What are some of the physical signs that have been associated with hallucinogen ingestion?

Hyperglycemia, tachycardia, hyperthermia, paresthesias, mydriasis, rhabdomyolysis

What are some of the psychotropic effects?

Significant variation from person-to-person, but include visual and auditory hallucinations, time distortion, feelings of dissociation, synesthesia, intense color perceptions, feelings of ecstasy or terror

Name some natural hallucinogens.

Salvinorin A (*Salvia divinorum*), bufotenine (*Bufo alvarius*), mescaline (*Lophophora williamsii*), psilocin/psilocybin (*Psilocybe sp.*), lysergic acid hydroxyethylamide (*Ipomoea violacea*)

Name the household spice capable of producing hallucinations.

Nutmeg. The active chemical is myristicin.

What is a "bad trip"?

A terrifying or paranoid experience associated with the use of hallucinogens, often associated with the environment or mindset of the user.

How are these effects treated?

Primarily supportive with close monitoring of vital signs, IV fluids for rhabdomyolysis, and benzodiazepines for agitation. A quiet, dark, nonstimulating environment is recommended.

INHALANTS

What are inhalants?

A large group of substances whose vapors can be inhaled to produce a "high."

What are the general classes of inhalants?

1. Volatile hydrocarbons – paint thinners, paints, glues, degreasers, gasoline, felt-tip marker fluids, dry-cleaning fluids, refrigerants
2. Nitrites – cyclohexyl nitrite, amyl nitrite, butyl nitrite
3. Gases – nitrous oxide

What is the terminology for the various methods of inhaling?

1. Huffing – using an inhalant-soaked rag placed in the mouth or over the face
2. Sniffing or snorting – inhaling fumes directly from a container through the nose
3. Bagging – inhaling fumes from substances sprayed or deposited in a bag

What is the mechanism of action and onset for most inhalants?

While the exact mechanisms are poorly understood, most inhalants appear to work by modulating cell membranes, ion channels, and GABA receptors. Nitrites differ by causing peripheral vasodilation. Onset of inhalant action is within seconds with effects lasting only several minutes; thus, abusers use repeatedly over short periods of time.

What are the signs and symptoms of acute inhalant intoxication?

Slurred speech, euphoria, dizziness, hallucinations, delusions, ataxia, headache, lethargy, agitation, unconsciousness, seizures, respiratory depression, asphyxiation, coma, sudden death

Are there long-term effects with inhalant use?	Yes. Weight loss, muscle weakness, ataxia, mood instability, depression. Toluene and other organic solvents have been shown to cause cerebral atrophy and peripheral demyelination.
Chronic inhalation of what anesthetic may produce a peripheral neuropathy and vitamin B_{12} deficiency?	Nitrous oxide
Which volatile hydrocarbon is metabolized to carbon monoxide?	Methylene chloride
Which agents may produce methemoglobinemia?	Nitrites
What are slang terms for some common inhalants?	1. "Poppers" or "snappers" – amyl and butyl nitrite 2. "Whipits" – whipped cream aerosols
What is the term for a patient with sudden death from inhalant use?	Sudden sniffing death syndrome (SSDS)
Describe the proposed mechanism of SSDS.	Halogenated hydrocarbons sensitize the myocardium to endogenous cate-cholamines $\rightarrow \uparrow$ risk of VF
Why may toluene abuse result in metabolic acidosis?	1. Following acute abuse, toluene is metabolized to acidic metabolites (i.e., benzoic and hippuric acid) that result in an anion gap metabolic acidosis. 2. Following chronic abuse, toluene may induce a distal renal tubular acidosis and subsequent non-anion gap metabolic acidosis with hypokalemia.
Are there any specific antidotes or interventions?	Generally, treatment includes supportive care. Symptomatic methemoglobinemia induced by nitrites should be treated with methylene blue.

MARIJUANA

Marijuana is derived from what plant?	*Cannabis sativa*
How is marijuana consumed as a drug of abuse?	1. Inhalation (smoking) 2. Ingestion (often baked into brownies)
By which method is the onset of action most rapid?	Inhalation
What is the predominant psychoactive chemical in marijuana?	Delta-9-tetrahydrocannabinol (THC)
What is the mechanism of THC?	It binds to cannabinoid receptors (anandamide and palmitoylethanolamide) to modulate euphoric effects.
What is the origin of the name "anandamide"?	*Ananda* is the Sanskrit word for "bliss." Anandamide is an endogenous cannabinoid.
What are some common forms of cannabis?	1. Marijuana – leaves and flowers of *C. sativa* 2. Hashish – concentrated resin of *C. sativa* 3. Kief – marijuana mixed with tobacco 4. Bhang – marijuana and other spices boiled in milk 5. Budder – hashish whipped with butter
What is a "joint" or "reefer"?	Marijuana cigarette made by rolling marijuana in cigarette papers
What is a "bong"?	A pipe used to smoke marijuana. Water is commonly used to "filter" the smoke.
How can marijuana be ingested?	1. Baked goods, commonly in brownies ("magic brownies" or "space cakes") 2. Infused into milk or tea ("bhang") 3. Infused into ethanol ("Green Dragon")
What is the approximate half-life of marijuana?	20–30 hrs

What are the short-term effects of marijuana use?

Euphoria, ↑ appetite, altered time perception, poor short-term memory, paranoia, lethargy

What are the signs of acute marijuana use?

Tachycardia, orthostatic hypotension, conjunctival erythema, ↓ IOP, slurred speech, ataxia

What physical findings are associated with chronic marijuana use?

"Amotivational syndrome," obesity, pulmonary disease

By what methods can recent marijuana use be detected?

1. Direct blood or urine detection (several hrs after use)
2. Detection of metabolites in blood or urine (24–36 hrs after use)
3. Hair analysis (weeks to months after use)

How long can marijuana be detected in the urine?

In chronic users, positive urine screens can occur for up to 1 month.

Describe the treatment of acute marijuana intoxication.

Due to low acute toxicity, few abusers present with a primary complaint of marijuana intoxication. Those that do have adverse symptoms likely have co-ingestions with more toxic drugs. Treatment consists of supportive care.

MESCALINE

What is mescaline?

Mescaline is a hallucinogenic alkaloid present in peyote that is structurally related to amphetamines and is a $5\text{-}HT_2$ agonist.

What is peyote?

The flesh of the spineless cactus *Lophophora williamsii*, whose crowns and seeds contain a considerable amount of mescaline. The crowns are dried and sold as "buttons."

What term is sometimes preferred over "hallucinogen"?

Psychedelic agent

Mescaline is similar to what other hallucinogenic agent?	LSD; however, mescaline is much less potent.
Mescaline is what structural type of hallucinogen?	Phenylethylamine
Describe the typical triad of peyote intoxication.	1. First – nausea and vomiting 2. Second – catecholamine surge 3. Third – hallucinations and a sense of depersonalization
Name the household spice that may produce a similar toxidromic triad as peyote when taken in excess.	Nutmeg
Name the psychedelic chemical in nutmeg.	Myristicin
List the clinical features of mescaline ingestion.	Nausea, vomiting, abdominal pain, CNS stimulation, mydriasis, nystagmus, headache, dizziness
Where is peyote found?	Southwestern United States and northern Mexico
How much mescaline does a peyote button contain?	~45 mg; 6–12 "buttons" are typically taken to produce hallucinations
How much mescaline is needed to produce a psychedelic effect?	A typical dose is 3–12 mg/kg, or 200–500 mg of mescaline.
What is the duration of action?	The initial uncomfortable physical effects may last ~2 hrs (GI symptoms and sympathomimetic symptoms), while hallucinations may last 6–12 hrs.
Describe the management of mescaline toxicity.	Supportive care. Death typically occurs from behavior, not direct toxicity.
When is the use of peyote legal?	For traditional use by Native Americans

NICOTINE

How may people become poisoned by nicotine?	1. Ingestion of chewing tobacco 2. Ingestion of cigarettes 3. Ingestion of or dermal exposure to nicotine-containing pesticides 4. Ingestion of or dermal exposure to prescription nicotine-replacement products
What is the toxic dose?	Ingestion of as little as 2 mg can lead to GI upset, but 40–60 mg can be fatal if absorbed quickly.
Ingestion of how many cigarettes or cigarette butts is reason for concern in a child?	Children who ingest 1 whole cigarette or 3 cigarette butts are likely to become symptomatic.
When is the usual onset of symptoms?	Symptoms usually occur within 30–90 min.
What are the symptoms of nicotine toxicity?	Activation of nicotinic receptors at autonomic ganglia (sympathetic and parasympathetic), along with end-organ effects (neuromuscular junction and CNS), produces nausea, vomiting, diarrhea, abdominal pain, salivation, diaphoresis, pallor, and agitation then lethargy. Initial elevation of heart rate, blood pressure, and respiratory rate may occur followed by subnormal values of each. CNS depression, muscle fasciculations, and seizures, followed by paralysis, may reflect severe toxicity.
How is nicotine toxicity treated?	1. Atropine – anticholinergic agent that can be used to treat symptoms such as bronchorrhea and cardiac depression (due to parasympathetic excess) 2. Benzodiazepines for seizures
What is "green tobacco illness"?	Tobacco workers with direct skin contact to moist tobacco leaves may absorb a significant amount of nicotine and become symptomatic.

OPIOIDS

What are opioids?	Naturally-occurring or synthetic drugs that have opium-like activity
How do opioids exert effects?	Agonists of opioid receptors in the central and peripheral nervous systems and the GI tract
What are the three main receptors activated by opioids?	Delta (OP1), kappa (OP2), mu (OP3)
What are clinical effects of opiate administration?	Analgesia, drowsiness, changes in mood (often euphoria)
What triad of symptoms strongly suggests opioid intoxication?	CNS depression, miosis, respiratory depression
Which opioids are not associated with miosis?	Tramadol, propoxyphene, meperidine
What are the cardiovascular effects of opioid overdose?	Hypotension and bradycardia (may be mild or absent)
What are the dermatologic symptoms of opioid intoxication?	Flushing and pruritus (variably present)
What are other respiratory effects of opioid intoxication?	Respiratory depression, bronchospasm, and noncardiogenic pulmonary edema. Fentanyl administration may be associated with chest wall rigidity.
What are the GI effects of opioid intoxication?	Nausea, vomiting, constipation
What is the cause of most opioid-related deaths?	Respiratory depression resulting in anoxia
How do opiates cause respiratory depression?	Direct effect on brainstem respiratory centers (through mu and delta receptors)

What are the primary metabolites of heroin?

1. 6-monoacetylmorphine
2. Morphine

What paralytic infection is associated with the use of black tar heroin?

Wound botulism (*Clostridium botulinum*)

Which opioid has cardiac fast sodium channel blocking properties?

Propoxyphene and its metabolite norpropoxyphene, both of which cause QRS prolongation

Which opioid has a unique interaction with monoamine oxidase inhibitors (MAOI)?

Meperidine – may result in serotonin syndrome

What is the opioid antagonist that is used to treat acute toxicity?

Naloxone, which competitively binds opioid receptors

What is the normal elimination half-life of naloxone?

30–60 min

What medical condition results in prolongation of the elimination half-life of naloxone?

Renal failure

What are "body packers"?

Individuals who swallow wrapped packets of illicit drugs or insert such packets into body orifices. Most are asymptomatic but can have acute intoxications with rupture of the packets. If suspected, abdominal radiographs may be obtained, but packets present are not always radio-opaque. Consider whole bowel irrigation with polyethylene glycol (PEG-ELS). Surgical indications include bowel obstruction or intestinal perforation. Continuous infusion of naloxone may be indicated with rupture of heroin packets.

What are "body stuffers"?

Individuals who swallow poorly wrapped or un-wrapped drugs, usually in an attempt to avoid arrest. There is generally more likelihood of becoming symptomatic secondary to the exposure to the intestinal lumen.

PHENCYCLIDINE (PCP)

What is PCP?

Synthetic piperadine derivative that works as a dissociative anesthetic and is considered a hallucinogen

Why is PCP unlike other hallucinogens?

It causes marked sympathomimetic activity and agitation in addition to hallucinations.

What drug is structurally similar to PCP?

Ketamine

What is the mechanism of action of PCP?

1. Glutamate antagonism at the NMDA receptor – leads to loss of pain perception with minimal respiratory depression
2. Reuptake inhibition of serotonin, dopamine, and norepinephrine
3. Modulation of sigma opioid receptors

How can phencyclidine be administered?

Ingestion, injection, sniffing, smoking

What are the onset and duration of action of PCP when smoked?

Onset is 2–5 min with "high" at 15–30 min and duration of 4–6 hrs. Return to baseline may take 24–48 hrs.

What is the street name for the most common preparation of PCP?

"Angel dust"

What is a typical dose of PCP?

1–6 mg can cause disinhibition and hallucinations, while 6–10 mg causes toxic psychosis.

Why is PCP often unknowingly ingested?

It is easy and inexpensive to make, so is often used as an adulterant of other drugs. For example, a marijuana joint may be dusted with PCP to create a "Wicky Stick."

List some clinical effects of an acute PCP ingestion.

Nystagmus (horizontal then vertical or rotary), hallucinations, delusions, agitation, hypertension, tachycardia

For which psychiatric condition may acute PCP intoxication be mistaken?

Schizophrenia

List some medical complications of PCP overdose.

Coma, seizure, rhabdomyolysis, renal failure, hyperthermia, intracerebral hemorrhage (due to hypertension), trauma

Does a positive PCP urine toxicology screen mean acute ingestion?

No. Chronic users can test positive for weeks following last use. Dextromethorphan, diphenhydramine, and ketamine may produce false positive urine PCP screens.

How long after acute use is PCP able to be detected in the urine?

1–5 days

What is the treatment for PCP overdose?

Generally supportive. Benzodiazepines are indicated for agitation and psychosis. Aggressive cooling may be needed for hyperthermia.

Why are pharmaceutical interventions preferred over physical restraints for violence and agitation?

Limits muscular activity and the development of rhabdomyolysis

Chapter 4

Environmental and Industrial Toxins

ACIDS

What are some common acids and common uses of these acids?

Used in disinfectants, cleaners, glues, batteries, polish, photographic solutions, among many others. Some of the most common acids include acetic acid, boric acid, carbolic acid, chromic acid, formic acid, hydrochloric acid, oxalic acid, nitric acid, phosphoric acid, and sulfuric acid.

How do acids cause tissue damage?

Acids (hydrogen ions) desiccate tissues by drawing water out of cells to form hydronium ions (H_3O^+), which results in coagulative necrosis and eschar formation. Depending upon the severity of the exposure, eschars can prevent the deeper penetration of acids, causing superficial damage to the tissues.

What are some factors that determine the severity of an acid injury?

pH, volume, concentration, duration of contact, titratable acid reserve

What types of burns are typically caused by ingestion of acid?

Mucosal burns to the mouth, esophagus, and the lesser curvature of the stomach. Acid-induced pylorospasm may spare the duodenum but lead to acid pooling in the stomach and subsequent gastric perforation.

How do acidic and alkali injuries differ?

In mild and moderate acid burns, there is less damage because acids precipitate and coagulate, acting as a mechanical barrier to further penetration. Severe acidic burns can penetrate the self-limited tissue barriers and cause more extensive damage. Alkalis cause saponification of membranes, which allows for rapid and extensive burns through tissues.

Describe the clinical presentation of an acid ingestion.

1. Upper respiratory – stridor, drooling, respiratory distress
2. GI – oropharyngeal pain and burns, odynophagia, nausea, vomiting, abdominal/chest/epigastric pain
3. Severe injury can manifest with hypotension, metabolic acidosis, DIC, mediastinitis

How should a patient with acid ingestion be managed in the emergency department?

1. Supportive care – give water or milk to dilute, especially with powder or granular preparations. It is important to make sure the patient can swallow without difficulty.
2. Decontamination with an NG tube and gentle suction is controversial.
3. Endoscopic evaluation as needed
4. Emergent laparotomy for suspected perforation
5. AVOID cathartics, neutralization, induced-emesis, activated charcoal, steroids

Who should undergo endoscopy?

Anyone with stridor, pain, vomiting, or drooling. Esophageal or gastric injury is not ruled out by the absence of oral burns.

Why should hydrofluoric acid (HF) burns be managed differently than other acid burns?

HF is a weak acid that easily crosses membranes and causes deeper tissue damage. Fluoride ions chelate calcium and magnesium and form deposits. Dysrhythmias may develop secondary to hypocalcemia or hypomagnesemia. Treatment for superficial injuries involves topical calcium gluconate gel. Deeper wounds with systemic symptoms may require intra-arterial calcium gluconate with additional IV calcium and magnesium replacement.

How should ocular acid injuries be managed?

Copious irrigation with normal saline is the mainstay of therapy. Several liters of irrigation are usually needed to raise the pH back to 7.40. Fluorescein exam should be done to confirm that a normal pH is achieved. An ophthalmology consult is warranted for corneal involvement.

AMMONIA

What products contain ammonia?	Fertilizers, refrigerants, household and commercial cleaning solutions, explosives
Are aqueous solutions of ammonia acidic or alkaline?	Alkaline
Combination of ammonia with what compounds will produce chloramine gas?	Solutions containing chlorine or hypochlorite
In what two forms is ammonia available?	Gas and aqueous solution
What is the mechanism of toxicity of ammonia?	When ammonia gas contacts moist surfaces (i.e., mucous membranes), ammonium hydroxide is formed, yielding a corrosive effect. Ammonia solutions skip the first step of dissolution in water and are directly caustic.
On what organ systems will ammonia gas have its effects?	Integumentary, ophthalmic, respiratory (upper > lower tract injury)
How does skin exposure manifest?	Mild to severe burns depending on concentration and duration of contact
How much more concentrated are commercial cleaning solutions compared to household versions?	2.5–6 fold more concentrated. Household cleaning solutions contain 5% to 10% ammonia, while commercial cleaning solutions contain 25% to 30%.
Are household solutions (dilute) typically associated with significant injuries?	No. They can only cause harm if a massive amount is ingested.
What signs and symptoms are seen with eye exposure to ammonia gas or solution?	Immediate pain, redness, conjunctivitis, lacrimation, blistering to full-thickness burns, blindness

How does inhalation of ammonia gas present clinically (in order of exposure severity)?

1. Immediate burning of nose and throat with resultant cough
2. Upper respiratory tract injury may result in airway obstruction, presenting as stridor, hoarseness, wheezing, and "croupy" cough.
3. Lower respiratory tract injury manifesting as wheezing or pulmonary edema

What symptoms are seen with ingestion of ammonia solutions?

Immediate oral/pharyngeal pain, which may progress to dysphagia, difficulty handling secretions, and chest/abdominal pain. Esophageal or gastric injury is not ruled out by the absence of oral burns.

What life-threatening event can occur with ingestion of concentrated solutions?

Esophageal or gastric perforation

List a long-term sequela of ammonia ingestion.

Esophageal and/or gastric scarring causing stricture and chronic dysphagia

How is ammonia gas inhalation treated?

1. Remove from exposure immediately and administer supplemental O_2.
2. Observe for signs of airway compromise, and initiate intubation early.
3. Administer bronchodilators for wheezing.
4. Treat pulmonary edema by avoiding excessive fluid administration and adding PEEP as needed to maintain $PaO_2 \geq 60$–70 mm Hg.

How is ingestion of aqueous ammonia solution treated?

1. Give water or milk orally to dilute the ammonia if early after the ingestion and the patient is able to swallow without difficulty.
2. Gastric suction with an NG tube may be beneficial early after ingestion when large amounts have been taken. Use a small, flexible tube to avoid worsening of mucosal injury. Never force the tube, and only use if the patient can tolerate it.

3. If a solution ≥10% has been ingested or if dysphagia, drooling, or pain is present, flexible upper endoscopy is warranted.
4. Chest and abdominal radiographs
5. AVOID induced emesis, activated charcoal, and neutralization with acid.

How is eye exposure treated?

Copious irrigation with several liters of normal saline to lower the pH back to 7.40. Fluorescein exam should be done after normal pH is achieved. An ophthalmology consult is warranted for corneal involvement.

ANTISEPTICS AND DISINFECTANTS

Define "antiseptic."

An antimicrobial agent applied to vital tissues to exert "cidal" (i.e., kills the microorganism) or "static" (i.e., halts the growth of the microorganism) effects.

Define "disinfectant."

An antimicrobial agent applied to nonliving surfaces. They may be "cidal" or "static."

Where is chlorhexidine found?

1. Dental rinses, including mouthwashes
2. Skin cleansers
3. Cleaning solutions

What are the toxic effects of chlorhexidine?

Irritation and corrosive injury to the oral and esophageal mucosa may occur after ingestion. Hepatic injury has been reported following ingestion. Dermal absorption is minimal, but skin irritation may occur.

Systemic absorption or ingestion of what antiseptic agent may cause a low or negative anion gap?

Iodine or iodophors. These agents may cause a falsely elevated serum chloride on some analyzers, resulting in a decreased anion gap.

Where is glutaraldehyde found?

1. Hospital equipment disinfectants
2. Tissue preservatives
3. Topical antifungal agents

What are the toxic effects of glutaraldehyde?	1. Skin irritation 2. Respiratory tract irritation 3. Repeated exposure may result in contact dermatitis.
Where is hydrogen peroxide found?	1. Dental products 2. Skin cleansers 3. Hair products 4. Earwax irrigants 5. Industrial oxidizing solutions
How many milliliters of oxygen are released from 1 mL of 35% (concentrated) hydrogen peroxide?	100 mL
What are the toxic effects of hydrogen peroxide?	Hydrogen peroxide breaks down readily to water and oxygen. When ingested, the production of oxygen gas can cause distension, perforation, and even gas embolization.
What specific therapies may be used to treat hydrogen peroxide poisoning?	Gastric aspiration with an NG tube may help prevent gas formation and embolization. Hyperbaric oxygen therapy may be used to treat gas embolization.
Where is potassium permanganate found?	1. Dilute antiseptics 2. Swimming pool, fish tank, and well water purification/decontamination products 3. Industrial oxidants
What are the toxic effects of potassium permanganate?	Acute toxicity is primarily a corrosive injury. Secondary to strong oxidative effects, methemoglobinemia may also occur.
What complications can occur following chronic potassium permanganate exposure?	Manganese toxicity characterized by parkinsonian symptoms, also known as "manganese madness"
How is hypochlorite used?	1. Household bleach (sodium hypochlorite) contains ~5% hypochlorite

2. Industrial strength disinfectants in 20% solutions

What is the primary toxicity of hypochlorite exposure?

Corrosive injury

What are the acute effects of phenol ingestion?

Phenol is a caustic agent that may result in oropharyngeal and esophageal burns. Systemic symptoms include seizures, lethargy, hypotension, and coma.

Name the organomercury compound used as a topical antiseptic.

Mercurochrome

How does mercurochrome toxicity occur?

Systemic mercury toxicity may occur after ingestion or from repeated exposure to compromised skin.

What are the key features of formaldehyde ingestion?

Caustic injury to the stomach, including possible gastric necrosis and perforation. Systemic absorption results in the metabolism of formaldehyde to formic acid, resulting in an anion gap metabolic acidosis.

What are typical effects of dilute antiseptic ingestions?

GI (i.e., vomiting and diarrhea)

How is antiseptic or disinfectant ingestion treated?

1. Removal of the offending agent with decontamination
2. Supportive care
3. Mild irritation is self-limited, but more corrosive agents may require endoscopy
4. Hyperbaric oxygen (HBO) therapy for gas emboli following hydrogen peroxide ingestion

How is decontamination performed following acute ingestion of corrosive agents?

Dilute with milk or water

What should not be given following ingestion of corrosive agents and why?

1. Proemetics, as they exacerbate erosive injury

2. Activated charcoal is contraindicated and will obstruct endoscopic evaluation.

How are eyes and skin decontaminated?

1. Remove contaminated clothing
2. Irrigate with copious amounts of water

ASBESTOS

What is asbestos?

Naturally occurring silicate fibers that are chemically inert but have been implicated in carcinogenesis and, once inhaled, can remain in the lungs for a lifetime

What type of asbestos fiber is considered the most injurious?

Amphibole, particularly crocidolite

What is the major concern with asbestos?

Inhalation of asbestos fibers >5 μm can lead to pulmonary fibrosis and cancer (i.e., mesothelioma).

Why are fibers smaller than 5 μm not implicated in the pathogenesis of lung fibrosis and cancer?

They are removed from the lungs by macrophages.

What populations are most likely to be exposed to asbestos?

Most exposure is work-related, and a high incidence of exposure is known to occur in insulation workers, asbestos-cement workers, shipyard workers, and plumbers.

What is the average time after exposure for clinical presentation?

15–20 yrs

List some clinical manifestations of asbestos exposure.

Asbestosis, pleural disease (e.g., pleural thickening/plaques/effusions), lung cancer, mesothelioma (pleural and peritoneal)

What is asbestosis?

Progressive interstitial pulmonary fibrosis, leading to a restrictive pattern with compromised gas exchange

What is seen on CXR?	X-ray changes are dependent on the stage of disease; commonly seen are small, irregular opacities in the mid and lower lung fields, thickening of the pleura, pleural plaques, and calcifications. Later stages may show progression to involvement of the upper lung fields.
Why should you encourage asbestos workers to stop smoking?	The relative risk for development of lung cancer approximately doubles for asbestos and smoking combined. The effects of this combination are synergistic.
What antidotes are available for asbestos exposure?	None
What advice would you give someone who will be working in an asbestos environment about treatment?	Emphasize avoidance of exposure. Protective equipment should be worn to prevent inhalation. Although fibers are not absorbed transdermally, inhalation from the skin may occur, so attention should be paid to cleansing the skin after exposures.

AZIDE

How is sodium azide used commercially?	It is commonly used as the propellant agent in automobile airbags. Azide may also be used in military explosives, as a reagent/preservative in laboratories, and as an herbicide/fungicide.
What is the route of toxicity for sodium azide?	Inhalation, ingestion, dermal, IV (uncommon route)
How is sodium azide eliminated?	Metabolized hepatically, then excreted renally
What is the mechanism of toxicity of sodium azide?	Azide inhibits the function of cytochrome C oxidase by binding irreversibly to the heme moiety in a process similar to that of cyanide, thereby inhibiting the formation of ATP.
What are acute effects of sodium azide toxicity?	Hypotension, dysrhythmias, pulmonary edema, headache, syncope, CNS depression, nausea, vomiting, diarrhea

What is the clinical presentation of an inhalation exposure?	Hypotension, tachypnea, conjunctival erythema, nasal mucosal irritation, pulmonary edema, respiratory arrest
Which is the most commonly reported effect, irrespective of route of exposure?	Hypotension
What metabolic abnormality is expected to be present after exposure?	Anion gap metabolic acidosis
Are enhanced elimination methods available for sodium azide?	No
Is a specific antidote available for sodium azide?	No
What precautions should be taken when treating patients?	Azides are converted to hydrazoic acid in acidic environments; exposure to vapors from emesis may result in bystander toxicity. Hydrazoic acid appears to have similar anti-metabolic properties to azide. Contact of azides with metals may result in spontaneous explosion.
What treatments should be undertaken for patients who have ingested sodium azide?	Supportive care

BENZENE

What is benzene?	A volatile aromatic hydrocarbon that is widely used as a solvent in industrial processes and can be found in a variety of plastics, dyes, rubbers, and pesticides. It is also a byproduct in the burning of organic compounds and is therefore a component of cigarette smoke.
How are people exposed to benzene?	Usually by inhalation or ingestion, but dermal absorption is possible

What is the clinical presentation of a person with acute benzene poisoning?

Acute toxicity is similar to other solvent syndromes, including dizziness, nausea, vomiting, headache, possible seizures, and coma. Benzene may also result in acute hemolysis. Dermal exposure may result in chemical burns. Inhalation or aspiration can lead to chemical pneumonitis, potentially progressing to ARDS.

What are the symptoms of chronic exposure?

Long-term benzene exposure is known to cause bone marrow suppression and hematologic pathology, including aplastic anemia, myelodysplastic syndromes, and leukemia. Benzene is a known carcinogen (IARC group I). Effects on human fertility are unknown, but menstrual irregularities and ovary shrinkage have been reported. Secondary to the carcinogenic risk, workplace exposure is limited to 0.5 ppm per 8-hr day.

Describe the mechanism of toxicity.

Benzene is metabolized in the liver, primarily by cytochrome P450. This forms multiple metabolites including benzene oxide, phenol, and reactive oxygen species. These metabolites are directly cytotoxic and may form protein and DNA conjugates that promote carcinogenicity.

What is the antidote?

None. Additionally, hemodialysis and hemoperfusion are ineffective.

What is the recommended treatment?

Supportive care. Consider placement of an NG tube with aspiration of gastric contents if the patient presents promptly after benzene ingestion. Oxygen is the preferred treatment for acute solvent exposure. Avoid sympathomimetics, as benzene may cause myocardial sensitization to catecholamines.

What tests should be ordered?

Check a CBC with differential to evaluate for hemolysis or bone marrow effects. Reticulocyte count may also be useful if anemia is found. Electrolytes, LFTs, and

RFTs should be ordered. Order a CXR as needed for evaluation for potential pneumonitis. Urine phenol levels are useful to monitor for or detect chronic exposure. Acute exposures may be confirmed by blood testing for benzene and its metabolites.

BORIC ACID, BORATES, AND BORON

How toxic are boron, boric acid, and borates?

Borates, boranes, and boric acid are chemical compounds of the element boron. Generally, borates and boric acid have low toxicity, usually developing after repeated exposures. Boranes are much more toxic and may produce both acute and chronic poisoning.

What are the routes of exposure?

Exposure to boric acid is primarily through the oral route; however, repeated contact with abraded or compromised skin may result in toxicity. Boranes may be toxic through ingestion, inhalation, or dermal exposure.

What is the mechanism of toxicity of borates?

Unknown

How is boric acid speculated to cause toxicity?

It is likely a metabolic poison.

Where are boric acid and borates found?

Pesticides (e.g., roach powder), skin lotions, medicated powders

Where can boranes be found?

Boranes are primarily used in the commercial/industrial setting. They are found in herbicidal and bactericidal agents, in fuels, and in various manufacturing processes.

What are the adverse effects of boric acid and borates?

Mucous membrane irritation, nausea, intractable vomiting, diarrhea, abdominal pain, and skin erythema. Seizures, alopecia, and renal failure have also been reported.

Describe the typical skin finding associated with boric acid toxicity.	Diffuse erythema that involves the palms and soles, which later desquamates, and is described as a "boiled lobster" appearance
What is the characteristic color of diarrhea and emesis produced by boric acid ingestion?	Blue-green
What other ingestion may cause a similar emesis finding?	Copper sulfate
Describe the toxicity of borane exposure.	Acute inhalation primarily produces pulmonary irritation; however, pulmonary edema may occur. CNS depression and seizures have been reported as have cardiac and hepatic toxicity. Concentration and personality changes, along with hepatic and renal damage, may occur after chronic exposure.
What methods can be used to detect boric acid, borates, or borane exposure?	Predominantly by history. Blue-green color of diarrhea or emesis may be helpful. Serum/blood levels are not widely available and are of little clinical utility.
How are these exposures managed?	1. Antiemetic therapy with nonsedating agents 2. Fluid and electrolyte repletion 3. Treat seizures with benzodiazepines. 4. Local wound care for potential skin exfoliation 5. Evaluate for hepatic or renal damage.
Are there any available antidotes or enhanced elimination methods?	There are no antidotes. Hemodialysis is effective and may be considered after large exposures.

BROMATES

What are the common forms of bromate?	Potassium bromate and sodium bromate
What is potassium bromate commonly used for?	1. Flour enhancer in the baking industry

2. Neutralizing solution for cold wave home hair permanents and professional solutions

What are the signs and symptoms of acute bromate poisoning?

1. GI distress (i.e., nausea, vomiting, diarrhea)
2. CNS depression
3. Anemia from intravascular hemolysis
4. Acute renal failure (acute tubular necrosis), which may be irreversible
5. Sensorineural hearing loss (irreversible)

What hematological effects may bromates cause?

Methemoglobinemia and hemolysis, secondary to their oxidizing ability

Chronic exposure to bromates is thought to cause what cancer?

Renal cell carcinoma

What are useful tests when evaluating a bromate-toxic patient?

CBC, ABG with co-oximetry to evaluate for methemoglobinemia, electrolytes, BUN, creatinine, audiometry to evaluate for hearing loss

How should bromate ingestions be treated?

1. Supportive care
2. Consider gastric lavage with 2% sodium bicarbonate to prevent the formation of hydrobromic acid.
3. Consider administration of IV sodium thiosulfate.
4. Consider early hemodialysis in large ingestions.

In theory, what does the sodium thiosulfate do?

Reduces bromate to bromide (less toxic)

BROMIDES

What are some of the pharmaceutical agents in which bromide may be found?

Brompheniramine, dextromethorphan, halothane, pancuronium, pyridostigmine, scopolamine

Historically, how was bromide used?

As a sedative and antiepileptic agent

By what mechanism does bromide exert its physiological effects?

Displacement of chloride ions in cellular processes

Acute ingestion of bromide causes what signs and symptoms?

Severe GI distress and CNS depression

What laboratory abnormality may be found with bromide toxicity?

Pseudohyperchloremia

Elevated bromide levels will do what to the anion gap?

Because bromide resembles chloride, it may falsely elevate the chloride on some analyzers and may decrease the anion gap.

What is "bromism"?

Neurologic and dermatologic changes seen with chronic bromide intoxication

What are the neurological features of "bromism"?

Behavioral changes (e.g., depression, dementia, delirium), psychosis, hallucinations, tremor, ataxia, slurred speech, hyperreflexia, lethargy

What are the dermatological features of "bromism"?

1. Acneiform eruptions on face and upper trunk (most common)
2. Erythema nodosum-like lesions on the lower extremities
3. Pemphigus-like vesicles
4. Morbilliform dermatitis

What is another name for the dermatological features of "bromism"?

Bromoderma

Why are activated charcoal and other GI decontamination methods not useful for bromide ingestions?

1. Bromide is rapidly absorbed.
2. Charcoal does not bind bromide.

How is bromide eliminated from the body?

By the kidney – providing exogenous chloride may help clear bromide from the body.

What enhanced elimination methods are effective for bromide?	1. IV normal saline to optimize chloride repletion 2. IV furosemide may be helpful to enhance excretion but has not been shown to improve clinical outcome. 3. Hemodialysis is effective but reserved for severe intoxication.

CAMPHOR

What is camphor?	Volatile aromatic compound (essential oil) initially isolated from the *Cinnamomum camphora* tree
What are the major uses of camphor?	1. Liniments and decongestant ointments 2. Plasticizers 3. Preservatives in pharmaceuticals and cosmetics 4. Mothballs
What are the signs and symptoms of camphor intoxication, and how long is the onset of action?	Initially, GI complaints (e.g., nausea and vomiting), tachycardia, confusion, agitation. Eventually, CNS and respiratory depression and seizures may develop. Camphor may be evident on the breath. Onset of toxicity is rapid, usually within 1 hr of exposure.
Describe the manifestations of dermal toxicity.	Prolonged exposure may result in dermal and mucous membrane irritation and mild burns. Systemic toxicity may result from large mucous membrane exposure.
What is the mechanism of camphor toxicity?	Largely unknown. Camphor may halt cellular respiration or interact with cell membrane channels.
What oral doses of camphor may be toxic in adults and children?	As little as 1 g of camphorated oil may cause severe toxicity.
How are patients with camphor toxicity managed?	Primarily supportive care. Seizures should be managed initially with benzodiazepines.

Does activated charcoal or hemodialysis have any role in managing toxic camphor exposures?

Activated charcoal has unknown efficacy, and caution should be used secondary to the risk of aspiration. Hemodialysis is not expected to be beneficial.

CARBON DISULFIDE

What is carbon disulfide?

A volatile industrial solvent that readily evaporates when exposed to air. It also may be known as carbon bisulfide, carbon sulfide, or dithiocarbonic anhydride.

What are common uses and sources of carbon disulfide?

1. Cellophane, rubber, and rayon production
2. Insecticides/fumigants
3. Common laboratory solvent
4. Disulfiram metabolite

What are possible routes of exposure to carbon disulfide?

Inhalation, ingestion, absorption (dermal, ocular, mucous membranes)

What is the most common route of exposure?

Inhalation

What is the mechanism of toxicity of carbon disulfide?

Mechanisms are largely unknown. Dithiocarbamates, which chelate zinc and copper, are produced from metabolism of carbon disulfide. Carbon disulfide also binds sulfhydryl, amino, and hydroxyl groups. These effects may be partially responsible for the neurotoxicity seen with exposure. Finally, carbon disulfide inhibits dopamine beta-hydroxylase and interferes with catecholamine metabolism.

What is the approximate onset of action following an acute exposure to carbon disulfide?

Immediate, though carbon disulfide is rapidly metabolized

What are symptoms of an acute, high-level carbon disulfide exposure?

CNS excitation, followed by CNS depression (which may be profound), psychosis, mania, delirium, respiratory depression progressing to failure, eye/skin irritation

What symptoms are consistent with a chronic, low-level carbon disulfide exposure?

Peripheral neuropathy (predominantly of the lower extremities), fatigue, headache, personality changes, and memory loss are most commonly reported. Extrapyramidal symptoms (EPS) and atypical parkinsonism are also frequently reported. Other possible findings include optic neuritis, hearing loss, fatty liver degeneration, atherosclerosis, blood dyscrasias, dermatitis, renal damage, and reproductive problems.

What additional symptoms are associated with an ingestion exposure?

Irritation of the GI tract with associated abdominal pain, nausea, and vomiting

What additional symptoms are associated with a dermal exposure?

1. Severe mucous membrane and skin irritation, possible partial- and full-thickness burns
2. Ocular irritation with potential for corneal burns

What additional symptoms are associated with an inhalational exposure?

Upper respiratory tract irritation and bronchospasm

How is a carbon disulfide exposure detected?

No specific diagnostic test. Diagnosis relies on history and supportive presentation and is not based on blood/urine testing.

Are there any drugs or antidotes effective at treating a carbon disulfide exposure?

No. Management is supportive.

What are the treatments indicated for an acute exposure?

1. Placement of an NG tube for aspiration of gastric contents is appropriate for patients presenting promptly after liquid ingestion.
2. Copious irrigation for dermal and ocular exposures
3. Oxygen and bronchodilators may be needed for inhalational exposures.
4. Otherwise, general supportive care is indicated.

Are there any secondary contamination risks to healthcare providers?	Only in those exposed to liquid carbon disulfide, who may contaminate care providers through direct contact or vapor off-gassing

CARBON MONOXIDE

What is carbon monoxide (CO)?	A gas generated by the incomplete combustion of organic (carbon containing) compounds
Why is CO so dangerous?	Odorless, colorless, tasteless, nonirritating
What are common sources of CO exposure?	1. Gas appliances 2. Charcoal grills 3. Combustion engine exhaust (e.g., automobiles, boats) 4. Smoke from any type of fire 5. Cigarettes
How much stronger is CO's affinity for hemoglobin than oxygen?	240 times greater
CO's uptake into the body is dependent upon what factors?	1. Concentration of CO inspired 2. Patient's minute ventilation 3. Duration of exposure
What is the elimination half-life of CO when breathing room air, 100% oxygen, and under hyperbaric oxygen (HBO)?	1. ~320 min with room air (21% oxygen) 2. ~90 min with 100% oxygen at 1 atmosphere 3. ~20 min under HBO at 3 atmospheres
In what direction does CO shift the oxyhemoglobin dissociation curve?	To the left
Besides hemoglobin, where else does CO bind in the body?	1. Cytochrome oxidase 2. Myoglobin (both skeletal and cardiac)
What are the clinical signs and symptoms of CO intoxication?	Headache, nausea, vomiting, fatigue, dizziness, confusion, dyspnea, ataxia, chest pain, syncope, seizure, coma, dysrhythmia, hypotension, death

What syndrome can manifest days to weeks following a significant exposure to CO?	Delayed neuropsychiatric sequelae
Would a CO poisoned patient with normal respirations have a high, low, or normal pulse oximetry? Blood gas PaO_2?	Both would be normal
What hemoglobin type binds CO strongest?	Fetal hemoglobin
Name three chemical asphyxiants.	1. Cyanide 2. Carbon monoxide 3. Hydrogen sulfide
Typical hospital co-oximetry measures what 4 types of hemoglobin?	1. Oxyhemoglobin 2. Deoxyhemoglobin 3. Methemoglobin 4. Carboxyhemoglobin
Which would provide an accurate assessment of the CO concentration, an arterial blood gas or a venous blood gas?	Either
What is the primary treatment for CO intoxication?	Oxygen
What are the proposed mechanisms of HBO's efficacy for CO poisoned patients?	1. Increases the amount of oxygen dissolved in the blood 2. Dissociates CO from all heme moieties 3. Causes cerebral vasoconstriction, thereby ameliorating reperfusion injury 4. Impairs leukocyte adherence
HBO should be considered for patients with what clinical findings?	1. A history of loss of consciousness 2. Severe neurologic findings (e.g., coma or seizures) 3. Persistent findings despite 100% oxygen therapy

4. Symptomatic pregnancy
5. CO level >40%

CARBON TETRACHLORIDE

What is the mechanism of carbon tetrachloride toxicity?

Carbon tetrachloride (CCl_4) metabolism through the cytochrome P450 system creates free radicals that cause nephrotoxicity and hepatotoxicity. Similar to halogenated hydrocarbons, carbon tetrachloride may produce CNS depression and sensitize the myocardium to endogenous catecholamines.

How is carbon tetrachloride used?

Primarily as a reagent in the production of other chemicals. Use has been limited secondary to the toxicity of this compound. It was formerly used in fire extinguishers, as a fumigant, and as a solvent for dry cleaning.

What substance can potentiate the nephrotoxic and hepatotoxic effects of carbon tetrachloride?

Ethanol particularly increases hepatotoxicity. These effects are further pronounced with long-term use.

What are the routes of exposure for carbon tetrachloride?

Inhalation, ingestion, dermal

How is carbon tetrachloride metabolized and excreted?

1. Nearly half of the absorbed carbon tetrachloride is excreted unchanged via the lungs.
2. The remainder is metabolized to the trichloromethyl free radical via the cytochrome P450 enzyme system (primarily via 2E1).

Carbon tetrachloride may be partially metabolized to what anesthetic agent?

Chloroform (Cl_3CH)

What are signs and symptoms of exposure to carbon tetrachloride?

Irritation of mucous membranes/eyes/skin, nausea, vomiting, confusion, dizziness, headache, cardiac dysrhythmias due to increased myocardial sensitivity to catecholamines, CNS depression

What is the potential delay to onset of hepatotoxicity and nephrotoxicity?

1–4 days

Name the hepatic zone most prone to damage from carbon tetrachloride.

Zone 3 (centrilobular)

What is considered a lethal level of exposure?

Ingestion – as little as 5 mL may be lethal
Inhalation – air concentrations as low as 160–200 ppm may be lethal

How can exposure to carbon tetrachloride be detected?

For occupational purposes, levels may be obtained in urine, blood, and expired air, though they are of minimal clinical utility. Abdominal x-rays may show this radiopaque substance when ingested. A history of exposure associated with a consistent clinical picture remains the cornerstone of diagnosis.

Is carbon tetrachloride a human carcinogen?

Possibly (IARC Group 2B)

Why is epinephrine relatively contraindicated after acute carbon tetrachloride exposure?

Increased myocardial sensitivity to catecholamines after carbon tetrachloride exposure may lead to cardiac dysrhythmias.

What can be used to treat carbon tetrachloride exposure?

N-acetylcysteine (NAC) may help prevent hepatic and renal damage after exposure. Otherwise, treat supportively.

Is gastric lavage with an NG tube indicated after ingestion of carbon tetrachloride?

Yes, if the patient presents promptly after exposure.

Are enhanced elimination procedures of proven clinical benefit?

No

CAUSTICS

What is a caustic agent?

An agent that causes corrosive injury upon tissue contact. Although other agents can cause corrosive injury, acids and alkalis are the predominant agents in this class.

What are examples of caustic agents?

1. Acids – hydrochloric acid (toilet bowl cleaner), sulfuric acid (drain cleaner and automobile battery fluid), phosphoric acid (metal cleaner)
2. Alkali – sodium or potassium hydroxide (drain cleaner, hair relaxer), calcium hydroxide (wet cement), sodium hypochlorite (bleach), ammonium hydroxide

What is the fundamental chemistry behind caustic agents?

1. Acidic agents donate protons in an aqueous solution.
2. Alkali (or basic) agents accept protons in an aqueous solution.

What is the pathology associated with an injury secondary to acid exposure?

Acids cause coagulation necrosis. This may cause eschar formation, limiting penetration and further damage.

What is the pathology associated with an injury secondary to alkali exposure?

Alkalis cause liquefaction necrosis. This can result in extensive penetration.

What are the toxic routes of exposure?

Inhalation, ingestion, dermal, ocular

What are common signs and symptoms after a caustic ingestion?

Oral/abdominal/chest/throat pain, vomiting, drooling, dysphagia, coughing and stridor, possibly progressing to airway obstruction

What are the clinical manifestations of an inhalational injury?

Mucous membrane irritation, stridor, bronchospasm, pulmonary edema

Why is it dangerous to mix ammonia and bleach (sodium hypochlorite)?

It will produce and release chloramine fumes, resulting in pneumonitis.

What are the clinical manifestations of a dermal or ocular injury?

Pain, erythema, and blistering. Ocular exposure can cause corneal ulceration and opacification → blindness.

How should a caustic ingestion be managed?

1. A small amount of water or milk can be given to dilute the agent; however, care must be taken to avoid inducing vomiting, as this will reexpose tissues and may cause aspiration.
2. Assess for any airway compromise.
3. Careful nasogastric aspiration of liquid caustics can be attempted.
4. Endoscopy if indicated
5. Surgical consultation for any signs of perforation

Should a neutralizing agent be given?

No. There is a risk of the exothermic neutralization reaction, causing a thermal injury.

What are the indications for endoscopy?

Any patient presenting with an oral injury, vomiting, drooling, dysphagia, stridor, or dyspnea

How long after an exposure should endoscopy be performed?

In mildly symptomatic patients, endoscopy is commonly performed between 12 and 48 hrs. Before 12 hrs, the burns may not have fully developed, and after 48 hrs, there is increased risk of perforation. In anyone with potential airway compromise, endoscopy should be performed emergently.

How are esophageal burns graded?

Grade 0 – normal esophagus
Grade 1 – edema and hyperemia involving mucosa without sloughing or ulceration
Grade 2a – noncircumferential loss of mucosa, variable loss of submucosa with possible extension into muscularis. Some muscularis remains viable, and periesophageal tissues are not injured.
Grade 2b – all the findings in 2a but circumferential
Grade 3 – Grade 2 findings plus deep ulceration, friability, eschar formation,

perforation; entire esophageal wall is necrotic with possible extension to periesophageal tissues

What is the purpose of endoscopy?

For prognosis. Grading the lesions predicts the likelihood of stricture development. Grade 0 and 1 lesions do not cause strictures, while grade 2b lesions can result in strictures in 71% of cases, and grade 3 lesions will cause strictures in almost 100% of cases.

Are steroids indicated to prevent strictures?

This is disputed. Theoretically, steroids can prevent strictures by limiting the inflammatory process; however, strong evidence of effectiveness is lacking, and steroid therapy can mask symptoms of perforation and infection. In animal models, steroids resulted in increased mortality.

How would you treat an inhalational injury due to chlorine gas?

1. Remove patient from the environment.
2. Treat bronchospasm with beta 2-adrenergic agonists.
3. Nebulized sodium bicarbonate may relieve symptoms.

How would you treat dermal or ocular burns?

Immediate copious irrigation. Ocular burns should be irrigated for ≥15 min, and pH should be measured to determine need for additional irrigation. Due to extensive penetration, alkali burns may require extensive irrigation.

CHLORATES

In what chemical forms are chlorates usually found?

Usually in the form of salts, with sodium chlorate ($NaClO_3$) and potassium chlorate ($KClO_3$) being the most common. These are strong oxidizing agents.

In what products can chlorates be found?

1. Herbicides
2. Used in the production of explosives, matches, and fireworks

What are the initial presenting symptoms of acute chlorate ingestion?

The chlorate ion is a strong mucosal irritant and causes nausea, vomiting, diarrhea, and abdominal pain, usually within 1–4 hrs after ingestion.

What are the most serious clinical features of chlorate ingestion?

1. Intravascular hemolysis
2. Methemoglobinemia that can lead to cyanosis, dyspnea, and coma
3. Acute renal failure
4. DIC

What lab abnormalities can be found in acute chlorate ingestions?

Hemolytic anemia, elevated methemoglobin levels (>10%), elevated serum creatinine, hyperkalemia secondary to gross hemolysis and renal failure

Why might an ECG be helpful in a chlorate-toxic patient?

To evaluate for signs of hyperkalemia, such as peaked T waves, widened QRS, and PR prolongation

What procedure can be performed to help enhance chlorate elimination?

Chlorates are freely dialyzable, and hemodialysis is recommended in severe toxicity, especially in the presence of coexisting renal failure. This therapy may prevent life-threatening hemolysis.

Is there an antidote for chlorate toxicity?

Some case reports advocate the use of sodium thiosulfate, either PO or IV (2–5 g in 200 mL of 5% sodium bicarbonate), which may inactivate the chlorate ion, although supportive therapy remains the mainstay of treatment.

Should methemoglobinemia caused by chlorate ingestion be treated with methylene blue?

Yes; however, methemoglobinemia from chlorate ingestion may be poorly responsive to methylene blue. One proposed mechanism for this is that chlorates may inhibit G6PD, an enzyme necessary for the production of NADPH, which is required for the reduction of methemoglobin by methylene blue.

CHLORINE

How is chlorine used commercially?

Chlorine has multiple purposes, including chemical manufacturing (e.g., plastics, pesticides, solvents); disinfection; bleaching; sewage treatment; and water purification (including swimming pools).

What is the name of the chlorine gas agent used by the military in World War I for chemical warfare?

Bertholite

What are the routes of toxicity for chlorine?

Inhalation, ingestion, dermal

What is the mechanism of toxicity for chlorine?

Chlorine is a very caustic and irritating substance. Contact with water on dermal or mucosal surfaces produces hydrochlorous and hydrochloric acid, resulting in oxidative and corrosive damage.

At what concentration of chlorine gas will effects begin to occur?

1 ppm

What are acute effects of chlorine toxicity?

1. Inhalation – nasal and oropharyngeal irritation, wheezing, cough, rhinorrhea, respiratory distress, syncope
2. Ingestion – burn injuries to oropharynx/esophagus/gastric mucosa, dysphagia, drooling, possible hematemesis, and esophageal/gastric perforation
3. Dermal – irritation of skin/eyes/mucosa, burn injuries

Is a specific antidote available for chlorine?

Nebulized sodium bicarbonate may be beneficial in acute inhalational exposure. While chemical neutralization is normally not recommended, the large surface area of the lungs dissipates heat quickly; consequently, no thermal injury appears to occur.

Are laboratory tests available for specific levels of chlorine exposure?

Electrolyte studies may reveal hyperchloremia and acidosis. An ABG may be needed to assess for hypoxia. Obtain a

CXR as needed for evaluation of pneumonitis and pulmonary edema.

What emergency measures should be taken for patients who inhale chlorine?

1. Remove patient from exposure.
2. Provide supplemental humidified oxygen.
3. Bronchodilators for respiratory distress symptoms (e.g., wheezing)
4. Nebulized sodium bicarbonate should be considered.
5. The patient may need intubation for impending respiratory failure.

What emergency measures should be taken for patients who ingest chlorine?

Have the patient drink modest amounts of water. Gastric aspiration with an NG tube may be useful for patients with liquid exposures presenting promptly after ingestion. Patients may need endoscopic studies to assess for mucosal damage.

What emergency measures should be taken for patients who experience dermal exposure to chlorine?

Remove contaminated clothing, and irrigate the skin with water to remove any remaining chlorine.

Are enhanced elimination methods available for chlorine?

No

CHLOROFORM

What are the physical properties of chloroform (Cl₃CH)?

Colorless liquid with a sweet odor

How was chloroform first used?

As an anesthetic agent

What are other names for chloroform?

Trichloromethane, trichloroform, freon 20, formyl/methane trichloride, methenyl/methyl trichloride

What is chloroform used for?

1. Refrigerant and aerosol propellants
2. Extractant solvent for rubber, resins, oils

3. Chemical analysis
4. General solvent for industrial products

What are the modes of exposure?

Ingestion, inhalation, dermal

What is the concern with ocular liquid exposure?

Corneal injury

What are the main effects of acute inhalation?

Initially, mucous membrane irritation. With increased doses, CNS depression, CV depression, and cardiac dysrhythmias may occur.

What are the effects of chronic inhalation?

Hepatic and renal damage

Describe the mechanism of hepatic and renal injury.

Hepatic metabolism (primarily CYP450-2E1) of chloroform generates free radicals such as phosgene (Cl_3CO) that damage proteins and nucleic acids.

What are the clinical effects of ingestion?

Nausea, vomiting, ataxia, headache, progressing to CNS depression. Dysrhythmias due to sensitization of the myocardium may occur, as may hepatic and renal damage.

What is the effect of cutaneous exposure?

Skin irritation, dermatitis, and defatting of the skin may occur.

Why do patients require close observation after an exposure?

Due to delayed hepatic and renal effects up to 48 hrs post-exposure

What is the therapy for acute exposure?

1. Removal from the source and decontamination.
2. NG tube aspiration may be used if the patient presents soon after ingestion.
3. N-acetylcysteine (NAC) has been used to help reduce hepatic and renal damage, but efficacy data is limited.
4. Supportive care is otherwise indicated.

CYANIDE

What are some sources of cyanide exposure?

1. Ingestion of cyanide salts (e.g., potassium cyanide (KCN), sodium cyanide (NaCN))
2. Smoke inhalation (e.g., produced by the burning of plastics)
3. Acetonitrile (e.g., found in artificial nail remover and metabolized to cyanide)
4. Pits or seeds from fruit in the *Prunus* species (e.g., apricots, cherries, peaches) contain amygdalin, which releases cyanide when ingested.
5. Cassava root
6. Sodium nitroprusside

What is the mechanism of cyanide toxicity?

Cyanide inhibits multiple enzymes. The most important toxic action is inhibition of cytochrome oxidase. Cyanide binds to cytochrome a_3, blocking oxygen utilization in the last step of cellular respiration. This causes a shift from aerobic to anaerobic metabolism, depleting ATP and causing lactic acidosis.

What are the potential routes of exposure?

Ingestion, dermal, inhalation, parenteral

What is considered a toxic dose of cyanide?

Oral – 200 mg of either the potassium or sodium salt is potentially lethal
Inhalation – >110 ppm over 30 min is life-threatening, while ≥270 ppm is immediately fatal

What are the signs and symptoms of cyanide toxicity?

1. CNS – anxiety, agitation, confusion, lethargy, and headache initially, with possible rapid onset of seizures and coma
2. GI – abdominal pain, nausea, vomiting
3. Skin – cherry-red color (due to increased oxygen saturation of cutaneous venous hemoglobin) is classically described, although not often seen

4. CV – initial hypertension, which can progress to cardiac arrest heralded by bradycardia and hypotension
5. Respiratory – initial tachypnea followed by bradypnea or apnea (CNS-mediated); acute lung injury also can occur

What changes are seen on lab tests?

1. ↑ lactate
2. ↓ pH
3. ↑ venous oxygen saturation (due to ↓ tissue extraction)
4. Elevated anion gap metabolic acidosis

How quickly does onset of symptoms occur?

Inhalation – within minutes
Ingestion – minutes to hours. Onset is delayed when metabolism to cyanide is required.

What does a cyanide antidote kit include?

1. Amyl nitrite pearls to be crushed and inhaled
2. Sodium nitrite to be administered IV
3. Sodium thiosulfate to be administered IV

How does the antidote kit work?

1. The nitrites induce methemoglobinemia. Because cyanide has a higher affinity for methemoglobin than cytochrome oxidase, cyanide will leave the mitochondria, allowing for resumption of oxidative phosphorylation.
2. Sodium thiosulfate acts as a sulfhydryl donor. This helps the enzyme Rhodenase convert cyanide into thiocyanate, which is eliminated in the urine.

What other antidote is available for treating cyanide poisoning?

Hydroxocobalamin

How does it work?

Combines with cyanide to form cyanocobalamin (vitamin B_{12}). This is nontoxic and renally eliminated.

What advantages does hydroxocobalamin have?

1. It does not induce methemoglobinemia, so it is safe to administer to victims of smoke inhalation.
2. It does not cause hypotension (possible with nitrites).

Does hydroxocobalamin have any adverse effects?

Yes. Although it is a safe antidote, it will cause red discoloration of the skin, mucous membranes, and urine. This typically resolves in 48 hrs. The discoloration of the serum may interfere with several laboratory tests.

Is activated charcoal effective in treating cyanide ingestion?

Although cyanide is poorly adsorbed by activated charcoal, the lethal dose of cyanide is quite small and may be sufficiently bound by a 1 g/kg dose. Gastric lavage is controversial due to risk of secondary exposure of healthcare workers.

DETERGENTS

What are detergents?

Amphipathic compounds (having both hydrophilic and hydrophobic ends) that reduce the surface tension of water, acting as surfactants

How are detergents used?

Household uses are most familiar, including laundry- and dish-cleaning agents, as well as surface-cleaning solutions. Some mouthwashes also contain detergents.

List four chemical classifications of detergents.

1. Nonionic
2. Anionic
3. Cationic
4. Amphoteric

What is the basic mechanism of toxicity?

Detergents act as irritants, adversely affecting the skin, the mucosa of the GI tract, and the eyes.

Which of these types is considered the most toxic?

Cationic surfactants, which have been reported to be corrosive at concentrations >7.5% and cause hematemesis, abdominal pain, and inability to swallow secretions. Large ingestions can cause systemic toxicity (i.e., hypotension, CNS depression, seizures, coma).

What other potentially toxic agents can household detergents contain besides the actual detergent?

Sodium hypochlorite (bleach), bacteriostatic agents, enzymes

Which household detergent is particularly dangerous?

Automatic dishwasher detergents have a high alkalinity and can cause severe corrosive injury.

What respiratory effects can occur due to detergent ingestion?

Aspiration can cause chemical pneumonitis and pulmonary edema. Also, inhalation of powdered detergent can cause edema of the vocal cords and epiglottis.

What metabolic disturbances occur with ingestions of phosphate-containing products?

Hypocalcemia and hypomagnesemia (phosphates bind divalent cations)

How is detergent ingestion treated?

1. Supportive care is generally sufficient.
2. Any patient who vomits should be observed for at least 6 hrs for signs of aspiration.
3. Endoscopic evaluation of upper GI tract may be needed for persistently symptomatic patients who have ingested automatic dishwasher detergent or cationic detergents with concentrations >7.5%.

Are there any techniques to reduce toxicity?

A small amount of water or milk can be given orally for dilution if the patient can take the liquid without difficulty. Such liquids should never be forced and could potentially increase aspiration risk.

What can be used to specifically bind phosphate in the GI tract?

Aluminum hydroxide

How should eye exposure be handled?

Flush with copious amounts of water or saline for 15–20 min. If corneal injury is expected, consult ophthalmology.

Granular detergents and automatic dishwasher detergents have a greater chance of causing injury.

DIMETHYL SULFOXIDE (DMSO)

What is dimethyl sulfoxide (DMSO), and where might it be encountered industrially?

1. Industrial solvent
2. Used in organic synthesis, as a metal-complexing agent, and as a paint stripper
3. Found in hydraulic fluid and antifreeze

Are there any approved medical uses for DMSO?

Yes, as a bladder instillate for the treatment of interstitial cystitis. It is also used as a vehicle for certain medications and is effective topically in treating extravasation injury from certain antineoplastic agents.

What is the mechanism of toxicity of DMSO?

Unknown, but may cause mast cell degranulation with histamine release. DMSO spilled on the skin or clothing may carry other toxic substances transdermally.

What are the clinical effects seen with toxic exposure to DMSO?

Common symptoms include skin rash and urticaria, irritation of mucous membranes/eyes/respiratory tract, garlic odor to breath, nausea, and headache. Following intravascular administration, hemolysis may occur. CNS depression has been reported. As DMSO is an efficient solvent, dermal exposure to this chemical may result in toxicity characteristic of any solute present.

Are there any specific tests helpful for diagnosis?

No. Diagnosis relies principally on history.

What treatments are available for DMSO toxicity?

1. No specific antidotes exist. Management is supportive.
2. Rapid decontamination is important, as DMSO is readily absorbed transdermally.
3. Enhanced elimination methods are of no proven clinical benefit.

DIOXINS

What is the most common route of exposure to dioxins in the United States?	Dietary ingestion; however, absorption may also occur through dermal and inhalational exposure.
What are the major food sources of dioxin contamination?	Meat, fish, dairy
What is a dioxin?	A member of a group of 75 distinct chemicals known as chlorinated dibenzo-*p*-dioxins that consist of two benzene rings connected by two oxygen atoms. The remaining binding sites bind up to 4–8 chlorine atoms. They are lipid soluble compounds and bioaccumulate; they also tend to persist in the environment.
How are dioxins formed?	1. Combustion of polychlorinated compounds (e.g., PVC, plastic) 2. Exhaust from diesel engines 3. Waste from coal-burning power plants 4. Production of chlorinated organic solvents 5. Component of cigarette smoke 6. Municipal waste processing
What are some infamous environmental disasters that involved dioxins?	1. German – Ludwigshafen BASF accident in 1953 2. Netherlands – Amsterdam Philips-Duphar Facility explosion in 1963 3. Japan – *Yusho disease* (rice oil) in 1968 4. England – Coalite explosion in 1973 5. Italy – Seveso Meda ICMESA plant disaster in 1976 6. Taiwan – *Yu-Cheng disease* (rice oil) in 1979 7. Vietnam – "Operation Ranch Hand" in the Vietnam War from 1962–1971
In what tissue type are dioxins most heavily concentrated?	Adipose tissue, due to high lipophilicity

What are potential health effects of dioxin exposure?

Carcinogenicity (IARC Group 1), hepatotoxicity, immunotoxicity, cytochrome P450 induction, reproductive and developmental abnormalities, dermatological lesions

How are dioxins speculated to cause their effects?

Bind the aryl hydrocarbon receptor, which helps to regulate gene expression and other regulatory proteins

What is the minimum toxic dose in humans?

0.1 μg/kg

What are acute symptoms of dioxin toxicity?

Myalgias, mucous membrane irritation, nausea, and vomiting are reported, although acute toxicity is limited, as no deaths from acute exposure have been reported.

What are late clinical effects of dioxin toxicity?

Chloracne (pathognomonic), hirsutism, hyperpigmentation, peripheral neuropathy, porphyria cutanea tarda, elevated triglycerides, liver cytochrome enzyme induction

What is chloracne?

Cystic acneiform lesions, predominantly on the face and upper body, that may occur 1–3 weeks after exposure to dioxins and related compounds and may last for decades

What substance, designed as a fat substitute, can substantially increase the fecal excretion of dioxins?

Olestra®

What vitamins may be of benefit in high doses following dioxin toxicity?

Vitamins A and E

What is the name of the infamous dioxin-containing herbicide used by the United States during the Vietnam War?

"Agent Orange" (2,4,5-T, a chlorophenoxy herbicide)

Who is a famous victim of dioxin poisoning?	Viktor Yushchenko, a Ukranian politician who was poisoned by 2,3,7,8-tetra-chlorodibenzo-*p*-dioxin (TCDD)

DISK BATTERIES

What are disk batteries?	Also called button batteries, they are flat, smooth, and typically 8–25 mm in diameter. They are commonly used in watches, hearing aids, and calculators.
What chemicals do disk batteries contain?	Alkaline sodium or potassium hydroxide, plus a heavy metal (lithium, mercury, zinc)
Why is ingestion of a disk battery an emergency?	If stuck in the esophagus, mucosal damage may begin almost immediately with associated morbidity and mortality reported.
How do ingested disk batteries cause tissue damage?	1. Pressure necrosis 2. Electrical current 3. Leakage of alkaline corrosives
Does heavy metal poisoning occur if a disk battery fragments in the GI tract?	No. The amount of heavy metal content is too low to cause significant toxicity.
Should emesis be induced in patients who have ingested disk batteries?	No. This is unlikely to cause expulsion of the battery and may lead to esophageal perforation, aspiration, or other complications.
What imaging is done in patients with suspected disk battery ingestion?	Plain radiographs of the entire respiratory and GI tracts
What is the treatment for a battery located in the esophagus?	Emergent endoscopic battery removal
What is the treatment for a battery located past the esophagus?	Asymptomatic patients may be allowed 10 days for passage before further imaging or treatment is needed.

How long does spontaneous passage of the battery take once past the stomach?

Most pass within 7 days; every stool must be examined for presence of the battery.

Can a retained disk battery cause esophageal perforation?

Yes. Burns can occur within hours, and perforation has occurred in as few as 6 hrs.

ETHYLENE DIBROMIDE

What is ethylene dibromide?

A colorless substance with a sweet chloroform-like odor. It is a liquid at room temperature, having a vapor pressure similar to that of water.

What are common uses of ethylene dibromide?

Formerly used as an additive in leaded gasoline. It is used as a pesticide and fumigant, although its use was banned in the U.S. in 1984. It is still used as a solvent, a chemical intermediate, and a gauge fluid.

What are possible routes of exposure to ethylene dibromide?

Inhalation (vapor is heavier than air leading to accumulation), ingestion, absorption (dermal, ocular, mucous membranes)

What is the mechanism of toxicity of ethylene dibromide?

It is an alkylating agent that causes inhibition of DNA activity. Also, hepatic metabolism of ethylene dibromide leads to production of free radicals and cytotoxic metabolites.

What are possible clinical effects of an ethylene dibromide exposure?

1. Dermal – erythema, edema, blistering
2. Ocular – chemical conjunctivitis
3. Pulmonary – cough, bronchospasm, pulmonary edema, acute lung injury
4. GI – abdominal pain, nausea, vomiting, diarrhea
5. Systemic – it has general anesthetic properties resulting in mental status changes that can cause sedation progressing to coma. Also, it can cause metabolic acidosis, coagulation

abnormalities, and hepatic and renal failure.

What is the expected onset for symptoms?

Often immediate; however, development of dermal ulcers and pulmonary edema may be delayed for 2–3 days.

When working with or responding to spills of ethylene dibromide, what chemical property must be considered?

It will penetrate protective clothing, including rubber, neoprene, and leather.

How is an ethylene dibromide exposure detected?

1. Reliable history of exposure with consistent signs and symptoms
2. Expired air, blood, or tissue detection is possible but not useful.
3. Serum bromide levels can confirm an exposure but do not predict clinical course.

Are there any drugs or antidotes effective in an ethylene dibromide exposure?

There is no proven antidote. Dimercaprol and acetylcysteine have been suggested for use, but there is no supporting data.

What treatments are indicated for an ingestion exposure?

1. NG aspiration may be considered for recent ingestions.
2. Activated charcoal is only indicated in the alert, cooperative ingestion patient.

What treatments are indicated for a dermal or ocular exposure?

Remove clothing and decontaminate as needed. Irrigate ocular exposures immediately with saline or water for 15 min.

What treatments are indicated for an inhalation exposure?

Administer supplemental oxygen, treat bronchospasm with inhaled beta 2-adrenergic agonists, and observe for development of pulmonary edema.

ETHYLENE GLYCOL

What is the most common source of ingestion of ethylene glycol?

Engine coolant (antifreeze), not to be confused with gas line antifreeze, which likely contains methanol

What are the early signs of acute ethylene glycol toxicity?

Signs of inebriation – altered metal status, nystagmus, ataxia, slurred speech

Does the urine of a patient poisoned with antifreeze fluoresce under a woods lamp?

Not necessarily. Although fluorescein is frequently added to antifreeze to aid in mechanics' search for leaks, observer interpretation and even the presence of urine (or gastric content) fluorescence are highly variable. Treatment decisions should be based on history and clinical indication of ethylene glycol poisoning.

What finding in the urine should raise your suspicion of ethylene glycol poisoning in the appropriate clinical setting?

Presence of calcium oxalate crystals

Ethylene glycol is metabolized to what clinically significant compounds? What is the significance of each?

Glycoaldehyde, glycolic acid, glyoxylic acid, and oxalic acid. The latter three contribute to clinical acidosis. Glycolic acid can lead to a false elevation in serum lactic acid when using some methods of analysis. Oxalic acid is responsible for urine calcium oxalate crystal formation, acute renal failure, and hypocalcemia (and its sequelae).

What is the rate limiting step in oxalic acid production?

Conversion of glycolic acid to glyoxylic acid

What metabolic state is expected from ethylene glycol poisoning?

High anion gap metabolic acidosis

Can a patient with a normal osmolar gap be ruled out for significant toxicity?

No. Ethylene glycol, but not its metabolites, contributes to the osmolar gap. Late in metabolism, when no parent compound is present, the osmolar gap may be normal. It is at this time that the anion gap should be elevated. Also, due to individual variations in normal serum osmolarity, a gap may appear "normal" but still hide a significant ethylene glycol level.

How do you correct for concomitant ethanol intoxication when calculating the osmolar gap?

Using the standard formula for a calculated serum osmolarity (Osm$_c$), the blood concentration of ethanol (mg/dL) divided by 4.6 (molecular weight of ethanol divided by 10 to correct for units) must also be added in to correctly calculate the osmolar gap:

$$\text{Osm}_c = 2[\text{Na}^+] + \frac{\text{BUN}}{2.8} + \frac{\text{glucose}}{18} + \frac{\text{ethanol}}{4.6}$$

From the osmolar gap, how do you estimate the concentration of ethylene glycol (in mg/dL) of a suspected ethylene glycol intoxicated patient?

Multiplying the osmolar gap by 6.2 (ethylene glycol's molecular weight divided by 10) will give a rough estimate of the ethylene glycol level in mg/dL.

What role do calcium oxalate crystals play in ethylene glycol toxicity?

Calcium oxalate crystals primarily deposit in the kidney, resulting in renal failure, but also may deposit in other tissues such as the brain and spinal cord. This may result in neurologic deficits.

What "antidotes" are used in the medical management of ethylene glycol toxicity?

Fomepizole or ethanol administration

What enzyme do these medications inhibit?

Alcohol dehydrogenase

At what ethanol level is the metabolism of ethylene glycol by alcohol dehydrogenase completely inhibited?

100 mg/dL

When should fomepizole or ethanol be discontinued?

Therapy should continue until serum ethylene glycol concentrations are <20 mg/dL.

Once alcohol dehydrogenase is inhibited, how are ethylene glycol and its metabolites eliminated?

Ethylene glycol is cleared by the kidneys with a half-life of >17 hrs.

What is the definitive therapy for ethylene glycol intoxication?

Hemodialysis

What are the indications for hemodialysis in ethylene glycol poisoning?

Consensus opinion supports hemodialysis if metabolic acidosis, end-organ toxicity, or renal failure is present. A serum ethylene glycol level >50 mg/dL or high osmol gap are relative indications for hemodialysis. The ultimate decision should be based on physician judgment.

What theoretical adjunctive therapies may prevent toxicity in ethylene glycol poisoned patients?

Thiamine and pyridoxine may aid in converting glyoxylic acid to metabolites less toxic than oxalic acid.

ETHYLENE OXIDE

What is ethylene oxide?

A colorless, flammable, and highly reactive gas. It is used to sterilize medical equipment and in the production of ethylene glycol, surfactants, and polyesters.

Does it have an odor?

Yes, it has a sweet, ether-like odor; however, it can cause olfactory fatigue, limiting one's ability to smell it. As a result, smell does not provide adequate exposure warning.

What is the mechanism of toxicity of ethylene oxide?

It is an alkylator of protein and DNA that has general anesthetic properties.

What are possible routes of exposure to ethylene oxide?

Inhalation, ingestion (unlikely, as ethylene glycol is a gas at room temperature), absorption (dermal, ocular, mucous membranes)

Are there any contamination risks to healthcare providers?

People can be exposed through direct contact while sterilizing equipment, cleaning spills, or opening packaged supplies.

What is the approximate onset of action after an acute exposure to ethylene oxide?

Immediate local and systemic symptoms are possible; however, respiratory and neurologic symptoms may be delayed for hours following inhalation.

What are possible effects of an acute ethylene oxide exposure?

Neurological symptoms range from drowsiness, confusion, ataxia, and headache to seizures, coma, and death. Ethylene oxide is a potent irritant and will cause irritation of the eyes, nose, and throat. It may also cause bronchospasm and delayed pulmonary edema.

What effects are possible with dermal exposure?

Ethylene oxide liquid can cause frostbite, and contact with aqueous solutions can cause erythema, edema, vesiculation, and desquamation; this can be delayed for hours.

Why is allergic sensitization an important concern in an ethylene oxide exposure?

Repeat patient contact with ethylene oxide-sterilized medical equipment may result in sensitization, causing an acutely life-threatening allergic reaction.

What systemic effects are possible after an exposure to an ethylene oxide/freon mixture?

Cardiac dysrhythmias

How is an ethylene oxide exposure detected?

Diagnosed clinically with a reliable history of exposure and consistent signs and symptoms

How is an ethylene oxide exposure managed?

1. Remove the patient from the environment. Rescue personnel should wear personal protective equipment, including self-contained breathing apparatus (SCBA) if necessary.
2. Patients must be decontaminated by removing clothing and washing exposed skin.
3. Thoroughly irrigate affected eyes, assess visual acuity, and examine for corneal injury.

4. Treat significant skin exposures with appropriate burn care.
5. There is no proven antidote. Treatment is supportive.

What additional treatments are indicated for an inhalation exposure?

1. Administer supplemental oxygen.
2. Treat bronchospasm with a bronchodilator.
3. Anticipate and treat pulmonary edema.

What are the possible effects of chronic exposure?

Sensory and motor peripheral neuropathy, cataracts, and increased risk of leukemia. Exposure may also be responsible for birth defects and spontaneous abortion.

FLUORIDES

What are some of the most common products which contain fluoride?

1. Hydrofluoric acid (HF) – used in glass and silicon etching
2. Chrome cleaning agents (ammonium bifluoride)
3. Toothpaste (sodium monofluorophosphate)
4. Insecticides
5. Dietary supplements (sodium fluoride)

By what routes can patients be exposed to fluorides?

1. Ingestion – corrosive effects causing nausea, vomiting, and abdominal pain. Fluoride is also passively absorbed from the GI tract, leading to systemic toxicity.
2. Dermal – irritation, edema, pain, potential systemic absorption
3. Ocular – corrosive injury
4. Inhalation – respiratory tract irritation, potential systemic absorption

How does dermal exposure to a dilute HF solution or ammonium bifluoride present?

There may be a delay of hours before symptom onset. Patient can develop significant pain despite a normal exam. Progressive erythema, followed by blanching and possibly necrosis, can develop. The pain is excruciating, and deep tissue injury can result.

What are the mechanisms of fluoride toxicity?	1. Direct binding to divalent cations (i.e., calcium and magnesium), which can lead to hypocalcemia or hypomagnesemia 2. Interference with enzyme systems, including the Na-K-ATPase, which may lead to hyperkalemia, and enzymes involved in the oxidative phosphorylation, which leads to ATP depletion and cell death 3. Concentrated HF will cause coagulation necrosis in addition to the systemic effects of absorbed fluoride.
What GI signs and symptoms are most commonly seen with fluoride toxicity?	Nausea, vomiting, abdominal pain, hematemesis, dysphagia
What neurologic effects are most commonly seen with fluoride toxicity?	Clinical manifestations of hypocalcemia (e.g., muscle spasms, tremors, headache, seizures, hyperreflexia)
What CV effects are most commonly seen with fluoride toxicity?	1. Effects of hypocalcemia/hypomagnesemia (i.e., prolonged QT interval) 2. Effects of hyperkalemia (i.e., peaked T waves, widened QRS complex, AV nodal block, bradycardia) 3. Ventricular tachycardia and ventricular fibrillation
What is the estimated toxic dose for fluoride ingestion?	5–10 mg/kg
What studies should be performed on patients with suspected fluoride toxicity?	1. Serum calcium, magnesium, and potassium levels to monitor for hypocalcemia, hypomagnesemia, and hyperkalemia 2. Serial ECGs to look for prolongation of the QT interval (i.e., hypocalcemia) and/or peaked T waves (i.e., hyperkalemia)
Is it possible to check a fluoride level?	Yes, it is possible to check both serum and urine fluoride levels, but these tests

are not readily available in most hospitals.

How do you treat systemic fluoride poisoning?

1. Correct electrolyte abnormalities with IV preparations of calcium and magnesium.
2. Correct acidosis with sodium bicarbonate.
3. Hemodialysis can be considered for critically ill patients that are refractory to other forms of treatment.

What measures should be taken after an oral ingestion of HF or ammonium bifluoride?

1. Gastric emptying via NG aspiration may be considered.
2. Administer calcium carbonate, magnesium/aluminum-based antacids or milk to bind the fluoride in the stomach.
3. Endoscopy is indicated for any clinical suspicion of corrosive injury.

How is a dermal exposure treated?

1. Thorough irrigation with water or saline
2. Topical calcium gel should be applied (7 g of calcium gluconate added to 150 mg of sterile water-based lubricant)
3. For pain refractory to above treatment, SQ, regional IV infusion, or intraarterial infusion of calcium gluconate may be effective.

Can calcium chloride be used as a substitute for dermal application, infiltration, or infusion?

No. It can cause tissue toxicity.

How should an ocular exposure be treated?

1. Immediate irrigation for at least 15 min with saline or water
2. Irrigation with a weak (1%–2%) calcium gluconate solution may be beneficial.
3. Ophthalmology consultation should be considered.

What therapy may be beneficial after an inhalational exposure to HF?

Nebulized 2.5% calcium gluconate

How much fluoride is contained in toothpaste?

1 mg of fluoride per gram of toothpaste. Toothpaste contains sodium monofluorophosphate which has low solubility and is generally less toxic.

How should ingestion of toothpaste, fluoride rinse, or fluoride supplements be treated?

Fluoride salts will be converted to HF upon entering the stomach. This can cause local irritation and systemic absorption. Ingestions estimated to have >5 mg/kg should be treated with oral administration of milk or other sources of calcium or magnesium.

Who may be considered for discharge from the hospital after fluoride ingestion?

Asymptomatic patients who have ingested <3 mg/kg of fluoride and who have been observed for 6 hrs post-ingestion.

FLUOROACETATE

What is fluoroacetate used for?

Formerly a rodenticide in common use in the U.S., this compound is now prohibited except for use as a coyote poison (to protect cattle and sheep). It is still used outside the U.S. for its original purpose. It is commonly known as "Compound 1080" or sodium monofluoroacetate (SMFA).

What is/are the route(s) of intoxication?

Inhalation and ingestion

What is the mechanism of toxicity?

It poisons the Krebs cycle. Fluoroacetate (in place of acetic acid) combines with coenzyme A to form fluoroacetyl CoA. The latter undergoes conversion to fluorocitrate (by citrate synthase), which subsequently occupies the citrate binding site on aconitase, rendering this enzyme inactive and compromising aerobic metabolism. Urea metabolism is also hindered due to the inability to make intermediates such as glutamate.

What are the signs and symptoms of fluoroacetate toxicity?

Initial symptoms include nausea, vomiting, diarrhea, and abdominal pain. CNS manifestations and life-threatening CV manifestations follow, including agitation, seizures, coma, hypotension, and dysrhythmias.

What laboratory abnormalities are commonly associated with fluoroacetate toxicity?

Increased anion gap metabolic acidosis with high lactate levels. Hypocalcemia and hypokalemia may also occur.

What is the mechanism behind fluoroacetate-induced hypocalcemia?

Citrate, the substrate immediately upstream from the inhibited enzyme (aconitase), accumulates and is freely available to bind nearby calcium ions.

What is the recommended treatment?

Supportive care. Consider activated charcoal and gastric lavage if available within 1 hr post-ingestion.

Are there any antidotes?

Ethanol and glycerol monoacetate have both been studied in animal models as potential suppliers of acetate to competitively inhibit the action of citrate synthase on monofluoroacetyl-CoA; however, human data is limited.

FORMALDEHYDE

List some common sources of formaldehyde.

Automobile exhaust, tobacco smoke, fertilizers, foam insulation, burning wood, disinfectants

What is formalin?

Formaldehyde aqueous solution; it commonly also contains methanol

What are two common uses of formalin?

1. As a disinfectant
2. As an embalming fluid (effects tissue fixation)

What is the metabolic byproduct and serum marker of toxicity following formaldehyde ingestion?

Formic acid

What acid-base disorder may result from formaldehyde ingestion?

Anion gap metabolic acidosis

What are the physical effects of prolonged or excessive formaldehyde exposure?

1. Exposure to formaldehyde gas can cause irritation of eyes/skin/mucous membranes with associated sneezing, laryngospasm, bronchospasm, and noncardiogenic pulmonary edema.
2. It is a potent caustic causing coagulation necrosis. When ingested, it can cause rapid and significant GI injury, including ulceration, bleeding, and perforation.
3. CNS depression can develop and progress to coma. Hypotension and shock can develop secondary to GI injury and profound acidosis.

What measures may aid in reducing injury from acute formaldehyde ingestion?

Dilution with water may reduce local injury, and gastric aspiration may lessen systemic absorption.

How is formaldehyde toxicity treated?

1. Supportive care
2. Folinic acid to help convert formic acid to nontoxic metabolites (carbon dioxide and water)
3. IV sodium bicarbonate to treat metabolic acidosis
4. Fomepizole or ethanol should be administered if there is suspicion of a significant co-ingestion of methanol.
5. Hemodialysis will remove formic acid, formaldehyde, and methanol.
6. Endoscopy is indicated to evaluate caustic injury.

What are the indications for dialysis following formaldehyde intoxication?

Development of metabolic acidosis

FREONS AND HALONS

What is freon?

Freons are a type of halogenated hydrocarbon, and they are a subclass of chlorofluorocarbons (CFC). They are colorless, odorless, and noncorrosive. They have historically been used as refrigerants, aerosol propellants, solvents, and as polymer intermediates in plastic manufacturing. Although their production has been stopped, freon is still available in older air-conditioners and refrigerators, and there is a considerable stockpile.

How does the primary exposure to freon occur?

Primarily through refrigerator and air-conditioner leaks, which can cause absorption or inhalation of freon. Also, it is commonly inhaled intentionally as a drug of abuse.

How is freon metabolized?

Freon is rapidly absorbed through the skin or by inhalation and rapidly excreted through exhalation. It is not metabolized by the lungs or kidneys.

What toxic effects do freons have?

1. Dermal/ocular – low concentration exposure can cause ocular/mucosal irritation. Skin contact with liquid freon or with freon escaping from a pressurized container can cause frostbite. Systemic absorption can cause CNS depression, headache, confusion, and dysrhythmias.
2. Inhalation – pulmonary irritation, bronchospasm, pulmonary edema
3. Freon is neither a carcinogen nor a teratogen.

By what mechanisms can freon cause pulmonary edema?

1. Mucosal irritation
2. Freons can produce toxic gases (i.e., phosphine and chlorine) when heated or by decomposition.

How do freons cause dysrhythmias?

They sensitize the myocardium to endogenous catecholamines, predisposing the patient to tachydysrhythmias and ventricular fibrillation.

How do freons induce AMS and coma?

Both as an asphyxiant (by displacing oxygen) and through a general anesthetic effect

How do you manage patients with a freon exposure?	1. Remove patient from the source. 2. Provide oxygen and respiratory support, if needed. 3. A calm environment should be provided, and adrenergic agents should be avoided. 4. GI decontamination is not warranted. 5. Treat frostbite with warm water immersion, tetanus prophylaxis, and analgesia.
What is halon?	A halogenated hydrocarbon, also known as bromochlorodifluoromethane, used in fire protection systems
How are individuals exposed to halon?	When fire protection systems are activated, halon is released as a gas. It is also abused as an inhalant.
What is the clinical presentation of a halon exposure?	Similar to freon, with bronchospasm, lightheadedness/euphoria, CNS depression, and palpitations. Fatalities can occur secondary to dysrhythmias or asphyxiation.
What is the management of a patient exposed to halon?	Same as for freon exposures
What poisonous gas can be produced when halon is heated?	Phosgene

GASES (IRRITANT)

What are irritant gases?	Gases that result in mucous membrane irritation on exposure, producing a characteristic syndrome of pharyngeal, nose, throat, and eye burning.
Where do people encounter toxic irritant gases?	Industrial settings, structure fires, hazardous materials spills, certain household cleaning products
How should irritant gases be classified?	By water solubility: 1. High solubility – ammonia, chlorine, formaldehyde, hydrogen chloride, nitric acid, sulfur dioxide

2. Low solubility – nitric oxide, nitrogen dioxide, phosgene

What is the "warning property" of an irritant gas?

The amount of initial irritation the gas causes. Gases with high warning properties tend to result in lower patient exposure, as patients flee the irritating effects.

Name the gases that are formed from the common mistake of mixing household bleach and ammonia.

Chlorine and chloramine gas

What are the effects of high solubility gases?

Immediate irritation of the mucous membranes of the eyes, nose, and throat

What are the effects of low solubility gases?

Because these gases are less soluble to the upper airway mucosa, they can be inhaled into the pulmonary alveoli and cause delayed-onset pulmonary toxicity.

What are the common signs of exposure to high solubility gases?

Conjunctivitis, rhinitis, burns, dry cough, wheezing, odynophagia

What are the complications of exposure to low solubility gases?

Pulmonary edema (commonly delayed) and damage to the lower respiratory epithelium

Are there long-term complications of irritant gas exposure?

Usually not; however, some gases (i.e., nitrogen dioxide, phosgene) may predispose to bronchiolitis obliterans and COPD.

What is the treatment for irritant gases?

1. Remove the victim from the exposure.
2. Observe the patient for delayed sequelae.
3. Maintain the airway, with intubation if necessary.
4. Assess pulmonary status with CXR, ABG, and PFTs.

GLYCOL ETHERS

What are glycol ethers?

A class of industrial compounds that are used in solvents; industrial and home cleaners; topical coatings (i.e., lacquers, paint thinners, latex paints); semiconductor manufacturing; and automotive antifreeze and brake fluids. Examples include diethylene glycol, ethylene glycol monobutyl ether, and ethylene glycol monomethyl ether.

How does exposure typically occur?

Ingestion, inhalation, dermal absorption

What pivotal role have glycol ethers played in pharmaceutical regulation?

The misuse of diethylene glycol (DEG) in 1937 in the drug "Elixir Sulfanilamide" marketed by a Tennessee company, caused the deaths of over 100 people, many of them children, in 15 states. This disaster led to the passage of the 1938 Food, Drug, and Cosmetic Act, which allowed the Food and Drug Administration (FDA) to regulate drugs and cosmetics. Additionally, safe labeling and premarket testing were required prior to mass-market sales.

How are glycol ethers metabolized?

Although knowledge of exact pathways is limited, glycol ethers appear to be predominantly metabolized in the liver, with some metabolism through alcohol and aldehyde dehydrogenase.

What is the clinical presentation of a patient with acute glycol ether toxicity?

Generally, acute exposure may manifest as nausea, vomiting, and abdominal pain followed by metabolic acidosis, renal toxicity, and CNS depression/neurotoxicity. Hepatotoxicity may also occur.

What are the signs and symptoms of chronic glycol ether toxicity?

Renal failure appears to be a prominent feature. Neurologic abnormalities, including lethargy/CNS depression, progressive paralysis, and seizures, may occur. Bone marrow suppression has also been reported.

What three features characterized DEG toxicity in the 2006 Panamanian outbreak?

1. Renal failure
2. Metabolic acidosis
3. Symmetric ascending paralysis

What is the mechanism of toxicity of DEG?

Not fully understood. DEG and/or its metabolite, hydroxy-ethoxyacetic acid, may cause the majority of the toxicity.

What is the management of patients with glycol ether poisoning?

1. Gastric aspiration with an NG tube may be beneficial if the patient presents immediately after ingestion.
2. 4-methylpyrazole (fomepizole) is currently of unknown efficacy, as it is typically not apparent whether the metabolites or the parent compound cause the majority of the toxicity.
3. After DEG exposure, patients with early hemodialysis appear to have the best outcome. This may also apply to other glycol ethers.
4. Otherwise, general supportive care is indicated.

HYDROCARBONS

What are hydrocarbons?

Organic compounds primarily containing carbon and hydrogen atoms. They are derived from plants, oils, animal fats, petroleum, natural gas, and coal and are used as solvents, degreasers, fuels, and lubricants.

How are patients poisoned by hydrocarbons?

1. Ingestion – GI absorption of aliphatic hydrocarbons is limited, and systemic toxicity typically is absent. Aromatic, halogenated, or otherwise substituted hydrocarbons are more prone to cause systemic absorption and symptoms. Both pose an aspiration risk.
2. Inhalation (fumes) – may cause CNS depression

3. Dermal/ocular – cause local irritation and potential systemic absorption
4. Injection (SQ, IM, IV) – may result in localized necrosis, pneumonitis

What are their mechanisms of toxicity?

1. Disruption of the alveolar surfactant layer following aspiration → alveolar collapse, V/Q mismatch, and hypoxia. Also, direct pulmonary injury causes pneumonitis and pulmonary edema. Hydrocarbons of low viscosity (e.g., gasoline, kerosene, mineral seal oil, furniture polish) pose a higher risk of aspiration as compared to high-viscosity hydrocarbons (e.g., motor oil, petrolatum jelly, mineral oil).
2. Systemic intoxication (often after absorption of lipid-soluble solvents) will cause inhibition of neurotransmission and, thus, a general anesthetic effect.
3. Sensitization of the myocardium to endogenous catecholamines, resulting in dysrhythmias
4. Subcutaneous inflammation, "defatting," and liquefaction necrosis

Which clinical entity causes the most morbidity and mortality?

Aspiration. Only a small amount is necessary to cause significant pulmonary injury.

What factors increase the risk of aspiration?

Physical properties of the hydrocarbon ingested (i.e., low viscosity and low surface tension) and a history of coughing, gagging, or vomiting.

How will hydrocarbon aspiration present?

Patients usually will develop coughing or choking within 30 min and may have a rapid progression of symptoms, manifesting with tachypnea, abnormal breath sounds, hypoxia, pulmonary inflammation/edema, and potentially respiratory failure. These can worsen over several days. If a patient is observed for 6 hrs without development of respiratory symptoms, a significant aspiration is unlikely.

Is a CXR taken on presentation to the ED after a possible hydrocarbon ingestion useful for prognosis?

No. Radiographic changes can be delayed for up to 24 hrs. Also, radiographic recovery will lag behind clinical recovery.

How should hydrocarbon aspiration be treated?

1. Administer supplemental oxygen.
2. Treat bronchospasm with inhaled beta 2-adrenergic agonists.
3. Maintain a low threshold for endotracheal intubation and positive pressure ventilation.

Should prophylactic antibiotics be administered for pneumonitis?

Routine use is not indicated. Abnormal lung auscultation, fever, leukocytosis, and abnormal radiographic findings are often presenting findings of simple hydrocarbon pneumonitis. Antibiotics should be considered with a rise in temperature or white cell count occurring 24 hrs post-exposure.

Should prophylactic steroids be administered for pneumonitis?

No

What clinical effects are seen after a hydrocarbon ingestion?

Nausea, vomiting, and hematemesis can be seen. Certain hydrocarbons pose a risk for systemic absorption.

What GI decontamination should be performed for hydrocarbon ingestions?

For agents with little or no systemic absorption (e.g., kerosene or furniture polish), GI decontamination should not be performed, as it will increase aspiration risk without affecting toxicity. For systemically absorbed hydrocarbons or those containing toxins, decontamination must be considered. NG aspiration of a liquid ingestion is reasonable, as is administration of activated charcoal. Ensure a well-protected airway.

How are injection injuries managed?

1. Proper wound care, analgesia, and tetanus immunization as indicated

2. Surgical debridement to remove necrotic tissue and limit hydrocarbon exposure must be considered. A hand surgery consult is mandatory for patients who have injured themselves with a high-pressure injector (e.g., grease gun), as tracking through fascial planes can lead to extensive injury and loss of function.

HYDROGEN SULFIDE

What is hydrogen sulfide (H_2S)?

A colorless, toxic gas typically formed by bacterial decomposition of proteins or during many industrial processes

What does hydrogen sulfide smell like?

Rotten eggs

Does the absence of the distinctive odor of hydrogen sulfide mean that it is not present?

No. Hydrogen sulfide causes olfactory nerve fatigue at concentrations of 100–150 ppm, and the ability to perceive this odor can subsequently be extinguished.

What are some occupations at risk for hydrogen sulfide exposure?

Agriculture, petroleum industry, sewer workers, leather tanning, rubber industry, mining (coal)

Hydrogen sulfide exerts its clinical effects by what mechanism?

Binds to the cytochrome oxidase a_3, thus inhibiting oxidative phosphorylation

How does hydrogen sulfide poisoning result in an anion gap acidosis?

Lactic acidosis due to anaerobic metabolism

What other gas can cause similar symptoms to hydrogen sulfide poisoning?

Cyanide can cause a similar "knock down" phenomenon. Methane is also found in sewer gas but has a slower onset.

What are the signs and symptoms associated with early, mild hydrogen sulfide toxicity?

Ocular and respiratory tract irritation can be noticed at levels of 50–100 ppm. Prolonged exposure to these levels can cause reversible corneal ulcerations ("gas eye") and possibly irreversible corneal scarring.

As levels rise to >250 ppm, there is risk of developing pulmonary edema.

When hydrogen sulfide concentrations reach >500 ppm, what effects may be seen?

Systemic toxicity, including:
1. CNS – headaches, confusion, dizziness, seizures, coma
2. GI – nausea and vomiting
3. CV – chest pain, bradycardia, dysrhythmias, hypotension

Above what level can hydrogen sulfide cause immediate death upon inhalation?

>700 ppm

What is the most important treatment for victims of hydrogen sulfide poisoning?

Move the victim(s) to fresh, uncontaminated air. It is important never to attempt a rescue unless rescue personnel are wearing a self-contained breathing apparatus (SCBA).

How else can hydrogen sulfide poisoning be treated?

1. Provide 100% supplemental oxygen.
2. Consider methemoglobin induction with nitrites (i.e., amyl nitrite and/or sodium nitrite).
3. Consider hyperbaric oxygen treatment.

In theory, how does methemoglobin help treat hydrogen sulfide poisoning?

Hydrogen sulfide will preferentially bind methemoglobin to form sulfmethemoglobin. This will remove hydrogen sulfide from cytochrome oxidase a_3.

In reality, what limits the usefulness of methemoglobin?

Hydrogen sulfide has a rapid onset of action and is only present in the blood for a short period of time.

Is sodium thiosulfate indicated for hydrogen sulfide poisoning?

No. It provides no benefit.

IODINE

What different forms of iodine exist?

1. Iodine – a divalent molecule (I_2), also known as elemental iodine or molecular iodine. It is corrosive due

to its cytotoxic and oxidant properties.
2. Iodide – negative ion (I⁻) of iodine that is nontoxic
3. Iodophors – iodine complexed to a carrier agent. These are less toxic, as the release of the corrosive elemental iodine is limited. Betadine® (povidone-iodine) is a well-known iodophor.

Where is iodine commonly found in healthcare settings?

Contrast dye, Betadine® (povidone-iodine solution), expectorants, iodoform gauze, vaginal irrigants, Lugol's solution

How much free iodine is available in a typical Betadine® solution?

In a bottle of 10% Betadine®, there will be ~1% free iodine.

What clinical manifestations can be seen after an ingestion of iodine?

These are primarily related to corrosive injury and can include vomiting, abdominal pain, diarrhea, and GI bleeding. This can lead to hypovolemia, shock, and edema of the pharynx and glottis, possibly requiring intubation.

What other routes of exposure are possible?

1. Topical exposure can cause corrosive injury to the eyes or skin. Repeated or prolonged topical exposure can lead to systemic absorption and toxicity.
2. Inhalation of iodine vapor can cause bronchospasm and pulmonary edema.

How does chronic exposure to iodine differ from acute toxicity?

Chronic exposures can cause hyperthyroidism, hypothyroidism, or goiter formation. Contact dermatitis and other hypersensitivity reactions involving the salivary glands and skin can be seen.

What laboratory findings are seen in iodine toxicity?

1. Hyperchloremia – due to iodine's interference with some chloride assays
2. Lactic acidosis
3. Elevated iodine levels – toxic levels can range from 7,000–60,000 μg/dL (normal iodine levels range from 5–8 μg/dL)

4. Elevated thyroid function tests (particularly in chronic exposures)

Describe the management of iodine toxicity from ingestion.

1. Supportive care for most cases of Betadine® ingestion
2. Significant volumes of ingestion may require NG tube aspiration
3. The toxicity from iodine found in Betadine® can be minimized by using cornstarch, starchy food, milk, or sodium thiosulfate to convert iodine to iodide.
4. Endoscopy is indicated if corrosive GI injury is suspected.
5. Hemodialysis is effective at removing iodine although not indicated in those with intact renal function.
6. Hypovolemia and shock may require aggressive fluid resuscitation.

What color is the aspirate following a Betadine® ingestion when mixed with cornstarch?

Blue-green

ISOCYANATES

What are isocyanates?

Liquid compounds that can volatilize when exposed to air and are commonly used in the production of polymers and other chemicals including foams, paints, fabrics, insulation, and pesticides.

What are usual routes of exposure to isocyanates?

Inhalation and absorption (skin or mucous membranes)

What is the approximate onset of action following an acute exposure to isocyanates?

Usually immediate; however, symptoms may be delayed up to 6 hrs.

What are symptoms of an acute isocyanate exposure?

Isocyanates are strong irritants causing ocular, dermal, and airway burning, as well as dyspnea with cough and wheezing. Patients may progress to acute lung injury and noncardiogenic pulmonary edema.

Are there any long-term effects of isocyanate exposure?

After chronic low-level exposures, patients may develop reactive airway disease. Following acute poisonings, patients may develop pulmonary hypersensitivity and chronic eye irritation.

What are the treatments indicated for an inhalation exposure?

Decontamination with copious irrigation for dermal and ocular exposure. Respiratory symptoms should be treated symptomatically with oxygen and nebulized beta 2-adrenergic agonists, as needed.

What is the mechanism of isocyanate toxicity?

Not well established but likely through direct irritation and involvement of cell-mediated immunity pathways

Does cyanide poisoning result from isocyanates?

No. Cyanide is not released through breakdown or metabolism of isocyanates.

Which industrial disaster led to over 2500 deaths following a community-wide methyl isocyanate gas leak?

The Union Carbide Plant disaster in Bhopal, India (1984)

ISOPROPANOL

In what products is isopropanol (isopropyl alcohol) found?

Rubbing alcohol (70% concentration), industrial solvents, window cleaners, antiseptic and disinfectant agents

Which is more intoxicating, isopropanol or ethanol?

Isopropanol is 2 to 3 times more intoxicating.

Why doesn't isopropanol cause an anion gap acidosis like other toxic alcohols?

Isopropanol is a secondary alcohol that is oxidized to a ketone, and not acidic metabolites.

What is the metabolite of isopropanol?

Acetone

Does isopropanol cause an elevated osmolar gap?

Yes, both isopropanol and its metabolite, acetone, increase the gap.

What is the classic clinical triad of isopropanol ingestion?	1. CNS depression 2. Fruity breath odor 3. Ketosis without metabolic acidosis
What is a GI complication of isopropanol ingestion?	Gastritis, possibly hemorrhagic in nature
What are the signs and symptoms of isopropanol ingestion?	Inebriation, vomiting, abdominal pain, respiratory depression, hypotension
Why is activated charcoal not useful for isopropanol ingestion?	Because of the rapid absorption of isopropanol
How do you treat isopropanol ingestions?	1. Airway evaluation and management 2. IV crystalloid for hypotension 3. Consider hemodialysis (rare)
When is hemodialysis indicated for isopropanol toxicity?	In the setting of unresponsive hypotension or continued clinical deterioration

METALDEHYDE

What is metaldehyde?	A cyclic polymer of acetaldehyde
How is metaldehyde chiefly used in the U.S.?	Primarily as a slug and snail poison but may also be found in some camping fuels
What are the metabolites of metaldehyde?	Acetaldehyde and acetone
Describe the mechanism of toxicity.	Largely unknown; however, acetaldehyde appears to have some role.
What is the toxic dose?	100 mg/kg can result in convulsions; >400 mg/kg can be fatal.
How will metaldehyde poisoning present?	Within 3 hrs of ingestion, toxicity may initially resemble a disulfiram reaction (i.e., acetaldehyde toxicity) with flushing, nausea, vomiting, and diarrhea. Larger doses can result in ataxia, lethargy, myoclonus, hyperthermia, and seizures.

What metabolic derangements are found with ingestion?	Anion gap metabolic acidosis
How should metaldehyde poisoning be treated?	Supportive treatment. Ondansetron may be used to alleviate nausea and vomiting. Benzodiazepines are utilized for seizures initially.

METHANOL

What are the common sources of methanol?	Windshield washer fluid, model airplane or racing fuel, solid camping or chafing cooking fuel, automobile fuel line antifreeze. In industry, methanol is commonly used as a solvent.
What are the routes of exposure to methanol?	Ingestion is most common, but exposures via inhalation (i.e., "huffing" and industrial accidents) have been reported.
What are common signs of acute methanol intoxication?	Similar to ethanol, methanol produces inebriation. Signs and symptoms include nystagmus, slurred speech, ataxia, and altered metal status.
What clinical features are unique to methanol poisoning?	"Snowfield" vision or complete blindness (may be the source of the adage "blind-drunk"). Optic disc hyperemia or pallor may be observed along with central scotoma. Hypodense basal ganglion lesions may be observed on neuroimaging.
Methanol is metabolized by alcohol dehydrogenase and aldehyde dehydrogenase to what respective compounds?	Formaldehyde and formic acid
What metabolic state is expected from methanol poisoning?	High anion gap metabolic acidosis with minimal lactate elevation
Does methanol intoxication produce an elevated osmolar gap?	Yes. Methanol contributes to serum osmolarity and is, therefore, expected to produce an elevated gap; however, due to

variations in normal serum osmolarity, a normal gap does not rule out toxicity.

How do you correct for concomitant ethanol intoxication when calculating the osmolar gap?

Using the standard formula for a calculated serum osmolarity (Osm_c), the blood concentration of ethanol (mg/dL) divided by 4.6 (molecular weight of ethanol divided by 10 to correct for units) must also be included to correctly calculate the osmolar gap:

$$Osm_c = 2[Na^+] + \frac{BUN}{2.8} + \frac{glucose}{18} + \frac{ethanol}{4.6}$$

From the osmolar gap, how do you estimate the concentration of methanol in mg/dL of a suspected methanol-intoxicated patient?

Multiplying the osmolar gap by 3.2 (the molecular weight of methanol divided by 10) will give a rough estimate.

What are the "antidotes" for management of methanol toxicity?

Fomepizole or ethanol administration

What enzyme is inhibited by these medications?

Alcohol dehydrogenase

At what ethanol level is the metabolism of methanol by alcohol dehydrogenase completely blocked?

100 mg/dL

When should fomepizole or ethanol be discontinued?

Therapy should continue until serum concentrations are <20 mg/dL.

Once alcohol dehydrogenase is inhibited, how are methanol and its metabolites eliminated?

Methanol has little renal elimination and is cleared primarily via respiratory vapor ($T_{1/2}$ = 30 − 54 hrs). Methanol and formic acid can be removed by hemodialysis.

What are the indications for hemodialysis in methanol poisoning?

Consensus opinion supports hemodialysis if metabolic acidosis, end-organ toxicity, or renal failure is present. A serum methanol level >25 mg/dL or a

high osmol gap are relative indications
for hemodialysis. The ultimate decision
should be based on physician judgment.

**What cofactor can be added
to aid in methanol
metabolism?**

Folinic acid may speed the formation of
nontoxic metabolites.

METHEMOGLOBINEMIA INDUCERS

**How is methemoglobin
formed?**

Ferrous (Fe^{2+}) iron in hemoglobin is
oxidized to ferric (Fe^{3+}) iron.

**What is the normal
methemoglobin
concentration in blood?**

1%. Although RBCs are continuously
exposed to oxidizing agents, there are
enzymes which reduce methemoglobin to
hemoglobin in order to prevent
methemoglobin accumulation.

What are these enzymes?

1. NADH methemoglobin reductase –
   >95% of methemoglobin reduction
2. NADPH methemoglobin reductase –
   <5% of methemoglobin reduction

**What characteristics do
substances that cause
methemoglobinemia share?**

They are oxidizing agents.

**What drugs classically cause
methemoglobinemia?**

1. Antibiotics – trimethoprim,
   sulfonamides, dapsone
2. Local anesthetics – cetacaine,
   benzocaine
3. Antimalarials – chloroquine,
   primaquine
4. Phenazopyridine
5. Nitrites – amyl nitrite, sodium nitrite
6. Silver nitrate
7. Nitroglycerin

**What substances cause
methemoglobinemia?**

Nitrates (well-water, prepackaged foods),
aniline dyes, chlorates, bromates, nitric
and nitrous oxide

**How does methemoglo-
binemia decrease oxygen
delivery?**

Methemoglobin does not bind oxygen
to the oxidized heme molecules. In
addition, methemoglobin will shift the

oxyhemoglobin dissociation curve to the left, making the remaining normal heme molecules less likely to release oxygen.

Why is pulse oximetry unreliable in patients with methemoglobinemia?

Methemoglobin interferes with absorption of light by the oximeter probe, causing it to be inaccurate. Oxygen saturation readings on pulse oximetry will not drop below ~85% even with methemoglobin elevations >70%.

What device measures oxygen saturation in the presence of methemoglobinemia?

A co-oximeter, which directly determines methemoglobin levels

What signs and symptoms occur with methemoglobinemia?

Although individual variations may be significant, the following is a guide:

Level 10%–15% – cyanosis may become evident and is unresponsive to supplemental oxygen, symptoms are only minor if present

Level 20% – exertional dyspnea, fatigue, headache, dizziness, tachycardia

Level >45% – confusion, metabolic acidosis, lethargy, seizures, coma

Level near 70% – potentially fatal

What simple bedside tests can detect methemoglobinemia?

1. Bubble 100% oxygen through a tube with patient's blood – if it remains dark, methemoglobin may be present.
2. Blow supplemental oxygen onto filter paper with a few drops of patient's blood – if it does not change color, methemoglobin may be present.

What is the first-line antidote for methemoglobinemia?

Methylene blue

How does methylene blue work?

Acts as an electron transfer intermediate for NADPH methemoglobin reductase. This greatly increases its activity.

Which precautions should be considered when administering methylene blue?

1. Do not administer to patients with known G6PD deficiency. G6PD-deficient patients have low NADPH concentrations and, therefore, methylene blue will be ineffective.
2. Methylene blue, itself, can induce methemoglobinemia in excessive doses (>5 mg/kg) and can result in subsequent hemolysis.

What are alternative treatments for patients unresponsive to methylene blue?

Hyperbaric oxygen and exchange transfusion

Does a patient need to be exposed to a xenobiotic to develop methemoglobinemia?

No. Infants <4 months old have reduced NADH methemoglobin reductase activity and can develop methemoglobinemia secondary to a variety of insults, including diarrheal illness, dehydration, acidosis, and small amounts of oxidizing agents.

METHYL BROMIDE

What is methyl bromide?

An extremely toxic fumigant gas used in pest control, as a soil sterilant, and as a chemical reagent. Secondary to its potential environmental and human toxicity, its use is being phased out.

What is the cellular mechanism of toxicity of methyl bromide?

Not fully understood, but appears to alkylate DNA and proteins → cell death

What are the two most common routes of exposure to methyl bromide?

Inhalation and dermal

What property of methyl bromide makes humans susceptible to exposure?

It is denser than air and, therefore, collects in low-lying areas. It may also collect in and around clothing, predisposing to dermal absorption.

Why is a warning indicator added to methyl bromide preparations?

It lacks irritative properties, so lethal exposures can occur without warning.

What substance is added to methyl bromide to serve as a "warning" indicator?

Chloropicrin, a lacrimator

Describe the effects of dermal exposure.

May result in localized skin irritation and breakdown. Erythema, dermatitis, and vesiculation have been reported in areas of contact. Systemic effects may manifest after dermal exposure.

What are the effects of acute methyl bromide inhalation?

Airway irritation, cough, and dyspnea may occur upon exposure. Initially, the irritative symptoms are attributed to the chloropicrin. Primary pulmonary manifestations of methyl bromide include pneumonitis, acute lung injury, and possibly pulmonary hemorrhage. Systemic effects also are common following inhalation.

What are acute systemic effects of methyl bromide toxicity?

Systemic effects usually manifest as nausea, vomiting, headache, confusion, CNS depression, tremor, and ataxia. Severe poisoning may result in seizures and coma.

What chronic effects may be seen with methyl bromide exposure?

Chronic effects may emerge from both chronic low-level exposure and as sequelae of acute poisoning. Patients may present with neuropathy, ataxia, dementia, visual disturbances, personality changes, or seizures. Unfortunately, these symptoms are long-lasting and often irreversible.

Are any laboratory tests useful for evaluation?

No specific labs are helpful. Bromide levels are difficult to obtain and are very nonspecific. Recommended testing would include general labs to evaluate organ system function and to rule out other items on the differential diagnosis.

Describe the treatment of methyl bromide poisoning.

Decontamination is important, as methyl bromide can accumulate in clothing and poses a further risk to the patient and caregivers. Treatment is otherwise supportive.

METHYLENE CHLORIDE

What is another name for methylene chloride?	Dichloromethane
What is its major use?	Primarily used as a solvent for chemical reactions. It is also used as an aerosol propellant, degreaser, and paint stripper.
What metabolite of methylene chloride may contribute to systemic toxicity?	Carbon monoxide. Hepatic biotransformation of methylene chloride occurs via two pathways: 1. Mixed function oxidase system of cytochrome P450 yields conversion to CO (primary route) 2. Cytosolic transformation (glutathione transferase-dependent) during which formaldehyde and formic acid intermediates are produced (low-affinity, high-capacity route).
What is the mechanism of toxicity of methylene chloride?	Dissolves fats, destroying epithelial cells. It also causes CNS depression and may sensitize the myocardium to endogenous catecholamines.
What are the modes of toxicity for methylene chloride?	Inhalation, ingestion, dermal
What are the clinical manifestations of an acute methylene chloride exposure by inhalation?	Nausea, vomiting, dysrhythmias, CNS depression, seizures, pulmonary congestion, hypotension, respiratory arrest
What are manifestations of ingested methylene chloride?	Corrosive burns to GI mucosa, nausea, vomiting, CNS depression, dysrhythmias, renal and liver impairment, pancreatitis
What labs should be used to monitor patients who have ingested methylene chloride?	Serial carboxyhemoglobin concentrations with co-oximetry, CBC, lipase, electrolytes, liver and kidney function tests
What methods are available to decrease absorption of ingested methylene chloride?	NG tube aspiration, if patient presents promptly after ingestion

Are methods available to increase elimination of methylene chloride?	No
What emergency treatments should be provided to exposed patients?	1. Remove patient from exposure. 2. Administer 100% oxygen. 3. Airway management and cardiac monitoring for dysrhythmias 4. Treat seizures with benzodiazepines.
How is an increased carboxyhemoglobin concentration treated?	100% oxygen is the treatment of choice
How is an acute lung injury from methylene chloride treated?	Initially, 100% oxygen is used. Bronchodilators are used for respiratory distress symptoms (e.g., wheezing). Aggressive airway management may be necessary.
How is a dermal exposure treated?	Removal of all clothing and copious irrigation of the skin with water

MOTHBALLS

What two chemicals are used to create mothballs?	1. Naphthalene (now rarely used) 2. Paradichlorobenzene
Which of these chemicals is more hazardous?	Naphthalene. Paradichlorobenzene rarely causes toxicity.
What essential oil was formerly used in mothballs but has since been abandoned due to its high toxicity?	Camphor
How do mothballs function?	Sublimation to a gas that is toxic to moths (and humans at high levels)
What physical effects indicate excessive inhalation?	Eye/nose/throat irritation, headache, confusion
What are clinical manifestations of naphthalene ingestion?	Initial acute symptoms are primarily GI. In larger ingestions, lethargy and seizures may occur. Delayed methemoglobinemia

and hemolysis can occur after even a single mothball is ingested.

Describe the mechanism of hemolysis and methemoglobinemia.

Metabolites of naphthalene are potent oxidizers. Oxidation of ferrous iron hemoglobin produces methemoglobin. Patients with G6PD deficiency are at increased risk for oxidative stress.

What laboratory tests are useful for mothball exposure?

Hemoglobin level, lactate dehydrogenase, indirect bilirubin, and peripheral blood smear may help diagnose hemolysis. Methemoglobin levels may be obtained from co-oximetry.

What are the effects of paradichlorobenzene toxicity?

Paradichlorobenzene is primarily nontoxic. Mucous membrane irritation may occur, as hydrochloric acid is produced when paradichlorobenzene decomposes.

What treatments are of benefit in acute mothball ingestion?

1. IV hydration or transfusion if hemolysis occurs
2. Methylene blue for symptomatic methemoglobinemia; use caution when administering to G6PD-deficient patients

Is activated charcoal effective in acute ingestion?

Effective for naphthalene, unnecessary for paradichlorobenzene

Which type of mothball floats in fresh water?

Camphor

Which type of mothball has a green flame when burned?

Paradichlorobenzene

What foods should be avoided following mothball ingestion?

Milk and foods high in fats/oils due to enhancement of absorption

NITRITES

How are nitrites commonly used?

1. Ethyl, amyl, and butyl nitrites are used as air fresheners and can be abused as inhalants.

2. Sodium and amyl nitrites are used as cyanide antidotes.
3. Nitrites are also used in the curing and preservation of foods.

What are the physiological effects of nitrites?

Vasodilation and methemoglobinemia, resulting in functional anemia and hypoxia

How do nitrites cause methemoglobinemia?

Nitrites oxidize ferrous (Fe^{2+}) iron to ferric (Fe^{3+}) iron in heme. This results in the inability of that heme molecule to bind oxygen appropriately.

How do overdoses of nitrites present?

Flushing, headache, hypotension, tachycardia, cyanosis

What tests can diagnose nitrite overdose?

A nitrite dipstick can be used to detect nitrites in serum. ABG with co-oximetry will detect methemoglobinemia.

What treatments should be used for nitrite toxicity?

1. Supportive care
2. Methylene blue to treat symptomatic methemoglobinemia; use caution in patients with G6PD deficiency
3. Fluids and vasopressors may be needed for hypotension.

NITROGEN OXIDES

What are nitrogen oxides?

Various oxidized species of nitrogen. The most common forms are nitric oxide (NO); nitrogen dioxide (NO_2); and nitrous oxide (N_2O).

What role does NO play in the body?

NO serves as one of the few gaseous signaling molecules, acting on the endothelium to produce vasodilation.

From what sources might someone be exposed to nitrogen oxides?

Environmental air pollution, smoke from structure fires, gasoline and propane engine exhaust, welding fumes, fermenting grain fumes

What is "silo filler's" disease?

Delayed-onset pulmonary toxicity experienced by farm workers who, upon entrance into a poorly ventilated silo, are exposed to high concentrations of nitrogen dioxide produced by fermenting grain. Symptoms are characterized by dyspnea, cough, and hypoxia with possible wheezes and rales on exam.

Describe the mechanism of nitrogen oxide toxicity.

On contact with respiratory tract mucosa, nitrogen oxides react to form nitrous and nitric acids, along with other reactive nitrogen species. These products cause both caustic injury and oxidative stress to the pulmonary mucosa.

What are the medical and industrial uses of nitrogen oxides?

1. Treatment of pulmonary hypertension by selective dilation of pulmonary vasculature
2. Treatment of neonatal respiratory distress syndrome
3. Manufacture of related chemicals (i.e., nitric acid, nitrosyl halides) and bleaching of rayon

What acute findings can be caused by nitrogen oxide poisoning?

Airway irritation and bronchospasm, causing dyspnea and hypoxia. Patients may develop noncardiogenic pulmonary edema, and methemoglobinemia may occur (rarely).

What chronic pulmonary conditions may develop after nitrogen oxide exposure?

Pulmonary fibrosis and brochiolitis obliterans

What happens to NO in the bloodstream?

Quickly reacts with hemoglobin to form nitrosylhemoglobin, which is subsequently oxidized to methemoglobin

Are there any tests recommended to detect nitrogen oxide poisoning?

No. The most likely indicator would be a history of exposure. Pulse oximetry, CXR, and pulmonary function tests are indicated, as is ABG with co-oximetry to assess concomitant methemoglobinemia.

What treatments should be performed in the event of nitrogen oxide poisoning?

1. Airway monitoring with intubation/ventilatory assistance, as necessary

2. Humidified oxygen and inhaled beta 2-adrenergic agonists for bronchospasm
3. Corticosteroids have no role in acute treatment.
4. Copious irrigation of mucous membranes and eyes with water or saline, if exposed
5. Methylene blue for symptomatic methemoglobinemia

Name some common sources of N_2O.

Surgical anesthesia, compressed gas containers (e.g., whipped cream, cooking spray), automotive nitrous systems

What is a "whipit"?

A prepackaged cartridge filled with N_2O, which is inhaled by an abuser for its euphoric effects

What CNS receptor does N_2O target?

It is a rapidly acting NMDA receptor antagonist.

What is the most common cause of death from acute N_2O exposure?

Asphyxia (inadequate O_2 supplied with N_2O)

What are the common clinical manifestations of acute toxicity?

Confusion, dizziness, euphoria, CNS depression, syncope. Acute toxicity is commonly related to asphyxia.

What essential vitamin is inactivated by chronic exposure?

Vitamin B_{12} (required for normal DNA and myelin synthesis)

List the clinical manifestations of chronic N_2O toxicity.

Bone marrow suppression (i.e., megaloblastic anemia, thrombocytopenia, leukopenia) and peripheral neuropathy

What studies are helpful in suspected N_2O toxicity?

CBC, vitamin B_{12} and folic acid levels, nerve conduction study, homocysteine and methylmalonic acid levels

How might a chronic N_2O abuser be identified?

Manifestations of vitamin B_{12} deficiency (e.g., anemia and peripheral neuropathy) with elevated homocysteine and methylmalonic acid levels but normal vitamin B_{12} and folate levels.

What treatments are available for managing acute toxicity?	Supportive care with attention to airway management
How is chronic N_2O toxicity treated?	Effects typically reverse 2–3 months after discontinuing exposure. Bone marrow suppression may be treated with folinic acid.

NONTOXIC AND MINIMALLY TOXIC HOUSEHOLD PRODUCTS

Are there any nontoxic substances?	No. Any substance can be toxic given a large enough exposure. It is the job of the healthcare provider to determine if an exposure has a minimal risk of causing harm.
What information must be available before determining an ingestion to be minimally toxic?	1. Accurate identification of the product, with complete ingredients from the package label or other current reference 2. A reasonable estimate of the maximum amount ingested 3. Description of the symptoms being experienced 4. Whether an ingestion of the suspected substance in the amount ingested has been reported to cause any significant adverse effects
What are some pitfalls that must be avoided when evaluating risk of toxicity of a household product?	1. Brand name products can have several formulations, and older versions may have more toxic ingredients. 2. Some products can pose a choking risk even though there is minimal systemic toxicity (e.g., silica gel packs). 3. There are many "sound-alike" products – obtain the exact spelling of the product. 4. It is possible that toxic substances have been stored in containers meant for another benign substance. 5. Failure to determine if there has been chronic exposure to the substance 6. Not considering the possibility of co-ingestions

7. Not inquiring about underlying medical issues

Why is it important to accurately determine whether a product, such as bleach, is meant for household use or obtained from an industrial setting?

Household products tend to have low concentrations of their toxic components. For example, household bleach contains <5% sodium hypochlorite, and household ammonia has 3% to 10% ammonia hydroxide and will usually not cause significant corrosive damage unless large quantities are ingested. In contrast, industrial strength products are often significantly more concentrated and may cause serious injury.

Hair straighteners contain what highly caustic chemical?

Sodium hydroxide (1%–3%)

Ingestion of household hydrogen peroxide dilutions (<9%) is usually nontoxic; however, commercial-strength hydrogen peroxide is readily available. What complications can its ingestion cause?

Significant caustic injury and potentially life-threatening systemic oxygen emboli

Long-term ingestion of 1 g of licorice can result in what electrolyte disturbance?

Hypokalemia

By what mechanism does the glycyrrhizic acid in licorice work?

Exhibits mineralocorticoid activity through its inhibition of 11-beta-hydroxysteroid dehydrogenase, which normally inactivates cortisol

OXALIC ACID

What are the forms of oxalic acid?

Solution and salts

For what is oxalic acid used?

Bleaches, metal and wood cleaners, rust removers, leather tanning

Name some plants that contain soluble oxalic acid.

Sorrel, unripe star fruit, rhubarb leaves

What are the modes of exposure?

Inhalation, ingestion, cutaneous, ocular

Describe the symptoms of cutaneous or ocular exposure.

Primarily irritation and burning; however, corrosive injury may occur in large exposures.

What are the concerns with large inhalational exposures?

1. Airway irritation and burns
2. Chemical pneumonitis
3. Pulmonary edema

What are some symptoms of systemic oxalic acid toxicity?

Initially, muscular weakness and tetany followed by possible cardiac dysrhythmias or seizures. Renal failure, focal neurologic deficits, or paralysis may result secondary to deposition of calcium oxalate crystals.

What is the mechanism of systemic oxalic acid toxicity?

Oxalic acid binds divalent metals, predominantly calcium. In the body, calcium oxalate crystals are formed and may precipitate in tissue and in the vasculature (most often the kidneys, brain, and spinal cord).

Describe ECG findings that may be present following oxalic acid ingestion.

Hypocalcemia may result in QT prolongation.

What laboratory tests are helpful after oxalic acid exposure?

Electrolyte and magnesium levels to evaluate for hypocalcemia and hypomagnesemia. BUN and creatine to evaluate renal function. Urinalysis may show large amounts of calcium oxalate crystals.

What is the treatment for systemic ingestion?

1. Oral calcium salts (i.e., calcium chloride, calcium gluconate, or calcium carbonate) may bind oxalic acid in the stomach and prevent absorption.
2. IV calcium solutions should be used to treat systemic hypocalcemia.
3. Aggressive hydration is warranted to avoid formation of calcium oxalate crystals in the renal tubules.
4. Monitor for dysrhythmias and seizures.

PENTACHLOROPHENOL AND DINITROPHENOL

What are the uses of pentachlorophenol?

Historically, pentachlorophenol (PCP) has been used widely in insecticides, fungicides, and herbicides; however, PCP is no longer publicly available and is restricted to use as a wood preservative for utility poles, railroad ties, and wharf pilings.

What are the uses of dinitrophenol?

Dinitrophenol (DNP) has been used as a pesticide, herbicide, and fungicide, as well as in the manufacture of certain types of dyes, explosives, and photograph-developing chemicals.

What illegal (in the U.S.) and dangerous use of DNP has made it more readily available to consumers?

Use as a weight loss supplement

What is the mechanism of toxicity of PCP and DNP?

Disruption of cellular respiration by uncoupling oxidative phosphorylation, resulting in decreased ATP production and generation of excess heat. DNP also oxidizes hemoglobin to methemoglobin.

Are PCP and DNP carcinogenic?

Based upon animal studies, the Environmental Protection Agency (EPA) has classified PCP as a probable human carcinogen, although human studies have not confirmed this claim. Minimal animal studies exist to support DNP as a carcinogen, so the EPA has not classified DNP as a potential carcinogen.

What are the major routes of exposure to pentachlorophenol and dinitrophenol?

Inhalation, ingestion, dermal

How does acute PCP or DNP overdose present?

Nausea, vomiting, headache, and lethargy, progressing to hyperthermia, seizures, and CV collapse. In addition, DNP may cause methemoglobinemia, hepatomegaly, liver failure, kidney failure, and yellowish skin discolorations.

How does chronic PCP and DNP toxicity present?

Profuse sweating, fever, tachycardia, and tachypnea are hallmarks of both acute and chronic exposure. In addition, chronic exposure may result in weight loss, flu-like symptoms, and in rare instances, damage to bone marrow. Chronic DNP exposure is also associated with lens changes, including glaucoma and cataracts.

What metabolic abnormality is expected after PCP and DNP toxicity?

High anion gap metabolic acidosis

How is the diagnosis of PCP or DNP overdose made?

Positive diagnosis is made based on a history of exposure and consistent clinical findings. PCP or DNP exposure should be considered in the presence of an unexplained uncoupling syndrome (e.g., tachycardia, tachypnea, hyperthermia, high anion gap metabolic acidosis). Blood levels are not easily obtained and are not indicative of the severity of PCP or DNP poisoning; therefore, they should not be used in diagnosis or management.

What treatments should be performed in the event of PCP or DNP overdose?

1. Supportive care
2. Aggressive cooling (both external and internal) may be needed to address extreme hyperthermia secondary to the uncoupling process.
3. IV fluid replacement as appropriate to prevent dehydration and circulatory collapse

PERCHLOROETHYLENE

What is another name for perchloroethylene?

Tetrachloroethylene, PCE, Perc

What is its major use?

Primarily used in industry as a solvent, a dry cleaning chemical, and a degreaser

How is perchloroethylene eliminated?

Hepatically metabolized, then renally excreted

What is the mechanism of toxicity of perchloroethylene?

Like other chlorinated hydrocarbons, perchloroethylene acts as an anesthetic. The resulting CNS and respiratory depression may quickly lead to death. There is very high CNS penetration. Also, perchloroethylene potentiates the pro-arrhythmic properties of catecholamines.

What metabolite may contribute to its CNS depressant effect?

Trichloroethanol – a similar metabolite of chloral hydrate

What are the modes of toxicity for perchloroethylene?

Inhalation, ingestion, dermal

What are the potential clinical manifestations of an acute perchloroethylene exposure by inhalation?

Airway irritation, headache, dizziness, nausea, vomiting, CNS depression, cardiac dysrhythmias, elevated liver enzymes

What are possible manifestations of ingested perchloroethylene?

Nausea, vomiting, diarrhea, abdominal pain, hepatotoxicity, CNS depression, cardiac dysrhythmias

What labs should be used to monitor perchloroethylene patients?

LFTs and RFTs, ABG, ECG, CXR

What are the effects of chronic exposure?

Perchloroethylene is listed as a probable carcinogen in humans (IARC Group 2A) and is a known carcinogen in animals. It also may result in hepatotoxicity.

Where are the predominant environmental sources of perchloroethylene?

The air and ground water near industrial and waste sites

Are methods available to increase elimination of perchloroethylene?

One study found increased elimination of ingested perchloroethylene via hyperventilation.

What methods are available to decrease absorption of ingested perchloroethylene?

Placement of an NG tube to suction if the patient presents promptly after ingestion of liquid

What emergency treatments should be provided to exposed patients?	1. Administer 100% oxygen, and aggressively manage the airway, especially for those with aspiration pneumonia 2. Intubation may be required for those with inhalational exposures showing respiratory depression. 3. Mechanical ventilation for pulmonary edema 4. Cardiac monitoring for dysrhythmias
How is a dermal exposure treated?	Remove all clothing, and irrigate the skin with copious amounts of water.

PHENOL

What is phenol?	Phenol (carbolic acid) is a caustic agent with potent antiseptic properties.
How can phenol be identified?	Appears as a transparent, light pink liquid with a characteristic aromatic odor
In what other compounds can phenol be found?	1. Cigarette smoke 2. Disinfectants 3. Oral/throat hygiene and anesthetic products in the form of lozenges, throat sprays, and mouthwashes 4. Pharmaceutical preservatives in some analgesic compounds, vaccines, and antivenom preparations 5. Skin products, such as lotions and nail cauterizers 6. Solvents 7. Wood preservatives
Can phenol still be found as a preservative associated with glucagon?	Yes, but it is now uncommon. In historical preparations, glucagon was commonly paired with a diluent preserved with phenol that was used in the reconstitution of glucagon powder. The concentration was only toxic to patients who were receiving multiple large dosages of glucagon, as occurs in the treatment of beta-adrenergic and calcium channel blocker overdoses.
What is phenol's mechanism of toxicity?	Rapid protein denaturation, cell wall disruption, and coagulation necrosis

What are the pharmacokinetics of phenol?	1. Absorption – lipid-soluble, rapidly absorbed through all routes
	2. Distribution – V_D is very large (actual value is unknown)
	3. Elimination – renal, half-life is 0.5–5 hrs
	4. Lethal dose – >1 g in adults. If a high concentration is used, death can occur within minutes.

What is ochronosis?

A discoloration of collagenous tissue following prolonged dermal exposure to phenol

In dark-skinned individuals, what unsightly condition may occur following prolonged dermal exposure to phenol?

Depigmentation

What are the typical patterns of clinical effects following inhalational and GI exposure?

1. Inhalation – coughing, stridor, distinct aromatic odor to breath, chemical pneumonia, respiratory arrest
2. Ingestion – abdominal pain caused by corrosive burns, nausea, vomiting, diarrhea, hematemesis, hematochezia
3. Both routes of exposure may progress to systemic toxicity characterized by AMS, hypotension, dysrhythmias, seizures, and death.

How does "phenol marasmus," or chronic phenol toxicity present?

Anorexia, brown urine, headache, myalgias, salivation, vertigo, weight loss

Is there a specific antidote available to reverse phenol toxicity?

No

What dermal decontamination procedures are beneficial?

Flushing with copious amounts of water is controversial. Studies have demonstrated that water irrigation may enhance the absorption of phenol through the skin by enlarging the surface contact of phenol with the skin; however, water is typically the only irrigant available. As a result, the following is recommended: immediately remove all contaminated clothing, irrigate with copious amounts of water, and (if available) swab with a 50% solution of polyethylene glycol (PEG-300 or PEG-400).

Should endoscopy be included in the patient's treatment regimen?

Yes, in patients with GI symptoms following oral ingestion

PHOSPHINE AND PHOSPHIDES

What is the difference between phosphine and phosphide?

Phosphine is a poisonous gas. The solid phosphide releases phosphine when exposed to moisture (including gastric acid).

What different types of phosphide exist?

1. Calcium phosphide – used in welding and in flares
2. Zinc phosphide – used as a rodenticide
3. Indium phosphide – used in semiconductor manufacturing
4. Aluminum phosphide – used in food and grain fumigation (potent inhibitor of *Aspergillus* species)

What smell is associated with phosphine gas?

Odor is similar to decaying fish.

Describe how these agents are used as rodenticides.

Solid phosphide pellets (zinc phosphide) are placed in likely rodent locations (i.e., "mole holes"). Contact with moisture or ingestion produces toxic phosphine gas.

What is the mechanism of phosphine toxicity?

Phosphine is a metabolic poison, blocking electron transport.

What are the symptoms of phosphine gas toxicity?

Dyspnea, hyperpnea, cough, dizziness, headache, vomiting, pulmonary edema, acute lung injury

What are the symptoms of phosphide ingestion?

Ingestion will more likely lead to systemic symptoms. Nausea, vomiting, and diarrhea may initially occur. Symptoms of phosphine gas toxicity occur subsequently due to secondary inhalation. Progression to seizures and multi-organ system failure may occur.

How is phosphine toxicity diagnosed?	Based on clinical history and associated symptoms. No blood level available.
Is there a risk to healthcare staff when caring for a patient who has ingested a phosphide?	Yes. Bystander toxicity may result due to off-gassing from gastric contents. Use caution!

PHOSPHORUS

What are the allotropes of elemental phosphorus?	1. White phosphorus, also known as yellow phosphorus 2. Red phosphorus 3. Black phosphorus
Which allotrope is the most toxic and is also combustible?	White phosphorus
What is the ignition temperature of white phosphorus?	30°C (86°F) in moist air. It may, therefore, spontaneously combust in varying atmospheric conditions.
What is the byproduct of white phosphorus oxidation (combustion)?	Phosphoric acid. This may result in pulmonary symptoms along with ocular and dermal irritation.
What is the toxic oral dose?	Fatal oral dose for white phosphorus is ~1 mg/kg
In what products is phosphorus used?	Fireworks/pyrotechnics, military ammunition, production of methamphetamine, organophosphorus compounds, match pads, fertilizer
What are the potential routes of exposure?	Inhalation, dermal, ocular, ingestion
What is the cellular mechanism of white phosphorus toxicity?	White phosphorus is a metabolic poison, disrupting electron transport.

Describe the toxicity of dermal exposure.

White phosphorus can cause both chemical and thermal burns.

What are the effects of acute oral phosphorus toxicity?

Mucosal injury with nausea, vomiting, and diarrhea may be followed by a quiescent phase progressing to renal, hepatic, and cardiac toxicity.

Chronic inhalational exposure of white phosphorus may lead to what complication?

Mandibular necrosis, also known as "phossy jaw"

What methods can be used to detect phosphorus exposure?

History of exposure. Hypocalcemia may occur, and phosphorus levels are variable and of limited utility. Spontaneous combustion of phosphorus in emesis or stools may result in a "smoking" appearance.

Describe the treatment of phosphorus toxicity.

Solid phosphorus on clothing or skin should be covered in water to prevent combustion. Ocular contamination should be treated with irrigation. Supportive care is the mainstay of treatment.

PHTHALATES

What are phthalates?

Dialkyl or alkyl aryl esters of 1,2-dibenzenecarboxylic (phthalic) acid that are used in industry as "plasticizers" to make vinyl compounds more pliable

Where are phthalates commonly found?

Cosmetics; plastic wrap; food packaging; medical devices (e.g., blood bags, PVC tubing, disposable syringes); building materials; industrial materials (e.g., rocket fuel, agricultural fungicides, solvents)

How does phthalate exposure commonly occur?

Leaching from the parent material (e.g., PVC tubing)

What are the 4 primary routes of exposure causing phthalate toxicity?

1. Inhalation – off-gassing of PVC flooring, leaching from intubation tubing, occupational exposure
2. Ingestion – food packaging/wrap, water supplies, children's plastic toys

3. Dermal – clothing, personal care and beauty products, occupational exposure
4. Injection

How do acute phthalate toxicities typically present?

Acute toxicity of phthalates is generally low. Early symptoms are route-dependent and include bronchitis, airway irritation, pulmonary dysfunction, dermatitis, and possible hepatitis. In severe poisonings, late symptoms can include stupor, convulsions, and coma for those phthalates that cross the blood-brain barrier.

What is the principle treatment for acute phthalate toxicities?

Dilution (specific to route of exposure) and removal from the source

Are phthalates water soluble?

Low molecular weight phthalates are water soluble; however, the hydrophobicity of high molecular weight phthalates causes them to partition into lipids (e.g., adipose tissue) with limited water solubility.

What is the most common phthalate to which people are exposed?

Di(2-ethylhexyl)phthalate (DEHP)

Which known DEHP metabolite is thought to be responsible for DEHP's toxicity?

Mono(2-ethylhexyl)phthalate (MEHP)

What are the concerns of chronic phthalate poisoning?

While data is limited, there are concerns over hepatocarcinogenicity, testicular lesions and atrophy, infertility (in both genders), teratogenicity, and thyroid toxicity.

POLYCHLORINATED BIPHENYLS (PCBS)

What are polychlorinated biphenyls (PCBs), and where might they be encountered?

Synthetic chlorinated organic compounds previously used for insulating electrical equipment and as components of inks, lubricants, and hydraulic fluid. Their production and use has been banned in the U.S. since the 1970s due to environmental and carcinogenic concerns.

How does the oxidation and chlorination state of these compounds affect their toxicity?

Oxidized PCBs and those with more chlorine are more toxic.

What are the modes of toxic exposure to PCBs?

Secondary to their marked lipophilic nature, PCBs may be absorbed by ingestion, dermal exposure, or by inhalation. They subsequently bioaccumulate in fat stores following repetitive exposure.

What are the clinical effects seen with toxic exposure to PCBs?

Acute toxicity predominantly results in irritation of eyes, skin, and throat. Chronic toxicity is more problematic secondary to teratogenic effects. Exposure may result in elevated hepatic enzymes, chloracne, and increased risk or carcinoma (IARC Group 2A). Maternal exposure may also result in fetal developmental abnormalities.

Are there any specific tests helpful for diagnosis?

No. Diagnosis relies principally on history but may be supported by the presence of chloracne in association with otherwise unexplained elevated liver enzymes.

Is there a specific antidote available in the treatment of PCB toxicity?

No specific antidotes exist. Management is supportive.

What substance, designed as a fat substitute, can potentially increase the fecal excretion of PCBs?

Olestra®

RADIATION (IONIZING)

What is radiation?

Radiation is the transfer of energy in the form of particles or waves. It is also known as electromagnetic radiation (EMR), a self-propagating wave in space with electric and magnetic components. EMR can be classified into types according to the energy of the wave.

What are the classifications of EMR in order of increasing energy?

Radio waves, microwaves, infrared radiation, visible light, ultraviolet radiation, x-rays, gamma rays, cosmic rays

What is ionizing radiation?

Ionizing radiation is a particle or wave containing enough energy (>30 eV) to remove an electron from the outer shell of an atom. It is released from an unstable atom that has an unequal number of electrons and protons, causing too much energy in the nucleus. This unstable atom releases excess energy in the form of radiation in order to achieve stability.

What are sources of ionizing radiation?

1. Alpha-particles, containing 2 protons and 2 neutrons each. They travel only a few cm in air and are stopped by a thin film of water, paper, and the cornified epithelial layer of the skin.
2. Beta-particles are electrons that travel approximately 20 cm in air. They can penetrate the cornea and lens of the eye and several centimeters into the skin.
3. Gamma/x-rays can travel great distances in air and are highly energetic, removing electrons form their orbits. They can easily penetrate deep tissue to cause both acute and chronic organ injury. They can only be stopped by many feet of concrete or dense metals such as lead.
4. Neutrons are particles with no charge, and they do not occur during natural nuclear reactions. They are produced during nuclear fission and by radiotherapy beams. They can cause damage from direct collision with other atoms and also by causing previously stable atoms to be radioactive. Highly penetrating and difficult to stop, the combination of water, paraffin, and oil must be used to shield them.

Are alpha- and beta-particles of no concern because they are stopped so easily externally?

No. They can be incorporated into the body after being ingested, inhaled, or absorbed through wounds. They can then transmit a great amount of energy over short distances throughout the body.

What is radioactivity?

A term used to describe the spontaneous decay or disintegration of an unstable atom. Different radioactive materials decay, or lose their strength, over different periods and are measured in half-lives $(T_{1/2})$.

How is radiation measured?

The two fundamental units are the Curie (Ci) and Becquerel (Bq). They reflect the number of disintegrations of the nuclei per second.

How is a radiation dose measured?

The Roentgen (R) is a measure of the ionization of air caused by ionizing radiation and cannot be used to describe dose to tissue. When radiation interacts with tissue energy, it is deposited, and the traditional unit is the Radiation Absorbed Dose (rad). The SI unit for dose is termed the gray (Gy), with a conversion of 100 rad = 1 Gy. Since the degree of energy transferred to tissue can vary by type of radiation (alpha imparting more energy than beta internally), the effective dose or extent of damage done to that tissue also varies. The Roetgen Equivalent Man (rem) is the unit of effective dose actually absorbed, taking biological effects into account. The rem and rad are related by the formula:

rem = [rad][Quality Factor]

The SI unit for rem is the Sievert (Sv), with a conversion of 100 rem = 1 Sv.

Do all tissues respond the same to equal doses of radiation?

No. Equal absorbed doses from different kinds of radiation do not necessarily produce the same biological effect.

What are the most radiosensitive mammalian tissues?

Cells with a high turnover rate – lymphocytes, spermatagonia, hematopoietic tissues, gastrointestinal epithelial cells

What are the most radioresistant mammalian tissues?

CNS, muscle, bone

What damage does ionizing radiation cause to biological systems?

Two theories exist to explain the manner in which radiation causes damage to a cell:
1. Indirect – the radiation transfers its energy to a nonbiologic molecule such as water, converting the water molecule to a free radical. This highly reactive molecule then causes damage to biologic molecules. Indirect effects are believed to be more common with most types of radiation.
2. Direct – the radiation transfers its energy directly to a biologic molecule, causing damage without an intermediate.

What are major cell targets of radiation damage?

1. Membranes – damage to proteins leads to alteration in the permeability of the membrane, resulting in leakage of catabolic enzymes from lysosomes
2. Cytoplasm – irradiated proteins can be inactivated, but the cell can produce more proteins as long as the genetic material coding for the protein is still intact
3. Nucleus – DNA damage is the most devastating to a cell. If the damage is repaired accurately, the cell will continue to function; however, if the damage is not repaired or the repair is incomplete, the cell may be functionally impaired or neoplastic changes may be induced through damage to regulatory or operator genes.

What are possible exposure routes of ionizing radiation?

1. External irradiation – when all or part of the body is exposed to penetrating radiation

2. External contamination – the physical presence of radiation or radioactive material on the surface of the body
3. Internal contamination – when radioactive material enters the body through the digestive tract, airways, or wounds. Radioactive materials are distributed throughout the body and are incorporated. Location can vary depending on chemical properties (e.g., I-131 is taken up by the thyroid during ablation therapy and utilized just as stable I-127).
4. Combined exposures – mixtures of the above

Is a patient who is exposed to external irradiation a hazard to healthcare workers?

No

What are the principles of external decontamination?

1. Prevent internal contamination
2. Reduce total patient exposure
3. Reduce attendant exposure
4. Prevent contamination of facility
5. Reduce skin exposure

Has a healthcare provider ever been injured by a contaminated patient?

Healthcare providers have NEVER been hurt caring for contaminated patients. The highest recorded dose was 14 mrem, measured by an ED provider caring for a contaminated patient.

What are the decontamination procedures?

1. Remove patient's clothing.
2. Wash patient with detergent and water, or have them shower.
3. Above steps are 95% effective.

How are wounds treated?

Any wound shall be assumed to be contaminated. Following each wound-specific treatment below, all wounds should be covered to prevent cross-contamination from other areas of the body.
1. Lacerations – gentle irrigation with copious amounts of water or saline, collect and save wound drainage

2. Foreign bodies – remove if clinically indicated, be sure to mark and save for later analysis
3. Puncture wounds – can be handled by simple scrubbing, do not mutilate tissue to decontaminate (incision/coring)
4. Thermal/chemical burns – normal burn care, some radionucleides may be absorbed and trapped in the eschar that will be removed later during routine burn care
5. Orifices – if possible, the patient should rinse the mouth with copious amounts of water, save all irrigation fluids for analysis
6. Ocular wounds – treat like any other eye exposure, primary consideration is given to locating and removing any foreign bodies. Secondary consideration is given to chemical contaminants, which unlike radioactivity, can cause immediate damage to the eye.

Is there a difference in acute vs. chronic exposure of the same dose?

Delivering the same total dose of radiation at a much lower dose rate over a long period of time allows tissue repair to occur. There is a consequent decrease in the total level of injury that would be expected from a single dose of the same magnitude delivered over a short period of time.

What is Acute Radiation Syndrome (ARS)?

Effects from high-dose radiation that develop over a period of hours to months after exposure to >0.7 Sv. Clinical effects of ARS are divided into several distinct stages and phases based on time and organ systems affected. The stages based on time are the Prodrome, Latent, Manifest illness, and Recovery or Death. The phases based on the clinical picture are the Hematopoietic, GI, and CNS/CV Syndromes, and are in order of increasing dose rate.

What is the hematopoietic syndrome?

Results from exposures of doses >0.7 Sv (or 100–800 Rem)

1. Prodrome – nausea, vomiting, anorexia with an onset of 3–24 hrs, severity increases with dose
2. Latent – mostly asymptomatic, except for mild weakness, hair/weight loss around 14 days; circulating cell lines become depleted
3. Manifest illness – bone marrow atrophy with reduced circulating blood cell numbers, hemorrhage and infection around 3–5 weeks
4. Treatment – prophylactic oral absorbable quinolone antibiotics to sterilize gram-negative gut flora, adding amoxicillin-clavulanate or cefixime for gram-positive coverage. If bleeding develops, transfusions of irradiated blood, blood products, and platelets should be administered. Consider CMV, HSV, fungal, PCP prophylaxis if appropriate. If the bone marrow does not recover spontaneously, it can be stimulated with growth stimulation factors, or transplantation may be required.

Are there any useful laboratory tests for the hematopoietic syndrome?

The absolute lymphocyte count is the most useful indicator of dose received. A 50% drop in lymphocytes within 24 hrs indicates significant radiation injury.

What is the GI syndrome?

Exposure to radiation in the 7–30 Sv (or >800 rem) can cause damage to mucosal epithelial and crypt cells lining the GI tract. The hematopoietic syndrome occurs concurrently, as the doses are well above those required to produce severe bone marrow depletion.

1. Prodrome – severe nausea/vomiting, possibly watery diarrhea and cramps, onset 1–4 hrs
2. Latent – malaise and weakness, onset 5–7 days

3. Manifest illness – return of severe vomiting, diarrhea with fever, progression towards bloody diarrhea, shock, and death
4. Treatment – consists of replacing fluid and electrolytes, antibiotics for infection, in addition to all the treatment required for the severe hematopoietic syndrome. Despite intensive treatment, patients are likely to die.

What is the CNS/CV syndrome?

Doses above 30 Sv (or >300 rem) will lead to damage to the relatively radioresistant CNS and CV system. Most of the damage is to radiosensitive vascular components supplying blood to the CNS. The heart and great vessels are more radioresistant than the capillaries.
1. Prodrome – rapid development (usually within 1 hr) of severe nausea and vomiting, confusion, ataxia, and prostration
2. Latent – a short period of a few hrs at most
3. Manifest illness –return of nausea, vomiting, and diarrhea. Confusion, seizures, AMS, respiratory distress, hypotension, and death will follow within a few hrs to days.
4. Treatment – despite the aforementioned treatments, this syndrome is essentially fatal

What are permissible annual radiation dose limits (rem)?

1. General public – 0.5
2. Occupationally exposed pregnant female – 0.5 (over term of pregnancy)
3. Radiation and emergency workers – 5
4. Lifesaving exposure limit – 25

Are we exposed to natural, background radiation in the U.S.?

Yes. The average American is exposed to 360 mrem (3.6 mSv) per year of background radiation composed of the types listed below (mrem):
1. Cosmic – 28
2. Terrestrial – 29

3. Radon – 200
4. Medical – 53
5. Commercial products – 10
6. Internal – 39
7. Other – 1

What are typical exposures from diagnostic radiographic exams (mrem)?

1. Head/neck radiographic – 20
2. Cervical spine – 20
3. Chest – 8
4. Upper GI series – 245
5. Barium enema – 406
6. CT (head and body) – 111
7. Dental – 10
8. Lumbar spine – 127
9. Hip – 83

What are commercial and/or other sources of radiation (mrem/yr)?

1. Smoke detector – 0.008
2. Nuclear power – 0.01
3. Computer screen – 0.1
4. Watching TV – 1
5. Airline trip from New York to Los Angeles – 2
6. Cigarettes, 1 pack/day – 7,000
7. Astronauts – 36,000

SMOKE INHALATION

What is the composition of smoke?

Smoke is a composite of vapors, gases, heated air, and small solid and liquid particles.

What is soot?

Aerosolized carbonaceous particulate matter

How are toxic combustion products classified? Give examples of each.

1. Simple asphyxiants – carbon dioxide
2. Irritants – hydrogen chloride, acrolein, phosgene, nitrogen oxides
3. Chemical asphyxiants – carbon monoxide, hydrogen cyanide, hydrogen sulfide

How do the different combustion products cause toxicity?

1. Simple asphyxiants – displace oxygen from the airways
2. Irritants – may cause direct corrosive effects, free radical production, and immune-mediated effects

3. Chemical asphyxiants – interfere with systemic oxygen utilization

What are some toxic products produced in fires and their antidotes?

1. Hydrogen cyanide – hydroxocobalamin and sodium thiosulfate. Sodium and amyl nitrite should be used with caution in smoke inhalation secondary to worsening methemoglobinemia.
2. Methemoglobinemia – methylene blue
3. Carbon monoxide – high-flow oxygen

What is the most important part of management in smoke inhalation victims?

Airway management with early endotracheal intubation, as needed. Patients may decompensate quickly secondary to increased airway resistance from intraluminal debris, mucosal edema, and bronchospasm.

What delayed pulmonary complications may occur following smoke inhalation?

Acute lung injury and ARDS

What diagnostic tests should be included in management?

ABG analysis with co-oximetry to assess for acidosis, carboxyhemoglobin, and methemoglobin. An elevated lactic acid may help diagnose cyanide poisoning. CXR will evaluate for pulmonary infiltrates or edema.

What problems can accompany the use of the traditional cyanide kit (amyl nitrite, sodium nitrite, sodium thiosulfate) when treating cyanide poisoning in a smoke inhalation victim?

The nitrite components of the kit produce methemoglobinemia, which may worsen the functional anemia if the patient has coexisting carbon monoxide poisoning.

STRYCHNINE

What is strychnine?

An alkaloid derived from the seeds of the *Strychnos nux-vomica* tree, indigenous to South East Asia and Australia. The pure form is an odorless, bitter, white crystalline powder.

Where has strychnine been found in the past?

1. Old rodenticides, laxatives, and homeopathic tonics that are no longer in use
2. As an adulterant in illicit drugs such as heroin and cocaine

How quickly is strychinine absorbed following ingestion?

Rapidly absorbed by the GI mucosa with onset of symptoms in 15–45 min

How is strychnine eliminated?

80% hepatic and 20% renal; elimination half-life = 10–16 hrs

What strychnine dose is considered lethal?

Any dose should be considered potentially serious, but any single ingestion of 1–2 mg/kg or a serum level of >1 mg/L is considered lethal.

What is strychnine's mechanism of toxicity?

Competitive antagonism of inhibitory spinal cord glycine receptor, resulting in neuronal excitability with consequent skeletal muscle spasm

How does strychnine toxicity clinically present?

1. Episodic, simultaneous tonic flexor and extensor muscle contraction with alternating periods of relaxation.
2. Opisthotonus
3. Full consciousness, though severe poisoning can cause respiratory insufficiency and lactic acidosis, which can cause CNS depression.
4. "Risus sardonicus," facial grimacing often accompanied by trismus

Are these muscle contractions considered seizures?

No. They originate in the spinal cord, not the cerebral cortex. Consciousness is not impaired, no postictal period will be observed, and patients should have recollection of the event.

Are there any special considerations for this type of toxicity?

Any type of intense environmental or sensory stimuli can potentiate an episode of muscle contractions. It is very important to keep the patient in a dimly lit, quiet environment.

What are the complications of a strychnine overdose?

1. Rhabdomyolysis with resultant myoglobinuria and acute renal failure
2. Hyperthermia due to excessive muscle activity
3. Lactic acidosis
4. Respiratory arrest

What infection can mimic strychnine poisoning?

Tetanus, which acts by inhibiting glycine release. Tetanus has similar signs and symptoms, although it develops more slowly.

What is the primary goal of treatment?

Supportive care – airway protection and control of muscle contractions

What methods are effective at managing the symptoms of strychnine toxicity?

1. Benzodiazepines to reduce muscular hyperactivity. Barbiturates are second-line agents.
2. Paralysis with *nondepolarizing* neuromuscular blockade and intubation if symptoms are refractory to treatment
3. Active cooling if the patient is hyperthermic
4. IV hydration to prevent renal failure secondary to rhabdomyolysis

Is there a specific antidote?

No

Are there any specific decontamination/elimination procedures that have proven to be effective or are contraindicated?

1. Do not induce vomiting or use gastric lavage. Besides aspiration risk, there is the risk of potentiating an episode of muscle contractions.
2. Acidification of urine and diuresis are not effective.
3. Activated charcoal will bind strychnine and is effective if given soon after ingestion.

SULFUR DIOXIDE

What is sulfur dioxide?

An irritant gas

Where might sulfur dioxide be encountered?

Released from natural fires, automobiles, paper manufacturing plants, power plants fueled by oil or coal, metal smelting facilities. In addition, it can be used as a food preservative, a disinfectant, a refrigerant, and a water dechlorination agent.

What is the mechanism of toxicity of sulfur dioxide?

Contact with moist surfaces (e.g., eyes, mucosa) yields sulfurous acid, which causes intense irritation, induces bronchoconstriction, and alters mucous secretion in the respiratory tract. Direct contact with liquid sulfur dioxide freezes exposed tissues.

How did sulfur dioxide gain its notoriety?

It is a major component of acid rain.

What are the clinical effects seen with toxic exposure to sulfur dioxide?

Rapid onset of irritation of mucous membranes/eyes/skin/respiratory tract, dyspnea due to bronchoconstriction and pulmonary edema, nausea, vomiting. Pulmonary symptoms may be delayed. Liquid sulfur dioxide causes frostbite injuries upon contact and may result in corneal necrosis, and possible blindness, following ocular exposure.

Are there any specific tests helpful for diagnosis?

No. Diagnosis relies principally on history of exposure with consistent symptoms.

What treatments are available for sulfur dioxide toxicity?

1. No specific antidotes exist. Management is supportive.
2. Removal of the agent is important, through decontamination and physical relocation. Irrigate skin and eyes with copious water.
3. Treat frostbite injury from liquid sulfur dioxide as a thermal burn.
4. Enhanced elimination methods are of no proven clinical benefit.

TOLUENE

What is toluene?

Highly volatile aromatic hydrocarbon

How is toluene used?

1. Solvent for paints, lacquers
2. Gasoline additive
3. Found in explosives, glues, dyes
4. Abused as an inhalant

What are the effects of acute inhalation?	Dizziness, ataxia, headache, nausea, vomiting, euphoria
Describe the primary mechanism of action.	Enhances the activity of the GABA receptor and may inhibit the NMDA receptor
What is the primary method of abuse?	Abuse occurs though inhalation, with "huffing" (i.e., placing a solvent-soaked rag over the mouth and nose and inhaling); "bagging" (i.e., inhaling the solvent from a bag); and sniffing (i.e., inhaling the solvent directly from the container) being the primary methods.

What are signs of chronic toluene abuse?

1. Weight loss, muscle weakness, ataxia, mood instability, depression
2. Progressive irreversible encephalopathy
3. Renal tubular acidosis
4. Peripheral neuropathies

Are there any ways to monitor toluene levels during intoxication?

1. Most levels are noncontributory during initial stabilization of a patient.
2. Toluene levels may be measured from venous blood. Hippuric acid levels can be obtained from urine samples.

What are two important parameters to monitor in exposures?

1. CPK (creatinine kinase) – rhabdomyolysis is common in chronic users
2. Electrolytes – severe hypokalemia, hypophosphatemia, and both anion gap and non-anion gap metabolic acidosis may occur. Bicarbonate therapy should be avoided in these patients because of hypokalemia.

How does toluene produce an anion gap metabolic acidosis?	Metabolites of toluene include benzoic acid and hippuric acid, which contribute to the acidosis.
What is the mechanism of non-anion gap acidosis?	Toluene and its metabolite hippuric acid may cause a renal tubular acidosis similar to the distal (or type 1) variety, with potassium wasting and hyperchloremia.

What interventions and monitoring are indicated with toluene exposure?	1. All patients should be decontaminated and placed on cardiac and respiratory monitoring. 2. Basic labs such as CBC, electrolytes, ABG, chest radiograph, creatinine kinase, and urinalysis should be obtained. 3. Metabolic abnormalities usually resolve within a few days of discontinuing the exposure.

TRICHLOROETHANE AND TRICHLOROETHYLENE

What are trichloroethane (TCA) and trichloroethylene (TCE)?	Chlorinated hydrocarbons that are typically used as solvents
Name some products in which these agents are found.	Due to their solvent properties, these agents are found in degreasers, glues/adhesives, and paint removers. They were formerly found in dry cleaning solutions and typewriter correction fluid.
What are the potential routes of toxic exposure?	Inhalation, ingestion, dermal
What is the mechanism of toxicity responsible for CNS depression?	Multiple mechanisms have been described, including GABA$_A$ stimulation and inhibition of voltage-sensitive calcium channels.
Why might these agents be abused?	They have properties similar to inhalational anesthetics and, when inhaled, may produce dizziness, ataxia, and euphoria.
What key features of metabolism are shared between TCE, TCA, and the commonly used sedative, chloral hydrate?	All have the metabolite trichloroethanol, a GABA$_A$ agonist that contributes to the CNS depressant effects
What chemical property facilitates its anesthetic action?	Lipid solubility

What are the clinical effects following an acute exposure?

Inhalation or ingestion may produce ataxia, dizziness, nausea, vomiting, headache, confusion followed by lethargy, seizures, dysrhythmias, and coma. Delayed hepatic and renal injury may occur.

How do these agents exert their CV effects?

Chlorinated hydrocarbons may cause myocardial depression by altering the myocardial cell membrane bilayer. They also sensitize the myocardium to endogenous catecholamines, resulting in dysrhythmias.

Which of these two agents was associated with trigeminal neuralgia?

TCE

What is "degreaser's flush"?

Exposure to TCE may cause inhibition of aldehyde dehydrogenase, leading to a disulfiram-like reaction following ethanol exposure.

What are the dermal effects of exposure?

Both agents are solvents, and contact with the skin may cause defatting and dermatitis.

Are these two agents considered carcinogens?

TCE is probably carcinogenic in humans (IARC Group 2A), whereas TCA is not classifiable as to carcinogenicity to humans based on the available evidence (IARC Group 3).

How is a toxic exposure diagnosed?

History of exposure and clinical effects. The parent compounds can be measured in expired air, blood, and urine. The urine can be tested for trichloroacetic acid, a metabolite of both of these agents.

Describe the method of treatment.

Treatment is primarily supportive. Dermal decontamination consists of copious irrigation with soap and water. Care should be used when administering catecholamines due to the possibility of inducing dysrhythmias.

Chapter 5   Heavy Metals

ALUMINUM

List sources of aluminum exposure.

1. Dermal exposure – antiperspirants, cosmetics
2. Ingestion – contaminated water, food containers, cooking utensils, antacids
3. Inhalation – mine workers, processors of aluminum silicate
4. Parenteral – total parenteral nutrition (TPN) solutions, IV drug abuse, dialysis patients

How is aluminum eliminated from the body?

Renally. The body absorbs <1% of ingested aluminum, and the kidneys readily eliminate it.

Describe the typical presentation of aluminum toxicity.

Patients can present with encephalopathy, microcytic hypochromic anemia, and/or osteodystrophy. Acute toxicity is rare and presents with abdominal pain, vomiting, confusion, dysarthria, myoclonus, asterixis, seizure, and coma. Cardiomyopathy has been reported.

What are the mechanisms of toxicity for aluminum?

1. Interference with synaptic transmission
2. Oxidative damage
3. Localization to bone with inhibition of calcium and phosphorus turnover
4. Disruption of parathyroid function

The findings on blood smears mimic poisoning with which other metal?

Lead

How does aluminum cause anemia?

1. Impaired heme metabolism, including ↓ Hgb synthesis
2. Hemolysis
3. Impaired iron metabolism and transport

256

What is dialysis encephalopathy?

Encephalopathy induced by aluminum in renal failure patients undergoing dialysis. This typically results from the use of aluminum-containing phosphate binding agents or aluminum-contaminated water (softened or untreated). The encephalopathy is partially due to aluminum inhibition of dihydropteridine reductase.

What is osteomalacic dialysis osteodystrophy?

Aluminum reduces vitamin D activity on bone → ↓ deposition of calcium in osteoid and subsequent osteomalacia. Hypercalcemia results. Bone pain, pathological fractures, and proximal myopathy may subsequently be seen.

Does vitamin D reverse this condition?

No. This disease is resistant to vitamin D therapy as long as aluminum is present because aluminum blocks the action of vitamin D.

What is Shaver's disease?

Aluminum dust exposure may lead to pulmonary complaints consisting of dyspnea, coughing, substernal chest pain, weakness, and fatigue. A pneumoconiosis can be seen with CXR findings consisting of bilateral lace-like shadowing, more frequent in the upper halves and lung root.

Are serum aluminum levels helpful in the diagnosis of aluminum toxicity?

Not routinely, as they only reflect the amount in the blood. Because most of the aluminum is deposited in bone and liver, these studies may not reflect the true body burden of aluminum.

What is the preferred chelating agent for aluminum toxicity?

Deferoxamine

How can serum aluminum levels be helpful?

Deferoxamine draws aluminum from bone into the intravascular space where it may be quantified by blood testing. This effect may take several days.

How is the definitive diagnosis made?	Iliac crest bone biopsy

How is aluminum toxicity treated?

1. Avoid further exposure.
2. Optimize renal function.
3. Chelation therapy with deferoxamine, in combination with hemodialysis or hemofiltration. Hemodialysis alone will not significantly reduce body burden, as it only removes the aluminum in the intravascular space while leaving the bone deposits to leach out over time.

Why is aluminum phosphide so toxic?

Aluminum phosphide is used as a rodenticide. Its toxicity is due to liberation of phosphine gas in the body. This will inhibit oxidative phosphorylation and hinder ATP production. The resulting clinical effects include abdominal pain, vomiting, hypotension, pulmonary edema, renal failure, and CV collapse.

ANTIMONY AND STIBINE

What is antimony?

Antimony is classified as a "metalloid" and is similar to arsenic in toxicity. Antimony is one of the oldest known medical "remedies," being used for epilepsy, leprosy, and leishmaniasis. It also has significant historical use as a poison. Today, it is still used in many industrial processes, often as an alloy, in flame-retardant material, and in antiprotozoal medications.

What antimony compound was once used as a medicinal "cure-all"?

Tartar emetic (antimony potassium tartrate). This compound is a potent emetic that is no longer used secondary to its considerable toxicity.

What are some of the more common applications of antimony?

1. Used in the production of rubber
2. Incorporated in plastics to act as a flame retardant
3. Used in metal alloys as a hardening agent and to prevent corrosion

4. Used in paints and dyes to provide color
5. Used in the production of safety matches
6. Found in certain antiparasitic medications

Which is more toxic, pentavalent or trivalent antimony?

Trivalent

What are the two most common routes of antimony poisoning?

Inhalation and ingestion

What is the mechanism of antimony toxicity?

Although the definite mechanism is not known, it is theorized that antimony acts by binding to sulfhydryl groups, which thereby inactivates certain enzymes. Antimony also acts as a direct irritant to mucous membranes.

Concerning inhalation, what air level of antimony is considered to be the workplace limit?

0.5 mg/m^3 8-hour time-weighted average. Levels >50 mg/m^3 are considered to be life-threatening.

What symptoms are seen with exposure to elevated levels of antimony dust / fumes?

Nausea, vomiting, headache, weakness, pneumonitis, anorexia, oropharyngeal irritation / bleeding, pruritic and pigmented skin pustules (antimony spots), conjunctivitis

Are fatalities from antimony poisoning common?

No, they are rare. There are several reported cases of sudden death in individuals exposed to antimony, presumably from a cardiotoxic effect. Antimony has also been implicated as a possible carcinogen (antimony trioxide – IARC classification 2B), contributing to some mortality.

Describe the toxic effects of acute antimony ingestion.

1. Severe nausea, vomiting, and diarrhea (often hemorrhagic in nature)
2. Abdominal pain
3. Hepatitis or renal insufficiency may occur

Name the ECG abnormality that may occur secondary to antimony toxicity.

QTc prolongation

What laboratory findings are observed with antimony exposure?

1. ↓ RBC count
2. ↑ LFTs, BUN, creatinine
3. Pancytopenia has been reported.
4. RBCs and Hgb in urine

What are antimony spots?

Pruritic papules progressing to pustules occurring most frequently in areas of sweating

Are any laboratory tests used to quantify antimony exposure?

1. Serum antimony levels are available but are rarely used because they are unreliable.
2. Urine antimony levels >2 mg/L are considered abnormal. Exposure to air concentrations >0.5 mg/m^3 will increase urine levels but cannot be used to accurately quantify exposure levels.

What is the treatment for antimony toxicity?

1. Remove the patient from the exposure.
2. Gastric lavage may be considered if the patient presents promptly to the emergency department.
3. Patients may need large volume fluid resuscitation secondary to massive GI fluid loss.
4. Monitor and replace electrolytes as needed.
5. There is no role for activated charcoal, as it does not effectively bind antimony.

Is there any antidote for antimony toxicity?

There is no specific antidote. Based on animal studies, chelation with agents such as dimercaprol (BAL), DMSA, and DMPS are expected to be beneficial, but human data proving their efficacy is limited.

Is hemodialysis an option?

No. Dialysis is not effective at removing antimony.

What is stibine?

Antimony hydride (SbH_3) is a colorless gas which is produced when antimony-containing compounds are heated or treated with acid. Stibine smells strongly of rotten eggs.

Where might exposure to stibine occur?

During mining operations or industry

What is the mechanism of stibine toxicity?

Stibine causes the hemolysis and is an irritant gas which can affect the CNS.

What air level of stibine is considered the workplace limit?

0.1 ppm per 8-hour time-weighted average. Levels >5 ppm are considered to be life-threatening.

What symptoms and conditions can be seen with stibine inhalation?

Nausea, vomiting, headache, weakness, jaundice, hemolysis, hemoglobinuria, renal failure

What laboratory findings are observed with stibine exposure?

Anemia with elevated RFTs, CPK, LDH, bilirubin, hemoglobinuria

What is the treatment for stibine exposure?

1. Remove the patient from the exposure.
2. Supplemental oxygen
3. Blood transfusions in cases of massive hemolysis
4. IV fluids and bicarbonate for rhabdomyolysis
5. Exchange transfusions may be necessary in some cases of massive hemolysis.

Is there any antidote for stibine toxicity?

No. Chelation therapy is not thought to be effective.

Is there any way to enhance the elimination of stibine?

No. Hemodialysis and forced diuresis are not effective at reducing stibine levels.

ARSENIC AND ARSINE

What are some sources of arsenic?	1. Groundwater 2. Wood preservatives 3. Semiconductors 4. Smelting/soldering 5. Animal feed 6. Pesticides 7. Moonshine 8. Folk / alternative medicines 9. Used therapeutically for acute promyelocytic leukemia
What is arsine?	Arsine (AsH_3) is a colorless, nonirritating gas with a garlic odor formed when metal alloys containing arsenic are exposed to acid. In addition, it is formed as a byproduct of semiconductor production, metal refining, soldering, and galvanizing operations.
What is lewisite?	A gaseous arsine derivative that has been used as a chemical warfare agent. It causes severe eye, skin, and airway irritation, possibly progressing to necrosis.
In the United States, what are the major sources of accidental arsenic and arsine exposures?	<u>Arsenic</u> – ingested through contaminated food or water. Inorganic arsenic is tasteless and odorless and is readily absorbed by the GI tract and mucosa. <u>Arsine</u> – unintentional inhalation by workers in industrial settings
Can arsenic intoxication occur due to consumption of seafood?	While blood and urine tests may register positive, the arsenic found in seafood / shellfish is organic in the form of arsenobetaine, which is nontoxic and easily excreted. Organic arsenic is also found in several antiparasitic medications.
What is the mechanism of toxicity of arsenic?	Once absorbed, the trivalent (arsenite) form of arsenic will inhibit key components of cellular metabolism, including the pyruvate dehydrogenase complex and the alpha-ketoglutarate dehydrogenase

complex → ↓ ATP production. Pentavalent arsenic (arsenate) is metabolized to arsenite and will independently disrupt oxidative phosphorylation by substituting for inorganic phosphate. Other mechanisms include oxidative damage and direct mucosal irritation (causing GI ulceration and respiratory tract / skin cancers). It is thought to disable DNA repair.

What is the mechanism of toxicity of arsine?

The primary effect of arsine is profound hemolysis with resultant anemia. An increase in intracellular calcium caused by a reaction product of arsine binding to heme is thought to be responsible. Renal tubular damage results from the deposition of hemoglobin, and severe hemolysis can disrupt oxygen delivery.

What is the clinical presentation of acute arsenic intoxication?

Phase 1 (within hours) – profound gastroenteritis (cholera-like) with resultant nausea, vomiting, watery diarrhea, and abdominal pain. The GI fluid losses, plus diffuse third spacing of fluids, lead to tachycardia, hypotension, and possibly hemodynamic collapse. Metabolic acidosis, rhabdomyolysis, and renal failure may occur.

Phase 2 (after 1 to 7 days) – initial GI symptoms and hypotension may resolve in 24 to 48 hrs. This presents with cardiovascular compromise, including congestive cardiomyopathy, cardiogenic and noncardiogenic pulmonary edema. The QT interval may increase, potentially causing torsade de pointes. During this phase, encephalopathy with delirium, agitation, or coma may develop, as may elevated transaminases and proteinuria.

Phase 3 (after 1 to 4 weeks) – begins with a sensorimotor peripheral neuropathy. Initially, it presents with painful dysesthesias in a stocking-glove pattern. Ascending sensory and motor deficits will ensue, possibly leading to quadriplegia and respiratory failure. Pancytopenia with basophilic stippling of RBCs may be seen in this phase.

What dermatologic signs are seen with acute arsenic poisoning?

A diffuse maculopapular rash, desquamation of the palms and soles, periorbital edema, and herpetic-like lesions. Mees' lines or white transverse striae on the nails may be observed 4 to 6 weeks postingestion.

What is the clinical presentation of chronic arsenic intoxication?

Dermatological signs become more prominent and include darkened skin with hypopigmented areas, hyperkeratosis, brittle nails, and Mees' lines. Peripheral neuropathy, headache, and confusion may also be apparent. Peripheral vascular disease (*Blackfoot disease*), hypertension, and malignancy can be caused by chronic arsenic exposure.

What is the clinical presentation of acute arsine intoxication?

There are no immediate symptoms during exposure. After a delay of 1 to 24 hrs, nonspecific symptoms including nausea, vomiting, abdominal cramping, fatigue, headache, and chills will present. Hemolysis occurs, resulting in hematuria, renal failure, flank pain, and hepatosplenomegaly. Jaundice may be seen by day 2, and cardiovascular collapse has been reported. The classic triad is abdominal pain, jaundice, and dark urine.

Although rare, what is the clinical presentation of chronic arsine intoxication?

Nonspecific constellation of anemia, nausea, vomiting, headache, dyspnea, weakness

How are arsenic levels measured?

Atomic absorption spectrophotometry on blood, urine, hair, or nail samples. Blood testing is unreliable due to rapid clearance, although urine testing is accurate with levels peaking 1 to 2 days postexposure. Hair and nail levels remain elevated for 6 to 12 months, depending on individual growth and removal patterns. A 24-hour urine collection is the preferred method of testing for arsenic.

Does an elevated arsenic level definitely confirm arsenic poisoning?

No. Organic arsenic from seafood can cause an elevated urine arsenic without causing toxicity. Also, contamination of hair samples is not uncommon.

How is the diagnosis of arsenic or arsine overdose made?

<u>Arsenic</u> – history of exposure with otherwise unexplained systemic manifestations including severe GI distress, peripheral neuropathy, and possible cardiac conduction problems. Elevated urine levels can help confirm the diagnosis.

<u>Arsine</u> – rapid onset of hemolysis, hemoglobinuria and ↓ urine output with a history of potential occupational exposure to arsine

What is the treatment for arsenic intoxication?

1. Supportive care, including aggressive IV hydration
2. Avoid phenothiazine antiemetics, as these may further prolong the QT interval.
3. For large, recent ingestions, consider gastric lavage. Activated charcoal is ineffective.
4. Cardiac monitoring for 48 hrs
5. Chelation therapy with IV unithiol (analog of dimercaprol) is indicated for large oral overdose. If venous access or unithiol are unavailable, administer IM BAL. Oral chelation with succimer or unithiol may be used once vitals stabilize and GI distress abates.

What is the treatment for arsine intoxication?

1. Remove patient from toxic environment, including removal of clothes and copious irrigation of skin.
2. Supportive care
3. Chelation is ineffective.

BARIUM

What barium compounds are harmful to humans?

Any soluble barium salt, most commonly barium chloride, barium carbonate, barium peroxide, barium nitrate, and barium chlorate

Is there any danger from barium-containing radiological contrast agents?

No. These contain barium sulfate, which is insoluble and, therefore, has minimal systemic absorption.

How do barium compounds enter the body?

Ingestion and inhalation of dust containing barium compounds

What are the possible etiologies of barium toxicity?

1. Intentional ingestion
2. Occupational exposures
3. Accidental ingestion, either due to substitution of a soluble barium salt (e.g., barium carbonate) for barium sulfate in radiological contrast, or eating contaminated food

What industrial processes can lead to exposure to barium compounds?

1. Barium mining and refining
2. Manufacturing – glass, matches, explosives, paint, rubber products
3. Combustion of fossil fuels
4. Found in rodenticides and depilatory products

What is the mechanism of toxicity of barium?

Competitive antagonism of potassium efflux channels → ↑ intracellular potassium levels and extracellular hypokalemia → ↑ membrane potential → cellular depolarization and subsequent paralysis

Does barium toxicity cause hypomagnesemia?

No. Toxicity is associated with hypokalemia but not hypomagnesemia.

What are the acute symptoms of barium ingestion?

Initial symptoms are abdominal cramping, nausea, vomiting, and watery diarrhea. Within minutes to hours, patients can develop ↑ muscle tone manifested as rigidity, myoclonus, and trismus, followed by weakness progressing to flaccid paralysis. Patients can suffer lactic acidosis, rhabdomyolysis, renal failure, respiratory arrest, and cardiac arrest.

What are the cardiac effects following high-dose barium ingestions?

1. Hypertension due to vasoconstriction may be seen initially.

2. ECG findings include QRS widening, U waves, AV dissociation, ventricular ectopy, torsade de pointes, and VF.

How is barium poisoning diagnosed?

Diagnosis is based on a history of exposure, combined with the triad of severe hypokalemia, GI distress, and weakness. No routine test is available, but levels can be obtained for confirmation.

Does the degree of muscle weakness correlate with the degree of hypokalemia?

No. The barium level more accurately reflects the degree of muscle weakness.

How is acute barium poisoning treated?

1. Potassium administration for those with significant hypokalemia
2. Oral administration of sulfates (e.g., sodium sulfate, magnesium sulfate) can cause precipitation of soluble barium, as barium sulfate limits absorption.
3. Hemodialysis can be considered to treat refractory hypokalemia.
4. Anticipate airway compromise and the need for mechanical ventilation.

What is baritosis?

A benign, reversible pneumoconiosis that results from inhalation of barium

Does barium bioaccumulate like other heavy metals?

No

BERYLLIUM

What is beryllium?

A light metal often used in the telecommunication and aerospace industries secondary to its strength and conductive properties

How does beryllium enter the body?

1. Inhalation of dust or fumes containing beryllium or beryllium compounds
2. Through compromised skin

What are the most likely sources of inhaled beryllium?

Occupational exposure, natural occurrence, tobacco smoke

What industrial processes can lead to exposure to beryllium compounds?

1. Beryllium mining, refining, alloy production, machining, reclamation
2. Manufacturing – electronic devices, telecommunications, aerospace industry
3. Combustion of fossil fuels

What are the acute effects of inhalation of high levels of beryllium?

Acute berylliosis, also known as acute beryllium disease

What are the signs and symptoms of acute berylliosis?

Acute respiratory effects are those of chemical pneumonitis, including airway irritation, cough, chest tightness, and dyspnea; this may progress to pulmonary edema, cyanosis, tachycardia, anorexia, and general malaise. Acute exposure may also produce dermal effects, including dermatitis, ulceration, and granulomas.

Describe the treatment of acute berylliosis.

Pulmonary symptoms are treated with systemic corticosteroids along with oxygen and respiratory support, as needed.

What are the effects of chronic exposure to beryllium-containing dust?

Chronic beryllium disease (CBD), or chronic berylliosis, is a T-cell-mediated immune reaction in the respiratory system as a result of chronic beryllium exposure. It is characterized by the formation of pulmonary and extrapulmonary granulomas (noncaseating). These can mimic sarcoidosis and tuberculosis.

What test has been developed to establish if a person is at risk for CBD?

A beryllium-specific in vitro lymphocyte proliferation test

What are the symptoms of CBD?

Progressive pulmonary disease that may be restrictive or obstructive in nature. The disease usually manifests as increasing cough and shortness of breath. Systemic symptoms are likely to occur and include anorexia, weight loss, fatigue, and arthralgias. In severe disease, the patient may develop pulmonary hypertension and cor pulmonale. CBD may also have dermal manifestations, including nodular granulomas and chronic dermatitis.

What is the treatment for CBD?

1. Oxygen therapy
2. Glucocorticoids may be beneficial, but data on efficacy is limited.

Is beryllium a carcinogen?

Epidemiological studies are highly suggestive that beryllium is a cause of cancer, particularly lung cancer. It has an IARC Group 1 classification.

What are the federal limits for beryllium exposure?

1. EPA – industrial release of 0.01 $\mu g/m^3$ of air, averaged over 30 days
2. OSHA – 2 $\mu g/m^3$ of workplace area for an 8-hour workday

BISMUTH

How does bismuth typically enter the body?

Ingestion

How is bismuth typically used?

Bismuth may be found in fire detection devices, ceramic glaze, hunting shot, medications, and cosmetics.

What are the most likely sources of ingested bismuth?

Bismuth-containing medications

What bismuth compounds are commonly found in drugs?

1. Bismuth subsalicylate (Pepto-Bismol and Kaopectate) – used for GI upset and diarrhea
2. Bismuth subgallate (Devrom) – used for ostomy care
3. Bismuth subcitrate (Pylera) – used for treatment of *H. pylori*

How was bismuth historically used in medicine?

Injection for treatment of syphilis prior to advent of antibiotics

What are the signs and symptoms of acute bismuth poisoning due to a significant ingestion?

Acute toxicity is typified by abdominal pain, nausea, and vomiting, along with oliguric renal insufficiency secondary to acute tubular necrosis.

What are the signs and symptoms of chronic bismuth poisoning?

The key finding in chronic bismuth toxicity is progressive myoclonic encephalopathy. This is characterized by poor coordination, loss of memory, changes in behavior, dysarthria, myoclonic jerks, and progressive lethargy. Chronic toxicity may also produce renal failure.

What gingival findings may be present in chronic bismuth exposure?

Blue-black discoloration of the gumline (bismuth lines)

What is the mechanism of bismuth toxicity?

While the mechanism is not fully known, bismuth is thought to bind sulfhydryl groups, altering enzymatic and protein function.

How is bismuth poisoning usually diagnosed?

1. History of exposure
2. Blood or urine testing is available to confirm exposure, but levels have not been correlated with outcome.
3. Abdominal x-ray may detect radiopaque material.
4. Salicylate level should be obtained in the case of bismuth subsalicylate exposure.

How is bismuth poisoning treated?

1. Primarily with supportive care
2. Benzodiazepines may be used for myoclonic activity.
3. BAL and 2,3-dimercapto-1-propanesulfonic acid (DMPS) have been used with some success as chelating agents; however, data regarding their efficacy is limited.

CADMIUM

How does cadmium typically enter the body?

Inhalation and ingestion

What are the most likely sources of inhaled cadmium?

1. Occupational exposure
2. Cigarette smoke
3. Burning of fossil fuels

In what industries are workers most likely to be exposed to cadmium?

1. Mining and smelting
2. Production of batteries (Ni-Cd)
3. Welding and soldering
4. Production of pigments, plastics, and other synthetics

At what doses has inhaled cadmium been found to be harmful?

1. Concentrations >1 mg/m^3 of air are likely to cause symptoms
2. Concentrations >5 mg/m^3 of air are likely lethal

How does acute inhalational cadmium poisoning present clinically?

1. Respiratory – cough, wheezing, dyspnea, possible pulmonary edema
2. Systemic – fever, chills, weakness
3. GI – nausea, vomiting
4. Other – chest pain, headache, metallic taste

For what disease is acute cadmium poisoning sometimes mistaken?

Metal fume fever

How is poisoning from inhalation of cadmium treated acutely?

Supportive care. There is no proven role for chelation therapy, and chelators, such as BAL, worsen toxicity.

What is the most common source of ingested cadmium?

Contaminated water and food (particularly shellfish, liver, and kidney meats)

How is acute poisoning from ingested cadmium salts likely to present clinically?

GI distress (e.g., nausea, vomiting, diarrhea, abdominal pain), hypotension, metabolic acidosis. Pulmonary edema and facial / pharyngeal edema have been reported.

How is poisoning from ingested cadmium usually treated?

Supportive care. Aggressive fluid resuscitation may be needed.

What are the effects of chronic exposure to cadmium?

Renal disease is a common finding, initially manifesting as proteinuria. Chronic lung disease may develop following inhalational exposure. Osteomalacia, osteoporosis, and bone pain may result from disturbances in calcium homeostasis.

Neurologic abnormalities, such as Parkinsonian symptoms, have been reported.

What environmental cadmium disaster highlighted the pathologic bone changes produced by this disease?

"Itai-Itai" or "ouch-ouch" disease occurred in Japan in the 1950s. It was named for the severe bone pain and pathologic bone fractures incurred by patients who had the misfortune of eating food and drinking water contaminated with cadmium from mining runoff.

Is cadmium classified as a carcinogen?

Cadmium is associated with lung cancer and is classified as IARC Group 1.

What is the mechanism of toxicity for cadmium?

Cadmium binds to sulfhydryl groups, affecting protein and enzyme function. It may also mimic calcium in cellular processes and interfere with cell-cell adhesion.

How is suspected cadmium exposure confirmed?

1. Blood tests may help determine exposure, but concentrations have limited utility in management.
2. Urine protein, along with serum BUN and creatinine assays, can determine extent of renal damage.

What limits has the federal government placed on allowable workplace exposure?

1. EPA – ≤5 ppb cadmium in drinking water
2. FDA – ≤15 ppm cadmium in food colors
3. OSHA – 100 $\mu g/m^3$ of workspace per 8-hour time-weighted average (TWA) workday (cadmium fumes),
   200 mg/m^3 of workspace per 8-hour TWA workday (cadmium dust)

CHROMIUM

What are the three most common oxidation states of chromium?

Elemental chromium (Cr^0), trivalent chromium (Cr^{3+}), hexavalent chromium (Cr^{6+})

Which oxidation state of chromium is believed to be harmful to humans?

Cr^{6+}, though at high levels, Cr^{3+} may be harmful as well

Which oxidation state of chromium is an essential nutrient?

Cr^{3+}, required for metabolism of glucose and fat

How does chromium enter the body?

Ingestion, inhalation, dermal exposure

Which method of exposure is most harmful?

Inhalation. Cr^{6+} is most efficiently absorbed through the lungs.

What are the most common sources of chromium?

1. Cr^{3+} – food and drinking water
2. Cr^{6+} – chromium dust, usually an occupational exposure

In which industries is one most likely to be exposed to chromium?

Mining, steel production, welding, chrome plating, chrome pigment production

What is the estimated fatal dosage of soluble chromium salts?

50–70 mg/kg

Describe the mechanism of Cr^{6+} toxicity.

Cr^{6+} has a substantial oxidizing potential. It is corrosive to mucous membranes, the airway, skin, and GI tract. Significant sequelae come from its ability to oxidize DNA, resulting in cellular apoptosis and mutagenic effects.

How does acute ingestion of harmful amounts of Cr^{6+} present clinically?

1. Burns and ulceration of mouth, pharynx and upper GI tract
2. Abdominal pain, nausea and vomiting, often hemorrhagic in nature
3. Possible renal, pancreatic, and hepatic damage

How does acute inhalational toxicity of Cr^{6+} present clinically?

Airway irritation, including oropharyngeal burning, rhinnorhea, cough, and dyspnea, with a possible progression towards pulmonary edema

What are "chrome holes"?

Perforations in the nasal septum and/or dermal ulcerations secondary to chronic Cr^{6+} exposure

What are the manifestations of chronic Cr^{6+} inhalation?	Chronic airway irritation, nasal septal perforations, chronic cough, dyspnea, reactive airway disease, restrictive lung disease
Is Cr^{6+} a carcinogen?	Yes. Cr^{6+} is a widely recognized carcinogen and has an IARC Group 1 classification.
How does skin exposure to Cr^{6+} manifest?	Acute exposure induces skin irritation and ulceration. Contact dermatitis or ulcerations may occur through repeat exposures.
Are any labs useful in chromium exposure?	Chromium levels can confirm exposure, but levels may be difficult to interpret and are of little clinical utility. Electrolytes, CBC, BUN, creatinine, transaminases, and urinalysis should be checked to evaluate effects of toxicity.

How is acute exposure to Cr^{6+} treated?

1. Supportive care
2. Dermal or ocular decontamination may be needed.
3. Aggressive fluid resuscitation may be needed.
4. N-acetylcysteine may be effective in increasing the excretion of chromium, although human data is limited.
5. Animal studies suggest ascorbic acid may help reduce Cr^{6+} to Cr^{3+}, thereby limiting its absorption, but human data is limited.

What limits has the federal government placed on workplace chromium exposure?

1. EPA – ≤100 ppb Cr^{3+} and Cr^{6+} in drinking water
2. OSHA – 500 $\mu g/m^3$ of Cr^{3+} compounds and 52 $\mu g/m^3$ of Cr^{6+} compounds in the workplace per 8-hour time-weighted average workday

COBALT

Where is cobalt most commonly used?	In industry to produce heat-resistant super alloys, which are used in the fabrication of jet engines. It is also an important component of some magnets.

What are the medicinal uses of cobalt?

1. Source of radiotherapy for cancer
2. To label vitamin B_{12} when employed in the Schilling test (used to diagnose intrinsic factor deficiency)
3. Manufacture of medical prostheses
4. Cobalt dichloride ($CoCl_2$) has (rarely) been given orally to patients for the treatment of refractory anemia (induces an erythropoietic response).

Is cobalt toxicity common?

No. It is exceedingly rare, as cobalt and its salts are relatively nontoxic by ingestion. Most cases of cobalt toxicity are related to occupational skin exposure and inhalation of cobalt dust.

Who is at risk for cobalt inhalation toxicity?

1. Hard metal workers (e.g., tungsten-carbide industry)
2. Diamond workers (e.g., diamond polishing)
3. Chemical refinery workers

What are the effects of cobalt inhalation?

1. Hypersensitivity-induced asthma
2. Interstitial lung disease (i.e., fibrosing alveolitis)

Describe the treatment of cobalt inhalation.

1. Remove the patient from the exposure.
2. Treat asthma with conventional measures (e.g., beta 2-adrenergic agonists).
3. Annual medical evaluation, including CXR, CBC, and thyroid function tests

What are the effects of skin exposure to cobalt?

1. Allergic contact dermatitis (erythematous maculopapular type)
2. Rare cases of orofacial granulomatosis, which has been described in association with delayed hypersensitivity

What is the treatment of cobalt skin exposure?

1. Remove the patient from the exposure, and remove excess cobalt from the skin.
2. Treat with traditional remedies for allergic contact dermatitis.
3. Skin patch testing with 1% $CoCl_2$ may be done to confirm sensitivity.

What is considered a toxic inhalational dose of cobalt?

Inhalation by experimental animal studies for 3 years indicated that 20 mg/m^3 of cobalt-containing dust resulted in granulomatous changes and pulmonary fibrosis.

What are the symptoms associated with acute cobalt ingestion?

Ingestion of cobalt salts may produce abdominal pain, nausea, vomiting, and diarrhea. Polycythemia has also been reported.

Is there any treatment for acute cobalt ingestion?

1. Supportive care is the primary treatment.
2. Chelation with calcium disodium EDTA has proven successful in animal studies.
3. *N*-acetylcysteine may improve both urinary and fecal excretion of cobalt, although data on human exposures is limited.

What is cobalt-beer cardiomyopathy?

In the 1960s, cobalt salts were added to beer to act as a foam stabilizer. Some heavy drinkers were estimated to have consumed up to 10 mg of cobalt per day, which was associated with the onset of an atypical cardiomyopathy. Clinical symptoms included acute-onset, left-sided heart failure, followed by right-sided heart failure, cardiomegaly, hypotension, and cyanosis. Mortality rate was estimated to be 30% to 50%. Although it was never definitively shown that cobalt was responsible, when cobalt was removed from the brewing process, no new cases of associated cardiomyopathy developed.

COPPER

Who is at risk for copper toxicity?

1. People who live near or work at copper-producing facilities, such as mines, smelters, or refining facilities

2. People with copper pipes or who are drinking from / cooking with copper-lined vessels
3. Vineyard workers exposed to copper sulfate and hydrated lime
4. Exposure to algaecides, herbicides, wood preservatives, pyrotechnics, ceramic glazes, electrical wiring, welding, or brazing with copper alloys

Describe the mechanism of copper toxicity.

Copper is a transition metal and is capable of generating oxidative stress. Effects on epithelia and mucous membranes are irritative and corrosive in nature. Redox reactions contribute to the majority of systemic copper toxicity, including renal and hepatic damage with hemolysis.

What is the clinical presentation of acute copper toxicity?

Ingestion (salts) – severe GI irritation, resulting in abdominal pain, nausea, vomiting, and diarrhea. Hematemesis is common. Oxidative damage contributes to renal and centrilobular hepatic injury. Hemolysis is common after copper salt ingestion. The combination of these symptoms may lead to intravascular volume depletion, lethargy, and CV collapse.
Inhalation (fumes) – airway irritation, cough, dyspnea, chest pain, fever, pneumonitis

What is characteristic about the emesis seen with copper toxicity?

Blue-green in color

What is chalcosis?

Penetration of metallic copper into cornea / vitreous humor resulting in conjunctivitis, eyelid edema, granulomas, and retinal detachment

What is Indian childhood cirrhosis?

Chronic copper toxicity, and subsequent cirrhosis, that developed in children who drank copper-contaminated milk due to the storing of milk in brass containers (leaching of copper)

What is vineyard sprayer's lung?

The development (Portugal, 1960s) of granulomas, pulmonary fibrosis, and lung cancer in workers who utilized a fungicide vineyard spray consisting of copper sulfate.

Describe the manifestations of chronic copper poisoning.

Wilson's disease is an inherited disorder of copper metabolism that may result in behavioral and movement disorders; it is not a true exogenous copper poisoning, however. Little data exits on chronic exogenous copper poisoning. Most cases occur in the developing world in children exposed to copper-contaminated milk or water. In these cases, progressive hepatic cirrhosis is reported.

Chronic inhalational exposure may result in pulmonary fibrosis. Associations have been made between chronic copper inhalation and adenocarcinoma of the lung, hepatic angiosarcoma, and hepatic cirrhosis.

Is copper a carcinogen?

While copper has been associated with hepatic angiosarcoma and adenocarcinoma of the lung, the IARC does not include copper in the list of known carcinogens.

What labs are useful in the initial presentation of acute toxicity?

CBC, electrolytes, BUN, creatinine, transaminases, fractionated bilirubin, type and screen for severe hemolysis. Serum or whole blood copper levels may aid in sub-acute management of copper toxicity but are unlikely to influence acute management.

How is toxic copper ingestion treated in the emergency department?

1. Aggressive fluid resuscitation and electrolyte repletion for massive GI fluid losses
2. Blood transfusion for severe hemolysis
3. BAL chelation therapy is likely beneficial in severe poisoning, although data is limited.

How is toxic copper inhalation treated in the emergency department?	Inhalational exposure is generally self-limited. Supportive care with oxygen and nebulized beta 2-adrenergic agonists is indicated.
Describe the treatment for chronic exogenous copper poisoning.	Removal from the source of exposure is the primary treatment. Chelation therapy and other modalities that are used to treat Wilson's disease have not been studied for exogenous copper exposure.

GALLIUM

What are the common uses of gallium?	In semiconductors, metal alloys, and high temperature thermometers. Medically, gallium is used for radiologic studies. It has also been used to treat arthritis and has been studied for use in treating hypercalcemia and certain cancers.
Describe the manifestations of ingestional or inhalational gallium exposure.	While data is limited, gallium appears to have low toxicity through either route.
What form of gallium is used therapeutically?	Salt forms (e.g., gallium nitrate, gallium citrate) are used for radiological studies.
How is gallium administered therapeutically?	IV
What are the acute symptoms of parenteral gallium nitrate toxicity?	Primarily nausea and vomiting
What is the major adverse effect of acute gallium nitrate toxicity?	Renal toxicity
What therapy is needed to prevent or minimize acute renal failure with gallium nitrate toxicity?	Fluid therapy and osmotic diuresis

What electrolyte abnormalities may be expected with gallium nitrate toxicity?	Hypocalcemia and hypophosphatemia. Bicarbonate may also be reduced during acute toxicity.
What is the toxic dose of gallium?	Unknown. Patients using other nephrotoxic drugs (e.g., aminoglycosides), may have nephrotoxicity with lower doses of gallium.
What is the mechanism of toxicity of gallium?	While the mechanism is not fully known, hypocalcemia is caused by inhibited bone resorption.
How is gallium eliminated?	Renally
How should a gallium overdose patient be treated?	Supportive treatment. Aggressive fluid hydration and osmotic diuresis is warranted to prevent acute renal failure. Also, electrolyte disturbances may need to be corrected.

GERMANIUM

What is germanium used for in industry?	1. Semiconductor material for transistors 2. Camera lenses 3. Precious metal alloys
What is the major risk with industrial exposure?	Inhalation injury
Describe the effects of inhalational germanium exposure.	Airway / eye / mucous membrane irritation, along with cough and possible dyspnea
What are the symptoms of germane gas (GeH_4) inhalation?	Germane gas acts similarly to arsine and stibine gas, producing acute hemolysis. CV, renal, and hepatic dysfunction may also occur.
Describe the symptoms of oral germanium exposure.	Acute toxicity appears to be low. Manifestations may include nausea, vomiting, and abdominal pain.

What are the manifestations of chronic germanium exposure?

Chronic ingestion of germanium is more problematic. Renal insufficiency, myopathy, and transaminitis are the most commonly reported symptoms. Deaths have been reported from chronic germanium supplementation.

Who is most likely to develop germanium toxicity?

Those taking germanium health supplements (i.e., HIV patients)

How is germanium excreted?

Renally

What is the treatment for germanium toxicity?

Removal from the source of exposure and supportive care

GOLD

Is gold exposure toxic?

Yes, on a chronic level

Who is at risk for gold toxicity?

Patients being treated for rheumatoid arthritis with gold compounds

What gold compound is used to treat rheumatoid arthritis?

Gold sodium thiomalate

What are the most common manifestations of gold toxicity?

Dermatitis and renal disease

How does gold toxicity present?

Integumentary complaints are common, ranging from skin erythema to severe exfoliative dermatitis. Similar reactions are noted on the mucous membranes. Chronic exposure may produce a gray-blue pigmentation of the skin and mucous membranes, especially in sun-exposed areas. Thrombocytopenia, aplastic anemia, encephalitis, peripheral neuronitis, hepatitis, and pulmonary infiltrates have all been reported, but tend to be rare findings.

What is chrysiasis?

A permanent dermatological condition caused by the chronic ingestion of gold. This consists of a skin pigmentation that is uniformly grayish blue and is usually limited to sun-exposed portions of the body. It may involve the conjunctivae but usually spares the oral mucosa.

What is a nitroid reaction?

An uncommon reaction that can occur minutes after gold injection and consists of a sensation of warmth and skin flushing

How are the kidneys affected by gold toxicity?

Proteinuria, microscopic hematuria, and membranous glomerulonephritis may occur. All are reversible with cessation of treatment.

What is the treatment?

Cessation of gold compound therapy with symptomatic care

If conservative treatment fails, what is the next step?

Antihistamines and glucocorticoids can be used to treat skin and mucous membrane lesions. Dimercaprol, *N*-acetylcysteine, and D-penicillamine have all been shown to enhance elimination of gold from the body but are rarely used and have not been demonstrated to improve patient outcome.

IRON

What are the clinical uses of iron?

As a nutritional supplement, notably used for treating anemia and in prenatal vitamins

How do you calculate the amount of iron ingested per unit of body weight?

$$\frac{[\text{Total \# of tablets}][\text{weight (mg)}}{\text{per tablet}][\text{\% elemental Fe per tablet}]}{[\text{patient weight (kg)}]}$$

How much elemental iron does each formulation contain?

1. Ferrous gluconate (12%)
2. Ferrous lactate (19%)
3. Ferrous sulfate (20%)
4. Ferrous chloride (28%)
5. Ferrous fumarate (33%)

What is the toxic dose of iron?

≥10 mg/kg – GI effects
≥40 mg/kg – systemic effects possible
>60 mg/kg – potentially lethal

How is iron normally absorbed and utilized by the body?

10% enters mucosal cells of the small bowel where it is bound by ferritin (storage molecule). Transferrin carries iron to the liver, where it is stored until needed for biosynthesis. Unneeded iron is eliminated when the intestinal cells slough off. This limits absorption.

How does iron exert its toxic effects on the body?

1. Local GI effects are due to corrosion and include hemorrhagic necrosis, perforation, and infarction.
2. The local corrosive effect on the GI mucosa causes unregulated passive absorption of iron.
3. Systemic effects are mediated by free radical-induced tissue damage. The excess iron, unbound to transferrin, will cause oxidative damage to multiple organ systems.
4. Anion gap metabolic acidosis, due to disruption of oxidative phosphorylation, and hypovolemia secondary to third-spacing of fluids. The generation of protons from conversion of ferric iron to ferrous iron is life-threatening.
5. Coagulopathies may manifest due to iron-mediated inhibition of proteases necessary in the hemostatic pathway.

How does acute iron overdose present?

<u>Stage 1</u> (30 min to 6 hrs) – GI symptoms of nausea, vomiting, abdominal pain, and diarrhea. This can progress to hematemesis and hematochezia.
<u>Stage 2</u> (4–12hrs) – referred to as the latent stage. GI symptoms resolve, giving the impression of improvement; however, hypoperfusion and metabolic acidosis are developing. Patients will appear lethargic and have tachycardia or metabolic acidosis.

Stage 3 (12–24 hrs) – rapid clinical decline, progressing to severe metabolic acidosis and shock. Accompanied by possible coagulopathy, coma, and multisystem organ failure. Death due to iron intoxication occurs most frequently during this stage due to circulatory collapse and acidosis.

Stage 4 (12–96 hrs) – hepatotoxicity due to absorbed iron causing oxidative damage resulting in periportal hepatic necrosis. Can result in hepatic failure.

Stage 5 (2–4 weeks) – late scarring of the GI tract, causing pyloric obstruction, bowel obstruction, or hepatic cirrhosis

Do all patients experience all five stages?

No, many patients will not. Some will only suffer GI distress. Those with large ingestions can progress to stage 3 within several hours. Also, there is no universal agreement on the number of stages or the times assigned to those stages.

How is the diagnosis of iron overdose made?

1. History is most important.
2. If patient denies overdose but suspicion is high, abdominal radiograph can locate radiopaque iron tablets in the stomach. Significant ingestion is unlikely in the presence of a normal abdominal x-ray and a lack of GI symptoms.
3. Serum iron levels – significant toxicity with levels >500 μg/dL

When should a serum iron level be drawn?

Ideally, at 2 to 6 hrs post-ingestion when serum levels peak. Due to redistribution, serum levels drawn more than 8 to 12 hrs post-ingestion do not reflect the total body burden.

Should you wait for a serum iron level before initiating treatment?

No. Treat the patient according to their clinical situation.

Is the total iron-binding capacity (TIBC) useful for determining toxicity?

No. Also, in the past it was believed that a WBC >15,000 and a serum glucose >150 mg/dL would correlate with a serum iron >300 μg/dL. Recent studies do not support this.

What treatments should be performed for iron toxicity?

1. Supportive care with particular attention paid to aggressive hydration
2. Whole bowel irrigation should be considered if iron tablets are visible on abdominal x-ray.
3. Chelation therapy with deferoxamine is indicated for shock, AMS, metabolic acidosis, or a serum iron >500 μg/dL. Ensure hemodynamic stability prior to deferoxamine administration, as hypotension is common with this agent.
4. Avoid activated charcoal, as it is ineffective and potentially harmful (can exacerbate GI effects).

Ipecac is no longer recommended in the routine treatment of any poisoning, but why is it particularly ill-advised after an iron ingestion?

Vomiting and GI upset are useful in predicting if a toxic amount has been ingested. Ipecac will cloud the clinical picture.

LEAD

What is the mechanism of lead toxicity?

Lead binds sulfhydryl groups, which interferes with enzymes and structural proteins. Lead also chemically resembles calcium. It appears to interfere with calcium homeostasis and calcium-dependent signaling and metabolic pathways. This includes disrupting mitochondrial processes and interfering with the cellular second messenger signaling cascade.

What are common sources of lead exposure?

1. Lead-based paint
2. Contaminated soil
3. Water contaminated by lead-based plumbing

4. Emissions created by leaded gasoline (less common in United States due to EPA regulations)
5. Lead dust and fumes in the industrial setting
6. Food stored in lead-soldered cans
7. "Moonshine" whisky
8. Firearms training or bullet cartridge reloading

Which occupations have the highest risk of lead exposure?

Those involving burning, cutting, or welding of lead or lead-containing materials

What are the routes of exposure?

1. Inhalation (most rapid)
2. Ingestion (absorption is facilitated by young age and diet deficient in calcium, iron, and/or zinc)
3. Transdermal (least efficient, but organic absorption > inorganic absorption)

What are the general signs and symptoms of toxic lead exposure in adults?

Severe (whole blood lead level (BLL) >100–150 μg/dL) – encephalopathy (i.e., coma, seizures, delirium, signs of ↑ ICP), foot / wrist drop, abdominal pain (lead colic), vomiting, anemia, nephropathy

Moderate (BLL >80 μg/dL) – headache, memory loss, fatigue, irritability, insomnia, ↓ libido, muscle pain / weakness, abdominal pain, anorexia, weight loss, nephropathy (if chronic exposure), mild anemia

Mild (BLL >40 μg/dL) – fatigue, moodiness, hypertension, ↓ interest in everyday activities

Are children more or less sensitive to lead exposure?

More sensitive. The "classic" adult symptoms tend to develop at lower BLLs.

What subtle clinical presentation of lead poisoning is easy to dismiss as "normal" childhood behavior?

Constipation and abdominal pain

What age group is most severely affected by lead poisoning?

1 to 6 years old

What is the concern with even mildly elevated BLLs in children?

Lead affects neurocognitive development, and BLLs seem to inversely correlate with IQ.

How is lead detected in the body?

A BLL is the best way to detect and measure the amount of lead in the body. Capillary BLLs are often used for screening but may be easily contaminated from external sources. Venous BLLs should be drawn to confirm elevated capillary BLLs.

What other laboratory tests may be useful in the assessment of lead-poisoned patients?

A CBC may show a microcytic anemia with basophilic stippling on peripheral blood smears. Erythrocyte protoporphyrin levels may be elevated as a result of the inhibition of key enzymes in the heme biosynthetic pathway.

Does ingested lead show up on x-ray?

Yes, recently ingested lead, such as paint chips or solid objects, can be detected on x-ray.

What other radiographic evidence may help with the diagnosis?

Dense radiopaque metaphyseal lines ("lead lines"), especially at the wrists and knees, may indicate chronic lead exposure in children.

What is the current "action" level defined by the CDC for pediatric lead exposure?

10 μg/dL. Close observation, education, and follow-up evaluation should be arranged for children with confirmed BLLs at or above this level.

How is symptomatic lead poisoning treated?

1. Two options are available – chelation with $CaNa_2EDTA$ and dimercaprol (BAL) for severe poisoning with encephalopathy or with succimer (DMSA) PO for patients able to tolerate oral medication. Consultation with a toxicologist is recommended due to the complexity of this treatment.

2. Consider whole bowel irrigation if lead foreign bodies can be visualized in the GI tract on radiograph.
3. Endoscopic removal is indicated for lead foreign bodies retained in the stomach or esophagus.
4. Surgical removal is indicated if the lead object poses the threat of prolonged retention.

At what BLL do current recommendations advise starting chelation therapy in asymptomatic children?

45 μg/dL

What is another essential component of management for patients with elevated BLLs?

Patient or parent education on sources of lead in the environment and physician follow-up. An environmental survey may be necessary and will depend on local health department regulations.

Should retained lead foreign bodies in tissue (e.g., bullets) be removed?

Current evidence suggests removal of only those foreign bodies that are bathed in fluid (such as synovial fluid or CSF). Tissue foreign bodies tend to cause fibrosis and do not cause significant or long-term elevations in lead levels.

LITHIUM

What is the ionic charge of lithium?

Lithium is an alkali metal in Group 1 of the periodic table. It has a single valence electron, which it readily loses to become the positively charged cation Li^+.

What important elements share a similar valence with lithium?

Sodium and potassium

Lithium is usually administered orally as a salt in combination with what anion?

Lithium carbonate (Li_2CO_3). Lithium citrate and lithium orotate are also used.

What is the mechanism of action of lithium?

While exact mechanisms are unknown, lithium appears to modulate the release of serotonin and norepinephrine.

What are four medical indications for lithium use?

1. Bipolar disorder
2. Depression (often in combination with antidepressants)
3. Prevention of migraine and cluster headaches
4. Treatment of thyroid storm in patients with iodine allergy

What are four nonmedical uses of lithium?

1. Batteries
2. Mixed with alloys of aluminum, cadmium, and copper to make aircraft parts
3. Lithium chloride (LiCl) is a dessicant.
4. Lithium hydroxide (LiOH) is used to scavenge carbon dioxide in submarines and spacecraft, forming lithium carbonate.

Use of lithium, especially in combination with other serotonergic agents, may lead to what hyperthermic syndrome?

Serotonin syndrome

What are four groups of medications that can increase the risk of lithium toxicity?

1. Diuretics
2. NSAIDs
3. Tetracyclines
4. Phenytoin

What are the clinical findings of acute lithium toxicity?

Initial findings manifest as GI symptoms, including nausea, vomiting, and diarrhea. This is followed by CNS symptoms, including tremor, nystagmus, fasciculations, ataxia, hyperreflexia, lethargy, seizures, and coma.

What model of distribution helps explain the delayed CNS findings?

The two compartment model

What ECG findings occur with lithium toxicity?	1. Flattened or inverted T-waves 2. ST depression
What are the signs of chronic lithium toxicity?	CNS symptoms predominate and include fatigue, ↓ concentration, dysarthria, and ataxia, as well as acute toxicity findings such as tremor, seizures, and coma.
What is the most common renal complication of chronic lithium therapy?	Nephrogenic diabetes insipidus
What serum lithium concentration is considered therapeutic?	0.7–1.2 mg/dL
How is lithium eliminated from the body?	Renally
What is the effect of hyponatremia or dehydration on lithium clearance?	The kidney confuses lithium for sodium, and while trying to retain sodium, will also reabsorb lithium.
What is the effect of a high serum lithium concentration on the anion gap?	A decreased anion gap may be seen with lithium toxicity because lithium is an un-measured cation that may induce renal retention of chloride or bicarbonate, which are both measured anions.
What is the role of activated charcoal in the treatment of lithium toxicity?	It is a poor binder of lithium and is not useful in isolated lithium ingestion; it should be given if there is a possibility of a recent co-ingestion.
Describe the treatment for acute lithium toxicity.	1. Optimize fluid and electrolyte (especially sodium) status to increase renal excretion of lithium 2. Whole bowel irrigation may be used to limit absorption. 3. Dialysis may be considered for severe neurotoxicity, but forced diuresis plays no role in treatment.
What is the treatment for chronic lithium toxicity?	Similar to that of acute toxicity; however, since CNS tissue concentrations are

likely to be higher and neurologic symptoms are likely to be more prominent, hemodialysis should play a greater role in treatment.

What is the role of dialysis in lithium toxicity?

Lithium is freely dialyzable; however, secondary to the two-compartment model of distribution, slow equilibration between the tissue and blood compartments may cause fluid and electrolyte shifts and require multiple runs of dialysis. Continuous renal replacement therapy may be a better option. Neither method has been conclusively demonstrated to improve outcome. Hemodialysis is indicated for severe neurotoxicity, renal failure, and an inability to tolerate sodium repletion. Other indicators for dialysis, such as blood lithium concentration, are less fixed, and clinical judgment should prevail.

MANGANESE

What is manganese?

Trace element that serves as a cofactor for many enzymes, including superoxide dismutase

What is manganese used for?

Alkaline batteries, some pesticides, decolorizing glass, fuel additive

Who is most likely to experience manganese exposure?

Welders, miners, dry-cell battery manufacturers

What are the most common routes of exposure?

Inhalation and ingestion

What organ is most severely affected by manganese exposure?

The brain

How is manganese excreted from the body?

Biliary elimination

What chronic disease is associated with elevated manganese levels?

Hepatic cirrhosis. Manganese levels are increased secondary to decreased elimination from the body.

What is the mechanism of manganese toxicity?

Largely unknown; however, toxicity may be related to alterations in iron or other essential element metabolism.

What are the signs and symptoms of manganese neurotoxicity?

Personality changes, memory loss, and parkinsonian symptoms. These symptoms are progressive and often debilitating. Psychosis and hallucinations have also been reported with high manganese levels, often referred to as "manganese madness."

Describe the classic walk associated with manganese toxicity.

A high-stepping, toe walk known as "cock walk" or "Hehnestritt," which was named after its resemblance to a German soldier's high-step march

What disease does manganese toxicity mimic?

Parkinson's disease

How does neuroimaging differ in manganese toxicity versus Parkinson's disease?

In acute manganese toxicity, lesions appear in the basal ganglia on T1 imaging. In Parkinson's disease, lesions are concentrated in the substantia nigra.

What are sources to test for manganese levels?

Blood levels are commonly used, but urine levels are also available. As manganese is rapidly cleared from the body, neither method detects remote exposure.

What is the treatment for manganese toxicity?

1. Supportive care with removal from the exposure source
2. Carbidopa / levodopa has variable efficacy in symptomatic improvement.
3. Chelation therapy may ↓ blood manganese levels but appears to do little to alter the course of the disease.

MERCURY

What are the three primary forms of mercury?

1. Elemental (metallic)
2. Inorganic

3. Organic (most commonly methylmercury)

What are the primary routes of toxic exposure from each form of mercury?

1. Elemental – inhalation
2. Inorganic – ingestion or dermal absorption
3. Organic – ingestion or dermal absorption

By what physiologic mechanism does mercury primarily cause toxicity?

Reacts with sulfhydryl groups, phosphoryl groups, amide groups, and carboxyl groups, causing nonspecific inhibition of enzymes, transport proteins, and structural proteins. Inorganic mercury also has a corrosive effect on the GI tract.

What catecholamine-secreting tumor derived from chromaffin cells does mercury toxicity mimic?

Pheochromocytoma. Mercury inhibits S-adenosyl-methionine, ultimately preventing catecholamine catabolism and causing sympathomimetic signs and symptoms.

List some common sources of mercury exposure.

Thermometers, sphygmomanometers, folk remedies, seafood, burning fossil fuels, mercury mining/smelting, manufacturing chlorine, electrical equipment, gold mining, dental amalgams

What sea animals have the potential for bioaccumulation of high levels of methylmercury?

Shark, swordfish, mackerel, tuna, tilefish, crab

How does the acute inhalation of elemental mercury vapors present clinically?

Fever, chills, nausea, vomiting, abdominal cramping, diarrhea, ↓ vision, metallic taste. Pulmonary edema or chemical pneumonitis may develop.

What are the clinical manifestations of elemental mercury ingestion (i.e., thermometer-based)?

None. Only an extremely small amount of elemental mercury is absorbed from the GI tract. If it becomes trapped in the GI tract (e.g., within a diverticula or appendix), however, mercury absorption can be increased.

Is it dangerous to spill elemental mercury?

Yes. A spill in a confined space can lead to significant levels of airborne mercury, resulting in chronic inhalation. It is especially important to avoid vacuuming the spill.

What are the clinical manifestations of inorganic mercury ingestion?

Oropharyngeal pain, hematemesis, hematochezia, intestinal necrosis, renal failure, shock

What are the clinical manifestations of organic mercury ingestion?

Primarily CNS manifestations – dysarthria, ataxia, constriction of visual field, hearing impairment, paresthesias. The onset is usually insidious, and effects are permanent.

What are the manifestations of chronic mercury toxicity?

Tremor, gingivostomatitis, hypersalivation, abnormal neuropsychiatric manifestations. Renal dysfunction ranging from proteinuria to nephritic syndrome may result.

What is erethism?

Erethism is the psychiatric constellation of chronic mercury toxicity, consisting of irritability, anxiety, insomnia, and pathological shyness.

What is acrodynia?

Also called "pink's disease," it is a rare reaction to mercury toxicity in children, manifesting as painful pink discoloration of the hands and feet accompanied by sweating, hypertension, neurological changes, photophobia, and a peeling rash.

What body fluids prove most accurate when measuring levels of toxic mercury?

<u>Elemental and inorganic</u> – whole blood levels in acute exposure, urine levels in chronic exposure
Organic – whole blood levels (limited renal elimination)

What pharmacological therapies are available for mercury toxicity?

<u>Inorganic</u> – chelation with PO succimer (DMSA) or IM BAL if unable to tolerate oral medications. DMPS is an IV compatible derivative of BAL, but is not FDA-approved in the United States.

Elemental and organic – oral succimer and *N*-acetylcysteine (organic mercury). Oral penicillamine is available, but profound GI side effects limit its usefulness. Avoid BAL when treating for these two types of mercury poisoning, as there are animal studies indicating that it can cause redistribution of mercury to the brain.

Are activated charcoal or gastric lavage effective in acute ingestion?

Yes. These should be considered for acute ingestion of inorganic or organic mercury.

Can dialysis increase the rate of mercury elimination?

No; although, it may become necessary if renal failure results from intoxication.

MOLYBDENUM

What is molybdenum?

An essential trace element necessary for the catabolism of purines and the sulfur-containing amino acids cysteine and methionine

What is the role of molybdenum in industry?

Used in heat-resistant steel alloys, welding, pigments, and some fertilizers

Which enzymes require molybdenum as a cofactor?

1. Xanthine dehydrogenase (used for purine metabolism to uric acid)
2. Xanthine oxidase (a form of xanthine dehydrogenase)
3. Sulfite oxidase (located in mitochondria, catabolizes cysteine and methionine, converts sulfite to sulfate)
4. Aldehyde oxidase (pyrimidine catabolism and biotransformation of xenobiotics)

How is molybdenum carried in the bloodstream?

Bound to alpha-macroglobulin and adsorbed to RBCs

How is molybdenum excreted?

In urine and bile

How does molybdenum poisoning usually occur?

Over-ingestion of dietary supplements

Describe the features of oral molybdenum exposure.	While data is limited, acute toxicity from oral exposure appears to be low. Chronic toxicity may induce xanthine oxidase and increase uric acid production, leading to the development of gout. Toxicity may also result in a hypochromic microcytic anemia.
What are the manifestations of inhalational molybdenum exposure?	Inhalational exposure may produce a syndrome similar to metal fume fever, characterized by headache, arthralgias, myalgias, weakness, fatigue, cough, and diarrhea.
What is the treatment for molybdenum poisoning?	Supportive care

NICKEL

What is the most common disorder following nickel exposure?	Nickel dermatitis
What organ systems are affected by systemic nickel toxicity?	Skin, pulmonary, neurologic, hepatic
Name two types of nickel dermatitis.	1. Primary – an eczematous allergic reaction following direct contact. Erythematous papules and vesicles may progress to lichenification.
	2. Secondary – widespread rash caused by ingestion, transfusion, inhalation, or implanted medical devices / orthodontic appliances
Primary nickel dermatitis is an example of what type of immune reaction?	Type IV hypersensitivity
Which nickel compound most commonly causes acute, generalized nickel toxicity?	Nickel carbonyl

What is nickel carbonyl?

A highly volatile liquid compound used in nickel refining and petroleum processing

Name the two metabolites of nickel carbonyl.

1. Carbon monoxide
2. Elemental nickel

Describe the manifestations of acute nickel carbonyl exposure.

Initial symptoms after inhalational exposure often produce nonspecific respiratory complaints, including airway irritation, cough, and dyspnea. Nausea, weakness, and headache may develop, as may chemical pneumonitis. Severe symptoms of inhalational or ingestional exposure include myocarditis, ARDS, and cerebral edema.

What are the effects of chronic nickel exposure?

Chronic airway irritation and mucosal atrophy may occur along with the development of reactive airway disease and pulmonary fibrosis. Nickel is listed as an IARC Group 1 carcinogen and is associated with nasal and pulmonary carcinogenesis with long-term exposure.

What are the recommended limits in workplace nickel carbonyl exposure?

OSHA – $<0.007\,mg/m^3$ per 8-hour time-weighted average workday

What are the recommended treatments for nickel dermatitis?

1. Exposure avoidance
2. Topical steroids
3. Oral antihistamines
4. Avoidance of exposure to stainless steel (controversial)

What are the recommended treatments for acute, generalized nickel toxicity?

1. Removal from the source and general supportive care
2. For liquid ingestion with prompt presentation to the ED, gastric aspiration with an NG tube may be attempted.
3. Chelation with diethyldithiocarbamate may also be warranted for severe poisoning.

What is diethyldithiocarbamate (DDC)?

A chelation agent with purported efficacy for nickel toxicity. While animal studies and human case reports appear to show some benefit with its use, no conclusive evidence is available to support its efficacy; however, it is still considered the chelator of choice for nickel toxicity.

PLATINUM

In what form are toxic levels of platinum most often ingested?

The antineoplastic drugs cisplatin, carboplatin, and oxaliplatin

What are common side effects of platinum-containing drugs?

Primarily GI – nausea, vomiting, diarrhea

What are the common end-organ manifestations of platinum toxicity?

1. Renal dysfunction (cisplatin)
2. Auditory impairment
3. Peripheral sensory neuropathy
4. Myelosuppression (carboplatin)

What determines the maximum dosing of cisplatin?

Nephrotoxicity

What determines the maximum dosing of carboplatin?

Myelosuppression

With what pathological processes are cisplatin's nephrotoxicity associated?

1. Acute tubular necrosis (distal convoluted tubule)
2. Chronic interstitial nephritis
3. Renal tubular abnormality (e.g., acidosis, hypokalemia, hypomagnesemia)

What are the primary goals in the treatment of a cisplatin overdose?

1. Renal protection
2. Platinum elimination

What treatments help achieve these primary goals?

1. IV normal saline 1–3 mL/kg/h for 6 to 24 hrs
2. Osmotic diuresis with an appropriate diuretic (e.g., mannitol). Furosemide may potentiate ototoxicity.

3. Plasmapheresis initiated immediately after overdose

4. Sodium thiosulfate can limit nephrotoxicity if given after an overdose.

What role does hemodialysis play in treating cisplatin overdose?

None. Hemodialysis has not been proven effective in treating platinum / cisplatin overdose.

What symptoms are associated with cisplatin neurotoxicity?

Loss of proprioception and vibration sense with relative preservation of pain and temperature sensation

What fluid and electrolyte disturbances are associated with cisplatin toxicity?

1. Hypomagnesemia
2. Hypokalemia
3. Hypocalcemia (secondary to hypomagnesemia)
4. Syndrome of inappropriate anti-diuretic hormone secretion (SIADH)

What is the primary hemato-logical disturbance seen with carboplatin toxicity?

Thrombocytopenia

Is there another route of exposure which causes toxicity secondary to platinum?

Yes. Platinum is used in multiple industrial settings. Inhalation of platinum by workers can lead to sensitization and development of dermatitis and bronchospasm.

RARE EARTHS

What are the rare earth elements?

A group of metals that includes the lan-thanoids (except promethium, plus scan-dium and yttrium) – lanthanum (La), cerium (Ce), praseodymium (Pr), neodymium (Nd), samarium (Sm), eu-ropium (Eu), gadolinium (Gd), terbium (Tb), dysprosium (Dy), holmium (Ho), er-bium (Er), thulium (Tm), ytterbium (Yb), lutetium (Lu), scandium (Sc), yttrium (Y)

What are the main industrial/ medical uses of the rare earth elements?

Professional and motion picture lighting, glass production, manufacture of other metals, electronic devices (e.g., microphones, speakers, television tubes), magnets, nuclear power technology, portable x-ray devices, other radiographic imaging

In general, how dangerous is exposure to the rare earth metals?

Generally, the rare earths are of low to moderate toxicity. Few are radioactive (see below), and few are associated with risks following exposure during medical procedures.

Which rare earth metal is considered highly toxic?

Ytterbium. Compounds of ytterbium can be irritating to the skin and eyes, and may cause birth defects following exposure during pregnancy.

Which rare earth metals are radioactive?

1. Europium
2. Scandium has a radioactive isotope (Sc-46)
3. Promethium (technically not a "rare earth")

In what medical setting is the rare earth element gadolinium used?

Gadolinium is contained in the contrast medium used in MRI.

What medical condition has been linked to gadolinium exposure through MRI contrast agent?

Nephrogenic systemic fibrosis

SELENIUM

What are common commercial uses of selenium?

Pigments and dyes, gun-bluing solution (selenious acid), electronics

What are medical uses of selenium-containing compounds?

1. Selenium sulfide is used to treat pityriasis versicolor, scalp dandruff, and seborrheic dermatitis of the scalp.
2. Selenium is used as an OTC dietary supplement.

Which selenium compound is most toxic?

Selenious acid. ~15 mL of gun-bluing solution may be fatal.

Describe the mechanism of selenium toxicity.

Little is known about the mechanism of toxicity. Selenious acid produces corrosive injury to the GI tract. Selenium may also produce systemic oxidative stress in overdose; it may disrupt cellular respiration and/or cause interference with protein synthesis.

How does dermal, ocular, or inhalational selenium exposure manifest?

Select selenium compounds (i.e., selenious acid, selenium dioxide, and selenium oxychloride) cause corrosive injury. Corresponding symptoms include ocular or dermal erythema, pain, and caustic burns. Pulmonary findings after inhalation include airway irritation, cough, dyspnea, and chemical pneumonitis.

What are symptoms of acute selenious acid ingestion?

Severe GI distress with nausea, vomiting and diarrhea. This may progress to lethargy, hypotension, and multisystem organ failure. Ingestion of selenium salts may present similarly, but symptoms tend to be less severe.

Describe the symptoms of chronic selenium exposure.

Hair and nail abnormalities, including brittleness and discoloration, are common. Skin erythema, blistering, and peripheral neuropathy may also occur.

What breath odor is associated with selenium ingestion?

Garlic

What is the nail finding that can occur with selenium toxicity?

Red pigmentation of the nail beds or Mees' lines (transverse lines on the nails)

How is selenium toxicity diagnosed?

Whole blood, serum, and urine selenium levels can be measured; however, these levels are not well correlated with degree of exposure or prognosis. Other laboratory evaluation should be determined by the degree of toxicity and the speculated organ systems involved.

What is the treatment for oral selenium toxicity?

Supportive care is the primary treatment. For patients presenting promptly after selenious acid ingestion, gastric aspiration with an NG tube may be beneficial.

What treatments may be helpful for dermal or ocular injury?

In addition to copious irrigation, a topically applied 10% sodium thiosulfate solution may help reduce corrosive selenium dioxide to elemental selenium, which is benign.

SILVER

What are some common sources of silver?

1. Colloidal silver (elemental silver in suspension) solutions found in alternative medicine dietary supplements
2. Electrical components
3. Photography

What are the medical uses of silver?

Silver has natural antimicrobial properties and, historically, was widely used for this purpose. Today, its use is more limited; it is commonly used as topical burn cream (silver sulfadiazine) and as a chemical cautery agent (silver nitrate).

What are the uses of silver oxide and silver nitrate?

1. Silver oxide is used to prepare other silver compounds and is the cathode in silver oxide batteries (often used in watches).
2. Silver nitrate is used as an antimicrobial in neonatal conjunctivitis, as a cauterizing agent, and in dentistry to assist in healing ulcers of the mouth. It is also used as a histological stain and in electron microscopy.

What are the most common acute manifestations of silver toxicity?

Mucosal irritation from exposure to silver oxide and silver nitrate

Describe the systemic manifestations of acute silver toxicity.

In very large ingestions or in intravenous dosing, silver has been shown to cause hepatic, cardiac, neurologic, and hematologic abnormalities; however, silver is considered to be essentially nontoxic.

Name the most common dermatologic manifestation of chronic silver exposure.

Argyria

What is argyria?

Local or generalized gray or blue-gray skin discoloration due to silver deposition within the skin from ingestion of elemental silver or silver compounds. Usually, ingestion is because of the touted antimicrobial properties of silver.

Is this condition reversible?

No, it is permanent. There is no known effective chelator.

What are the deleterious effects of argyria?

Cosmetic discoloration may lead to psychological stress. Otherwise, no harmful health effects are known.

THALLIUM

What is thallium?

It is a soft, gray, malleable metal that oxidizes when exposed to air. Thallium salts are extremely toxic, tasteless, odorless, and will dissolve completely in water, making it popular among poisoners.

Historically, what was the most common use of thallium?

As a rat poison and insecticide, but its use in the United States has ceased because of its high toxicity to humans

Are there other uses for thallium?

Yes. It is used in manufacturing lenses, semiconductors, infrared detectors, and alloys (due to its anticorrosive properties).

What is its mechanism of toxicity?

Exact mechanism is unclear. It may cause energy depletion by interfering with the Krebs cycle, glycolysis, and oxidative phosphorylation. Also, it may form complexes with sulfhydryl groups on enzymes, inhibiting function.

Which is more toxic, highly water-soluble compounds or compounds with low water solubility?

Highly water-soluble compounds (e.g., thallous acetate, thallic chloride) are more toxic than those with low solubility (e.g., thallic oxide, thallous iodide).

How does acute thallium toxicity present?

Thallium poisoning can result in many nonspecific clinical effects. This makes diagnosis difficult. GI complaints are often noted first and include abdominal pain and diarrhea, followed by constipation. Vomiting can occur but is usually not a major symptom. The most reliable early diagnostic feature of thallium poisoning is an extremely painful, rapidly ascending peripheral neuropathy. This can take from several days to 2 weeks to develop. Other neurological symptoms include weakness, tremor, cranial nerve palsies, optic neuropathy, seizures, coma, and death. Cardiac manifestations include hypertension, tachycardia, and nonspecific ST and T wave changes.

What is a distinctive feature of chronic thallium toxicity?

Hair loss with hyperpigmentation of the hair root; however, do not wait for this finding to consider thallium poisoning, as it may not be noticed for days to weeks and is not always present

What other dermatological finding can be seen?

Mees' lines, or transverse white lines across the nails. These will not be noted for at least 2 weeks.

What is the classic picture of thallium toxicity?

Gastroenteritis, painful peripheral neuropathy and subsequent alopecia

What radiological adjunct can be used to support acute thallium toxicity?

Abdominal x-ray. As thallium is radiopaque, plain films may be useful in acute ingestions. The sensitivity is not known if radiographs are obtained after symptoms develop.

What test can confirm the diagnosis?

A 24-hour urine thallium level

What is the antidote to thallium toxicity?	Prussian blue (ferric ferrocyanide, Radiogardase)
What is its mechanism?	Binds thallium ions and interrupts the enterohepatic recycling of thallium
What chelators are contraindicated in thallium toxicity?	Penicillamine and diethyldithiocarbamate, as they may augment CNS redistribution
What are other means to augment elimination of thallium from the body?	Activated charcoal
What distinguishes thallium poisoning from arsenic poisoning?	Arsenic poisoning has more pronounced GI symptoms, particularly copious diarrhea. Aresnic may also cause pancytopenia, whereas thallium does not.

TIN

What is tin most widely used for?	Plating steel cans for food preservation and as a protective coating for other metals
What special properties make tin great for storing food?	It is not easily oxidized and resists corrosion because it is protected by an oxide film.
What are other uses of tin?	Tin alloys are used in making bronze, soldering materials, and dental fillings, and it is found in toothpaste, perfumes, soaps, and additives. Organic tins may be used as fungicides, pesticides, and bactericides.
What is the most common route of tin exposure?	Ingestion of foods contaminated with tin compounds, especially large amounts of those stored in tin for long periods of time and in low pH conditions
What are other routes of exposure?	Inhalation of tin-containing particles or contact with the skin and mucous membranes
What are the effects of tin inhalation?	Acutely, tin salts and organotins produce irritation of mucous membranes and the

upper airway. Cough, dyspnea, and bronchospasm may develop.

What is stannosis?

A pneumoconiosis caused by chronic inhalation of inorganic tin

Describe the toxic manifestations of tin ingestion.

Ingestion of tin salts primarily produces GI symptoms, including nausea, vomiting, diarrhea, abdominal pain, and possible hematemesis. Usually, large amounts are needed to produce significant toxicity.

Do tin compounds cause dermal toxicity?

Organotins may cause corrosive skin injury, often presenting as erythema or dermatitis. Some organotin compounds may be dermally absorbed.

Describe the neurotoxicity associated with organotins.

Organic tin compounds are associated with CNS disease (e.g., delirium, encephalopathy, cerebral edema, cerebellar dysfunction) and peripheral polyneuropathy.

Which types of organotins are most associated with toxicity?

Triorganotins, including trimethyltin and triethyltin

What is the treatment for tin toxicity?

Inhalational exposure should be managed with oxygen and beta 2-adrenergic agonists, as needed. Ingestion of tin compounds is managed primarily with supportive care.

VANADIUM

In what industries is vanadium found?

Iron and steel industries, mining and processing of ores, production of chemical catalysts, boiler and furnace maintenance, pacemaker battery manufacturing

What is the most common type of vanadium exposure?

Vanadium pentoxide

What is the usual route of toxicity?

Inhalation of fine particulate matter. Direct ingestion is rare, and toxicity through this route appears to be limited.

How is vanadium excreted?	91% in the urine, 9% in the feces
What are the signs and symptoms of acute inhalational toxicity?	Mucosal irritation, cough, wheezing, dyspnea, and possible green-black discoloration of the tongue. Conjunctivitis may also be present secondary to ocular vanadium dust exposure.
What are the long-term effects of vanadium exposure on the lungs?	None. Airway disease is typically reversible, and no long-term changes in pulmonary function tests are seen.
What are the effects of vanadium ingestion?	Data is limited on oral exposures. Diarrhea, along with abdominal cramping, appears to be a common manifestation. Nausea and vomiting may also occur.
What is unique about pentavalent vanadium?	Vanadate (pentavalent vanadium) is one of the most potent known inhibitors of the Na-K-ATPase pump.
Does vanadium exposure pose a long-term health risk?	Vanadium is listed as a "possible human carcinogen," with an IARC classification of Group 2B.
What is the treatment of vanadium toxicity?	Supportive care, with oxygen and beta 2-adrenergic agonists as needed for pulmonary symptoms

ZINC

What is the typical use of metallic zinc?	Galvanizing steel and iron to prevent corrosion
What industries are associated with exposure to zinc?	Metal alloy manufacturing, petroleum refineries, paint and pigment manufacturing, cosmetics, woodworking, embalming, dentistry, military smoke bomb manufacturing, topical ointments in medicine
What zinc compound is most widely used?	Zinc oxide
What zinc compounds are associated with toxicity?	Zinc oxide and zinc chloride

What zinc compound is used as a common rodenticide?

Zinc phosphide

What is the most common route of exposure?

Ingestion of products containing zinc, followed by inhalation of dust and fumes containing zinc compounds. Dermal and mucous membrane exposure comes from aerosolized zinc compounds or topical ointments containing zinc.

What metal is the most common cause of metal fume fever?

Zinc.

What is metal fume fever?

A flu-like, febrile syndrome that may occur after inhaling fumes from heated metals. This typically occurs during welding.

What are the signs and symptoms associated with acute oral zinc toxicity?

Toxicity can present similarly to other corrosive metal salt exposures. Nausea, vomiting, diarrhea, hematemesis, and mucosal erosion have been reported.

Describe the manifestations of dermal and inhalational exposure.

Dermal or inhalational exposure to corrosive zinc compounds generally produces symptoms of local irritation. Pulmonary symptoms include airway irritation, cough, dyspnea, and chemical pneumonitis. Dermal exposure may produce dermatitis, erythema, and ulcerations.

Describe the effects of chronic zinc toxicity.

Anemia and myelodysplastic syndrome have been reported after long-term exposures. Both are reversible upon cessation of exposure. The pathogenesis is likely related to zinc-induced copper deficiency.

Are zinc levels useful for patient management?

Zinc levels may help confirm toxicity in cases of chronic exposure. Collection methods should be meticulous, as contamination can easily occur. Zinc and copper levels should be obtained together, as elevated zinc may cause copper deficiency. Zinc levels are unlikely to be helpful in acute poisoning because of the significant delay in receiving results.

What is the management for acute zinc toxicity?

1. Supportive care. Metal fume fever is self-limiting.
2. Pulmonary symptoms may be treated with oxygen and beta 2-adrenergic agonist therapy.
3. Aggressive fluid resuscitation may be needed following oral exposure, as GI losses may be significant.
4. Endoscopy for evaluation of the extent of corrosive injury.

METAL FUME FEVER

What is metal fume fever?

A febrile illness that develops after exposure to metal oxides

What is the route of exposure?

Inhalation of "fumes" that contain particulate metal oxides

What metal oxide is most strongly associated with metal fume fever?

Zinc oxide

What environments are associated with metal fume fever?

Occupations that involve the welding, melting, or cutting of metal, specifically galvanized or zinc-coated steel

What is the mechanism of toxicity?

The exact mechanism is not known but is suspected to be immune-mediated.

What are the signs and symptoms?

Flu-like symptoms including fever, chills, headaches, cough, dyspnea, fatigue, and myalgias that typically resolve within 36 hrs. Symptoms usually occur within 6 hrs of exposure.

Are there any helpful laboratory tests?

WBCs may be elevated. CXR is normal.

What are other names for metal fume fever?

Monday morning fever, brass foundry workers ague, brass chills, smelter shakes, zinc chills

Why is it called "Monday morning fever"?

After repeated exposure, patients develop a transient resistance to developing metal fume fever but rapidly become re-sensitized after cessation of exposure. Workers commonly develop symptoms again when returning to work after having the weekend off.

What is the antidote?

There is no antidote. After removal from the source, the symptoms are self-limiting. Treatment is supportive and aimed at symptomatic relief.

How is metal fume fever different from polymer fume fever?

Polymer fume fever is a similar flu-like illness developing after inhalation of fumes from fluorinated polymers. Unlike metal fume fever, patients with polymer fume fever are more likely to develop pneumonitis and acute lung injury. Infiltrates may be apparent on CXR. These patients do not develop the progressive acclimation that is characteristic of metal fume fever.

Chapter 6   Pesticides

FUNGICIDES

What are dithiocarbamates?

Commonly used fungicides. Unlike *N*-methyl carbamates, dithiocarbamates have no anticholinesterase activity.

By what mechanisms do dithiocarbamates cause toxicity?

1. Mucosal irritants
2. Metabolism produces carbon disulfide, causing headache, delirium, and encephalopathy.
3. Many of the dithiocarbamates will inhibit aldehyde dehydrogenase. This may cause a disulfiram reaction (tachycardia, hypotension, vomiting, tremor) if ethanol is ingested after exposure.

What neurological condition is caused by chronic exposure to maneb (manganese ethylene-bis-dithiocarbamate)?

Parkinsonism. This is caused by either chronic carbon disulfide exposure or toxicity from the manganese component.

What are organochlorine fungicides?

Also known as substituted aromatic fungicides. Important members of this class include pentachlorophenol, which is used as a wood preservative, and hexachlorobenzene.

What is the mechanism of toxicity for pentachlorophenol?

Uncoupling of oxidative phosphorylation, inducing a hypermetabolic state with fever, diaphoresis, tachypnea, tachycardia, and metabolic acidosis. As toxicity progresses, patients can develop AMS, coma, rigidity, seizures, and death.

How can human exposure occur?

Ingestion, inhalation, dermal. A number of infants were exposed to diapers and linens treated with pentachlorophenol and developed significant toxicity, including hepatosplenomegaly.

What condition can hexachlorobenzene cause?

Porphyria cutanea tarda, hepatomegaly, and hypertrichosis

What are organotin compounds?

Alkyl and aromatic derivatives of tin that are used as fungicides, preservatives for paints and fabrics, and antifouling agents for ships

What toxic effects do organotins have?

1. Tributyltin – potent skin and eye irritant, exposure can cause burns
2. Triphenyltin – also a dermal irritant, can cause headache, nausea, vomiting, blurred vision, and seizures. Hepatotoxicity is possible.
3. Trialkyltin – will readily cross the blood-brain barrier and cause neurotoxic effects, including tremor, headache, weakness, and paralysis
4. All organotins – immunotoxicity with decreased lymphoid tissue weight, lymphopenia, and altered immune function has been observed after organotin exposure in animal studies.

What clinical presentation can be seen after ingestion of a copper salt?

Corrosive effects on the GI tract. Ingestion may cause greenish blue emesis, abdominal pain, hematemesis, melena, hepatotoxicity, hemolysis, and methemoglobinemia.

What are examples of dicarboximide fungicides?

Vinclozolin and iprodione

What is the mechanism of toxicity of dicarboximides in humans?

Antagonistic binding at androgen receptors → ↓ protein synthesis for genes that require androgen binding for expression

What are the effects of prenatal exposure?

Hypospadias and cryptorchidism

What are examples of phthalimide fungicides?

Captan, folpet, captafol

What is another major use of phthalimides?	Synthesis of amines in the plastics industry
What is the mechanism of toxicity of phthalimides?	Inhibition of the cytochrome P450 system
What is the most commonly reported effect of phthalimide toxicity?	Reversible dermatitis
What are the prenatal effects of phthalimides?	There is concern they may be terato-genic, causing CNS and musculoskeletal defects. Phthalimides are analogs of thalidomide.
What are examples of strobilurins?	Azoxystrobin, pyraclostrobin, trifloxystrobin
What is the mechanism of action of strobilurins?	Inhibition of complex III of the oxidative respiratory system in mitochondria
What are the effects of strobilurin exposure?	Dermatitis and conjunctivitis predomi-nate. Patients can also suffer upper airway irritation, chest pain, or nausea after aerosol exposure. Strobilurins are not considered teratogenic.

HERBICIDES

CHLOROPHENOXY

What are chlorophenoxy herbicides?	A group of synthetic plant hormones, used as commercial and household herbicides, that selectively target broad-leaf plants
What is the prototypical chlorophenoxy herbicide?	Dichlorophenoxyacetic acid (2,4-D)
In what clinical situation is chlorophenoxy herbicide toxicity usually seen?	Intentional ingestion
Through what route does 2,4-D most efficiently enter the bloodstream?	Intestinal absorption (>90% of chemical ingested is absorbed). Transdermal absorption is low.

What increases dermal absorption of 2,4-D?	Sunscreen
What organ system is the primary target of 2,4-D?	CNS
What are symptoms of exposure to 2,4-D?	Marked irritation of the eyes, nose, and throat potentially lasting for days
Describe the manifestations of 2,4-D toxicity following ingestion.	Oropharyngeal burning followed by nausea, vomiting, and diarrhea. AMS, lethargy, and seizures may occur, along with cardiac dysrhythmias, in severe poisoning.
What abnormal laboratory values are associated with toxic 2,4-D exposure?	1. Elevated CPK 2. Myoglobinuria (with possible renal dysfunction) 3. Metabolic acidosis 4. Mild to moderate hepatic transaminase elevation
Can elimination of 2,4-D be enhanced?	Both urinary alkalinization and hemodialysis have been studied in 2,4-D poisoning, but neither treatment has been shown to improve patient outcome.
What chlorophenoxy herbicide used during the Vietnam War has been linked to chronic health problems?	2,4,5-trichlorophenoxyacetic acid (2,4,5-T), also known as "Agent Orange." The role of 2,4,5-T in long-term health problems is still uncertain but may be related to chemical contaminants, such as dioxins, and not the parent compound.

DIQUAT

What is diquat?	A fast-acting, nonselective herbicide
How is diquat used?	Applied directly to leaves and grass and is inactivated upon contact with soil
Who has access to diquat?	No formal license is required for use in the United States. It is found in several commercially available gardening products.

What are the major routes of entry to the systemic circulation for diquat?

Ingestion, inhalation, transdermal (poorly)

In what organ is diquat concentrated?

Kidney. Ingestion can lead to renal failure.

How does diquat toxicity differ from that of paraquat?

Following ingestion, there is no pulmonary involvement in diquat poisoning, as long as the patient does not aspirate. Paraquat, on the other hand, causes pulmonary injury.

With what pathological conditions is diquat ingestion primarily associated?

Renal failure

What are the initial symptoms associated with diquat ingestion?

GI distress (i.e., nausea, vomiting, abdominal pain) predominates, although symptoms vary in intensity with the dose ingested.

What are signs of diquat ingestion?

Corrosive GI injury, renal failure, myonecrosis, agitation, seizures, coma. Unlike paraquat, diquat does NOT cause pulmonary fibrosis.

How is diquat poisoning diagnosed?

1. History of exposure is most helpful.
2. Oral mucosal burns that may have a pseudomembranous appearance of the soft palate
3. CXR to rule out aspiration
4. Plasma and urine diquat levels are available from the chemical manufacturer.

What laboratory values are helpful in poisoning?

1. Electrolytes, BUN, and creatinine to assess for renal dysfunction
2. CPK to evaluate for myonecrosis

How is diquat ingestion treated?

1. Supportive care
2. Dermal and ocular decontamination through copious irrigation
3. Gastric aspiration with an NG tube may be indicated for early patient

presentation. Administer activated charcoal, bentonite, or fuller's earth if available and if the patient is able to swallow without difficulty (i.e., no signs of caustic injury).

What other treatments have been suggested for diquat poisoning?

Charcoal hemoperfusion or hemodialysis has been suggested in some reports, but no definitive scientific evidence is available.

PARAQUAT

What is paraquat?

A fast-acting, nonselective herbicide used for killing unwanted grass and weeds

How is paraquat used?

After topical application to weeds and grass, it distributes within the plant tissue, interrupting photosynthesis and generating free radicals. Paraquat is inactivated upon contact with soil.

Who has access to paraquat?

A license for use is required in the United States, so it is not often used for home gardening applications.

What is the mechanism of paraquat toxicity?

Generation of free radicals with subsequent damage to proteins, DNA, and cell membranes

What are the major routes of entry to the systemic circulation for paraquat?

Ingestion, inhalation, transdermal (poorly)

In what organs is paraquat most highly concentrated?

1. Lungs – selective alveolar cell uptake → necrosis and proliferation of connective tissue
2. Kidney
3. Liver
4. Muscle

How is paraquat concentrated in lung tissue?

Active transport by the polyamine uptake pathway keeps lung concentrations high.

What is a lethal oral dose of paraquat?

2 to 4 g of 20% solution (10 to 20 mL for an adult or 4 to 5 mL for a child)

What are the initial symptoms of paraquat ingestion?

Nausea, vomiting, abdominal pain, oropharyngeal pain. Symptoms vary in intensity with the dose ingested.

What are signs of paraquat ingestion?

1. Hours to days post-ingestion – corrosive injury to oropharynx and GI tract, renal failure, myonecrosis
2. Several days post-ingestion – progressive pulmonary fibrosis → respiratory failure (the major cause of death)

How is paraquat poisoning diagnosed?

1. History of exposure is most helpful.
2. Oral mucosal burns with a pseudomembranous appearance of the soft palate
3. CXR
4. Plasma and urine paraquat levels are not readily available but can be obtained through the product manufacturer.

How is paraquat ingestion treated?

1. Gastric aspiration with an NG tube should be attempted for patients presenting within a few hours post-ingestion.
2. Dermal and ocular decontamination, as needed, through copious irrigation.
3. Consider administration of activated charcoal, fuller's earth, or bentonite if the patient lacks significant signs of GI injury and presents early after ingestion.

What treatment is contraindicated for paraquat poisoning?

Oxygen, as it increases the production of free radicals

What other treatments have been suggested for paraquat poisoning?

Cyclophosphamide and methylpred-nisolone may improve outcomes in paraquat-poisoned patients, but no conclusive evidence is available to support their efficacy. Charcoal hemoperfusion and hemodialysis may also improve outcome if initiated early, but data on efficacy is limited. As paraquat has extreme toxicity and few treatment modalities are available, aggressive decontamination, as well as responsible use of the above unproven therapies, may be the patient's best option.

OTHER

What is the most widely used herbicide in the United States?

Roundup® brand weed killer

What is the active ingredient in Roundup?

Glyphosate

How does glyphosate inhibit plant growth?

Inhibition of plant-specific enzymes, resulting in disruption of aromatic amino acid production

What "inactive ingredients" are present in glyphosate-containing herbicides that may contribute to toxicity?

Surfactant, specifically polyoxyethyleneamine (POEA), which is included to allow passage through the waxy coating of leaves and is more toxic (lower LD_{50}) than isolated glyphosate. Because glyphosate targets a plant-specific enzyme, Roundup's adverse effects described in humans are due to the accompanying surfactant.

Through what route are glyphosate preparations most toxic?

Ingestion (often intentional). Direct oral mucosal injury is followed by adverse effects on CV, respiratory, renal, and hepatic function in select cases.

What are signs and symptoms of glyphosate toxicity?

Vomiting, diarrhea, oropharyngeal corrosive injury, metabolic acidosis, cardiogenic shock, cardiac dysrhythmias

How should glyphosate ingestion be treated?

Supportive care and decontamination. Consideration may be given to gastric suction with an NG tube if the patient presents promptly after ingestion.

What is atrazine?

A commonly used, nonselective herbicide in the chlorotriazine class

In what commonly used brands of home-use herbicides can atrazine be found?

Ortho Weed and Feed, Scott's Bonus Type S, Attrex, Atratol

Through what route is atrazine most toxic?

Ingestion. Transdermal and mucous membrane absorption is minimal.

What reported clinical effects are associated with atrazine-containing herbicide toxicity?

AMS, GI hemorrhage, metabolic acidosis, hypotension. As with glyphosate-containing compounds, effects from atrazine-containing compounds are thought to be mediated by other "inactive ingredients," such as surfactant.

How should atrazine ingestion be treated?

Supportive care with elective considera-tion for gastric aspiration by NG tube. Particular care should be taken to avoid pulmonary aspiration of the product, as many of the atrazine-containing products also contain a hydrocarbon solvent.

How is sodium chlorate used as an herbicide?

It is nonselective and may be applied to the plant or the soil, where it may remain for years. It is also used to remove moisture from crops before harvest.

What is the mechanism of toxicity of sodium chlorate in plants?

Oxidation of a necessary plant enzyme complex, rendering it inactive

Describe the mechanism of toxicity of sodium chlorate in humans.

Oxidation of heme complex ($Fe^{2+} \rightarrow Fe^{3+}$), creating methemoglobin. Oxida-tive stress may also result in intravascular hemolysis secondary to RBC membrane disruption.

Through what route is sodium chlorate most toxic?

Ingestion. While it may cause irritation to the skin and mucous membranes, it does not have significant dermal or mucous membrane absorption.

What are the early signs and symptoms of sodium chlorate ingestion?

GI distress (i.e., vomiting, diarrhea, abdominal pain)

What are the later signs of sodium chlorate ingestion?

Manifestations of hypoxia and hemolysis, including cyanosis, shock, cardiac dysrhythmias, hyperkalemia, renal failure, AMS, respiratory failure, acidosis, and jaundice. These manifestations may be delayed up to 48 hrs.

What is the treatment for sodium chlorate ingestion?

1. Supportive care is the primary treatment.
2. Methylene blue for symptomatic methemoglobinemia
3. Blood transfusions may be necessary for severe hemolysis.

What is the herbicidal mechanism of action of glufosinate?

Acts as a glutamate analog, incorporating itself into plant proteins and interfering with glutamine synthetase. This results in toxic ammonia levels, as the plant is unable to metabolize this substance.

What is the mechanism of toxicity of glufosinate in humans?

1. Disruption of ammonia catabolism, yielding elevated levels. Alternative metabolic pathways are available in humans, however, so small exposures may remain asymptomatic.
2. Inhibition of glutamate dehydrogenase → ↓ GABA → seizures and AMS

What are signs and symptoms of glufosinate toxicity?

Nausea, vomiting, AMS, respiratory depression, ataxia, seizures. Rarely, diabetes insipidus has been reported.

When do signs and symptoms of glufosinate toxicity become clinically apparent?

GI effects occur almost immediately; however, AMS may be delayed up to 8 hrs, and seizures may be delayed up to 24 hrs. Initial GI symptoms may be related to surfactant toxicity.

How is glufosinate toxicity treated?

1. Supportive care
2. Consider gastric aspiration with an NG tube if patients present promptly after ingestion.
3. Hemodialysis may also be considered for severe exposures but has not been definitively shown to improve outcomes.
4. Benzodiazepines for seizures

INSECTICIDES

CARBAMATES

What are the common carbamate insecticides?

Aldicarb, carbaryl (Sevin), pirimicarb (Aphox, Rapid), propoxur (Baygon), trimethacarb (Landrin)

What is the mechanism of action of carbamates?

Bind to a serine hydroxyl residue at the active site of the acetylcholinesterase (AChE) enzyme → active site is blocked → ACh breakdown ceases → ACh accumulates in the synapse → excessive cholinergic stimulation

Does "aging" occur with carbamates?

No. Carbamates bind to AChE reversibly, and aging does not occur (unlike organophosphates, which do cause aging).

What is a common mnemonic used to remember the cholinergic signs and symptoms of carbamate poisoning?

DUMBELS
Defecation
Urination
Miosis
Bronchorrhea / **B**ronchospasm / **B**radycardia
Emesis
Lacrimation
Salivation

Does this list include all the possible effects of carbamate poisoning?

No, it only includes muscarinic effects. The excess cholinergic stimulation will also stimulate nicotinic receptors, causing effects at the motor end plate (e.g., fasciculations, weakness, paralysis) and sympathetic ganglia (e.g., tachycardia, HTN).

What routes of exposure are possible with carbamates?

All routes of contact

Do carbamates penetrate the CNS?

Poorly; thus, patients with carbamate exposure have less CNS toxicity (rare seizures and coma) than patients with organophosphate exposure. However, patients may develop CNS effects secondary to hypoxia caused by bronchospasm and bronchorrhea.

What are treatments for acute carbamate exposure?

1. Removal from exposure source and clothing (avoid secondary exposure of healthcare workers)
2. Copious dermal irrigation with soap and water for cutaneous exposures
3. Consider activated charcoal for GI exposure.
4. Protect the patient's airway if necessary (use a nondepolarizing paralytic for RSI).
5. Atropine to resolve bronchospasm and pulmonary secretions
6. Pralidoxime is not indicated in pure carbamate poisoning, as AChE poisoned by carbamates does not undergo aging. It is reasonable to consider administration of pralidoxime to a patient presenting with cholinergic symptoms if the exact agent is not known.
7. Benzodiazepines for seizures

ORGANOCHLORINES

What are the common organochlorine insecticides?

Chlorobenzilate, dicofol (Kelthane), dienochlor (Pentac), endosulfan, lindane (Kwell), dichlorodiphenyltrichloroethane (DDT)

What is the mechanism of toxicity of organochlorines?

1. Disrupts normal axonal transmission, likely by opening sodium and potassium channels
2. Antagonizes GABA-mediated inhibition in the CNS → a hyperexcitable state in the CNS and PNS

What are the potential clinical effects following acute organochlorine exposure / toxicity?

Acute exposure causes CNS stimulation, resulting in paresthesias, ataxia, tremor / myoclonus, nausea, vomiting, and seizures.

What routes of toxicity are possible with organochlorines?

Ingestion, inhalation, dermal

How are organochlorines metabolized and excreted?

Most are metabolized by the liver and induce hepatic microsomal enzyme systems. Also, many are eliminated fecally, with some agents undergoing enterohepatic and enteroenteric recirculation.

What are the treatments for an acute organochlorine exposure?

1. Removal from exposure source and clothing (avoid secondary exposure of healthcare workers)
2. Copious dermal irrigation with soap and water for cutaneous exposures.
3. Cholestyramine (a nonabsorbable bile acid) may ↑ fecal elimination.
4. Benzodiazepines for seizures

Are there chronic health effects from organochlorines?

Extended exposure may produce chronic neurologic effects, including tremor, weakness, and ataxia. These effects were prominent among factory workers involved in the manufacture of the organochlorine chlordecone in Hopewell, Virginia; this became known as the "Hopewell epidemic."

What topical pediculicide is contraindicated in children secondary to its ability to cause seizures?

Lindane

Name the organochlorine that is credited for saving millions of lives worldwide and whose inventor won the Nobel Prize for his contribution to world health.

DDT

What is the name of the book that highlighted the adverse effects of DDT, coined the term *biocides*, and whose publication resulted in the subsequent ban on DDT use in the United States?

Rachel Carson's *Silent Spring*

ORGANOPHOSPHATES

What are the common organophosphate (OP) insecticides?	Acephate (Orthene), azinphos-methyl (Azinphos, Guthion), chlorphoxim (Baythion-C), chlorpyrifos (Dursban, Lorsban), diazinon, dimethoate (Cygon, DeFend), disulfoton (Di-Syston), ethoprop (Mocap), fenamiphos (Nemacur), fenitrothion (Sumithion), fenthion (Baytex), malathion (Fyfanon, Cythion), methamidophos (Monitor), methidathion (Supracide), methyl parathion (Penncap-M), naled (Dibrome), oxydemeton-methyl (MSR), phorate (Phorate, Thimet), phosmet (Imidan), profenofos (Curacron), terbufos (Counter)
What is the mechanism of toxicity of organophosphates?	Bind to a serine hydroxyl residue at the active site of the acetylcholinesterase (AChE) enzyme → active site is blocked → ACh breakdown ceases → ACh accumulates in the synapse → excessive cholinergic stimulation
What is a common mnemonic used to remember the cholinergic signs and symptoms of OP poisoning?	DUMBELS **D**efecation **U**rination **M**iosis **B**ronchorrhea / **B**ronchospasm / **B**radycardia **E**mesis **L**acrimation **S**alivation
Does this list include all the possible effects of organophosphate poisoning?	No, it only includes muscarinic effects. The excess cholinergic stimulation will also stimulate nicotinic receptors, causing effects at the motor end plate (e.g., fasciculations, weakness, paralysis) and sympathetic ganglia (e.g., tachycardia, HTN).
List the target organs of OP exposure and the associated clinical effects.	CNS – agitation, AMS, seizures, coma Eyes – miosis, lacrimation Mouth – salivation Lungs – ↑ bronchial secretions, bronchospasm

CV – tachycardia / bradycardia, QT interval prolongation
GI – diarrhea, emesis, ↑ motility
GU – urinary incontinence
Sweat glands – diaphoresis
Adrenals – ↑ catecholamines
Neuromuscular junction – fasciculations, weakness, paralysis

What is the mechanism of seizures from OP exposure?

Within the first 5 min, seizures appear to be due to cholinergic overstimulation, and atropine can abort or prevent seizures. After 5 min, other changes are noted, including a decrease in brain norepinephrine, an increased glutaminergic response, and the activation of NMDA receptors. At this point, both atropine and benzodiazepines are needed.

Why might seizure activity be missed in an OP-poisoned patient?

Nicotinic effects can progress from fasciculations to flaccid paralysis, resulting in nonconvulsive seizures. Any comatose OP-poisoned patient should be treated with benzodiazepines, as well as atropine, with emergent EEG monitoring.

What routes of exposure are possible with OPs?

All routes

What are the pharmacokinetics of OP exposure?

Absorption, peak effect, half-life, and elimination kinetics vary dramatically based on the specific OP, as well as on the route, dose, and rate of exposure (acute vs. chronic). For this reason, patients exposed to OP insecticides should be observed closely for at least 8 hrs after exposure for delayed effects.

What are treatments for acute OP exposure?

1. Removal from exposure source and clothing (avoid secondary exposure of healthcare workers)
2. Copious dermal irrigation with soap and water for cutaneous exposure
3. Consider activated charcoal for GI exposure.

4. Protect the patient's airway, if necessary (use a nondepolarizing paralytic for RSI).
5. Atropine titrated to the drying of pulmonary secretions and resolution of bronchospasm
6. Pralidoxime – 1–2 g IV over 10 min, repeated in 1–2 hrs. Alternatively, a bolus of 30 mg/kg, followed by an infusion of 8 mg/kg/hour, is advocated by the WHO.
7. Benzodiazepines to prevent and treat seizures
8. ECG to assess for QT prolongation

Why should one use a nondepolarizing neuromuscular blocker if intubating an OP-poisoned patient?

The effect of succinylcholine can be markedly prolonged due to inhibition of plasma pseudocholinesterase.

Is tachycardia a contraindication to atropine use in an acute OP exposure?

No. The tachycardia may actually improve due decreased activation of preganglionic nicotinic sympathetic nerve terminals, decreased release of norepinephrine from the adrenal glands, and alleviation of dyspnea and hypoxia.

How does pralidoxime work?

OPs form a covalent bond with the active site of AChE, preventing breakdown of ACh. Pralidoxime is attracted to the active site of AChE, and its nucleophilic oxime moiety will attack the phosphate atom of the OP. This will displace it from the active site, reactivating the enzyme.

What is "aging"?

"Aging" occurs when the OP forms an irreversible covalent bond with the AChE enzyme after losing an alkyl side chain. This permanently inactivates the AChE enzyme. This can take from <1 hour to several days, depending on the particular OP. Pralidoxime will have no effect on an aged AChE complex.

Why is it important to prevent aging?	Once aging occurs, the patient will not regain vital functions, such as muscle strength or respiratory drive, until new enzyme is synthesized. This may take weeks to months.
What lab test can confirm OP exposure?	Measurement of the activity of erythrocyte AChE and plasma pseudocholinesterase. Results are usually not available quickly enough to affect clinical decisions and are used only to confirm the diagnosis.
What is "intermediate syndrome"?	Development of profound muscle weakness 24–96 hrs after exposure to OPs. It occurs after resolution of the initial cholinergic syndrome. Patients present with weakness of neck flexion, cranial nerve palsies, and proximal muscle weakness. Respiratory muscle weakness may also occur, leading to respiratory insufficiency requiring intubation. Fasciculations and cholinergic signs will be absent.
How is intermediate syndrome treated?	There is no specific antidote. Atropine is not effective. With appropriate supportive care, recovery will occur in 5 to 18 days. Some experts believe adequate treatment with pralidoxime can prevent this.
What is OP-induced delayed polyneuropathy?	A rare disease characterized by leg cramping followed by progressive weakness and paralysis of the extremities (lower more than upper) that begins 1 to 4 weeks after OP exposure. The mechanism of this disease is thought to be related to phosphorylation and "aging" of a protein called neuropathy target esterase. As the condition progresses, flaccid paralysis can be replaced by hypertonicity with a spastic gait.

PYRETHRINS AND PYRETHROIDS

What are pyrethrins?	Active extracts from the *Chrysanthemum* plant. They are degraded by sunlight and

are commonly found in pediculicidal shampoos.

What are pyrethroids?

Synthetic analogues of pyrethrins. In comparison to pyrethrins, pyrethroids carry greater potency and have longer half-lives.

Explain the two groups of pyrethroids.

Type 1 – no cyano group. Examples include allethrin, cyfluthrin (Baythroid), and permethrin (Ambush, Dragnet, Nix, Pounce, Raid).
Type 2 – does contain a cyano group. Examples include cypermethrin (Barricade, Cymbush, Cynoff, Demon), deltamethrin, and fenvalerate.

What is the mechanism of action of pyrethrins / pyrethroids?

Disrupt sodium channel inactivation → prolonged depolarization → rapid paralysis of the insect nervous system. Humans are relatively resistant to these agents because of our ability to rapidly metabolize them.

What are the routes of absorption of pyrethrins / pyrethroids?

Ingestion, inhalation, dermal. Dermal absorption of pyrethroids can cause local paresthesias. Ocular exposure can cause pain, tearing, and photophobia.

What are the signs and symptoms of acute pyrethrin exposure?

1. Anaphylactic reactions are most common.
2. Inhalation may cause bronchospasm or induce an asthma attack.
3. Pyrethrins generally do not cause significant systemic toxicity.

What group is at particular risk for an allergic reaction from pyrethrin exposure?

Those with a ragweed allergy

What are the differences in clinical effects between type 1 and type 2 pyrethroids?

1. Type 1 – fine tremor, twitching and hyperexcitability, possibly leading to hyperthermia
2. Type 2 – hypersalivation, seizures, choreoathetosis, and sympathetic activation

Why are type 2 pyrethroids more toxic?

They cause a greater delay in sodium channel closure, producing a more sustained depolarization. They also inhibit chloride influx through the GABA receptor.

What are treatments for acute pyrethrin / pyrethroid exposure?

1. Skin decontamination with soap and water (avoid secondary exposure to healthcare providers)
2. GI decontamination with activated charcoal for recent ingestions
3. Benzodiazepines for seizures
4. Standard allergic reaction therapy (i.e., antihistamines, epinephrine, steroids)
5. Bronchodilators for bronchospasm / wheezing
6. Protect the patient's airway, if necessary. As with all pesticides, aspiration pneumonitis due to the hydrocarbon vehicle is possible, in addition to the effects of the individual toxins.

Pyrethroid toxicity mimics the effects of what other toxic agent?

Organophosphates. Type 2 pyrethroid toxicity can result in hypersalivation, seizures, and hypertension, resembling an acute organophosphate poisoning.

OTHER

Where is *N,N*-diethyltoluamide (DEET) commonly found?

Insect repellant

What is the mechanism of action of DEET on insects?

In theory, it blocks insect antennae receptors, which are used to locate hosts.

How does DEET toxicity occur?

Ingestion or prolonged exposure on covered or damaged skin

What are the signs and symptoms of DEET toxicity?

1. Mild skin irritation from prolonged dermal exposure
2. Nausea and vomiting following ingestion
3. Hypotension and tachycardia have been reported with heavy dermal or oral exposure.

4. Rarely, CNS depression, coma, seizures, and respiratory failure with excessive dermal or oral exposure

What is the treatment for acute DEET toxicity?

1. Removal from exposure source and clothing
2. Copious irrigation with soap and water for cutaneous exposures
3. Benzodiazepines for seizures

What is fipronil?

A broad-spectrum insecticide that antagonizes GABA receptors preferentially in insect nervous systems

Describe the effects of fipronil toxicity.

CNS depression, vertigo, weakness, and seizures have been described; however, human overdose data is limited.

What are avermectins?

As a group, these agents interact with both GABA and glutamate channels, resulting in paralysis of the target insect. Abamectin, ivermectin, and emamectin are commonly used insecticides.

Describe the manifestations of avermectin toxicity.

Coma and respiratory arrest have been reported, although human data is limited.

How does imidacloprid cause toxicity?

Nicotine receptor agonism. It is used as an insecticide and as a flea repellant.

What are the effects of imidacloprid toxicity?

While human data is limited, animal studies have shown effects of nicotine poisoning, including vomiting, muscle fasciculations, weakness, and paralysis. Symptoms in humans may also be related to solvents included in the product.

What is the general treatment for these insecticides?

1. Supportive care is the primary treatment.
2. Benzodiazepines for seizures
3. Dermal decontamination should be performed, if indicated.

RODENTICIDES

ALPHA-NAPHTHYLTHIOUREA (ANTU)

For what purpose is alpha-naphthylthiourea (ANTU) used?

As a rodenticide, sometimes used specifically against Norway rats. It was used widely in Britain in the 1940s and 1950s, but its use has now been all but abandoned because of the use of coumarin-derived rodenticides.

What are the manifestations of acute ANTU toxicity?

Toxicity appears to be limited, as no deaths have been reported following acute exposure. Following ingestion, patients may develop tracheobronchial hypersecretion requiring intubation.

Can exposure to ANTU result in carcinogenesis?

While ANTU has been associated with bladder carcinoma, especially when contaminated with beta-naphthylamine, no definitive evidence exists that it is carcinogenic. Therefore, it has an IARC Group 3 classification.

What organ is primarily affected by ANTU poisoning?

Lungs. Overall, ANTU is relatively selective for causing pulmonary symptoms.

Describe the mechanism of ANTU toxicity.

In animal studies, ANTU appears to damage pulmonary capillaries, leading to pulmonary edema and pleural effusions.

What are the signs and symptoms of ANTU poisoning?

Dyspnea, rales, cyanosis, and pulmonary edema / effusion may result after inhalation.

What are symptoms of chronic ANTU exposure?

Antithyroid activity and hyperglycemia have been reported.

Describe the management of acute ANTU exposure.

Supportive care. There is no specific treatment.

ANTICOAGULANTS

What is the mechanism of action of the coumarin-derivative rodenticides?

Inhibit the enzymes vitamin K 2,3-epoxide reductase and vitamin K quinone reductase, decreasing the availability of reduced vitamin K_1. Reduced vitamin K_1 is necessary to activate (by carboxylation) the vitamin K-dependent clotting factors II, VII, IX, X, and proteins C and S. Depletion of the clotting factors will cause coagulopathy.

What are the symptoms of rodenticide anticoagulant overdose?

All are related to inappropriate hemorrhage – gingival hemorrhage, spontaneous ecchymosis, hematuria, epistaxis, GI bleeding, intracranial hemorrhage

Are overdoses with anticoagulant rodenticides symptomatic immediately?

No. An increase in PT will not occur until active factors are decreased to 25% of normal. The factor with the shortest half-life is factor VII ($t_{1/2} = 5$ hrs); therefore, at least 3 half-lives (or 15 hrs) must pass before there is a detectable change in the measured PT (or calculated INR).

Do all rodenticides that are coumarin-based have equivalent toxicity to warfarin?

No. Long-acting anticoagulant rodenticides called "superwarfarins" are commonly used (e.g., brodifacoum, bromadiolone, coumafuryl, difenacoum).

What is an important chemical property of "superwarfarins," and what is a clinical consequence of this property?

"Superwarfarins" are lipophilic and have greater potency and longer half-lives than does warfarin. Typical half-lives of 42 to 51 days have been reported in humans, with some cases of anticoagulation lasting up to 1 year.

Does a single accidental ingestion of a "warfarin only" rodenticide usually produce bleeding?

No. There must be repeated ingestions over a period of time or a massive ingestion to cause clinically significant anticoagulation. An accidental exposure is rarely clinically significant. In contrast, ingestion of a "superwarfarin" rodenticide can produce coagulopathy following a single ingestion.

What are some important laboratory tests for assessing a patient with rodenticide anticoagulant poisoning?

PT is the best test to identify anticoagulant effect. PTT and thrombin time may be useful to evaluate for other causes of coagulopathy. Specific assays for "superwarfarin" molecules exist and can be ordered to confirm the diagnosis.

What are the antidotes to rodenticide anticoagulant poisoning?	1. Vitamin K_1 – phytonadione 2. FFP or whole blood to replace clotting factors in patients with active bleeding 3. Recombinant activated factor VII can be considered.
Should vitamin K_1 be given to every patient who has ingested a "superwarfarin"?	No. It should only be given if the patient develops significant prolongation of their PT, which may be delayed up to 48 hrs. If there is no elevation in the INR after 48 hrs, the patient will not develop toxicity and will not need treatment. The administration of vitamin K_1 prior to the development of coagulopathy can mask the toxicity and commit the patient to long-term vitamin K_1 treatment.
Are all forms of vitamin K effective at reversing the toxicity from coumarin-derived rodenticides?	No, only the K_1 form is effective. K_3 (menadione) and K_4 are provitamins which are slowly converted to the active form and are not effective as antidotes.

CHOLECALCIFEROL

What is another name for cholecalciferol?	Vitamin D_3. This is the same chemical produced when 7-dehydrocholesterol in the skin is exposed to sunlight.
What is the major clinical consequence of cholecalciferol overdose?	Hypercalcemia
Why is cholecalciferol used in rodenticides?	To induce hypercalcemia, resulting in death from metastatic calcifications in multiple organ systems
How is cholecalciferol metabolized?	1. Hepatic – converts cholecalciferol to 25-hydroxyvitamin D 2. Renal – converts 25-hydroxyvitamin D to 1,25-dihydroxyvitamin D (calcitriol) 3. Intracellular – calcitriol binds to its receptors → ↑ intestinal calcium absorption

When do the clinical manifestations of cholecalciferol overdose become apparent?

2 to 8 days following exposure. Data in human exposure is limited; however, no cases of severe toxicity or death have been reported in the literature.

What are the clinical manifestations of hypercalcemia?

1. GI – constipation (most common GI complaint), anorexia, acute pancreatitis
2. Renal – ↓ concentrating ability, acute renal insufficiency, nephrolithiasis
3. CV – shortened QT interval, HTN (due to renal insufficiency + peripheral vasoconstriction)
4. Musculoskeletal – weakness

What laboratory studies are essential for evaluation?

Electrolytes, including calcium, magnesium, and phosphorus. A normal calcium level at 48 hrs essentially excludes toxic ingestion. BUN and creatinine are helpful to evaluate renal function.

What are some treatments for acute cholecalciferol ingestion?

1. Standard treatments for hypercalcemia (i.e., IV fluids and loop diuretics to enhance renal calcium excretion)
2. Phosphate PO forms a nonabsorbable calcium-phosphate complex in the gut.
3. Calcitonin → ↑ renal calcium excretion and ↓ bone resorption
4. Bisphosphonates interfere with osteoclast activity and inhibit bone resorption.
5. Hemodialysis may be indicated for patients with renal failure or for severe toxicity.

SODIUM MONOFLUOROACETATE (1080)

By what other names is sodium monofluoroacetate known?

Compound 1080, SMFA

Is SMFA available as a rodenticide in the United States?

In 1972, it was banned as a rodenticide due to its high toxicity. Since that time, this ban has undergone several court challenges, resulting in limited availability for licensed pest control operators.

Other than as a rodenticide, where can SMFA exposure occur?

It is used today for coyote control. A commercially available "toxic collar" containing SMFA is placed on a sheep. The poison is released when the sacrificial sheep is attacked.

What are the main routes of SMFA toxicity?

Ingestion or inhalation

How does SMFA cause poisoning?

It poisons the Krebs cycle. Monofluoroacetate (in place of pyruvate) combines with coenzyme A to form fluoroacetyl CoA. The latter undergoes conversion to fluorocitrate (by citrate synthase), which subsequently occupies the citrate binding site on aconitase, rendering this enzyme inactive and compromising aerobic metabolism.

What are some clinical manifestations of SMFA poisoning?

Initial symptoms include nausea, vomiting, and abdominal pain. These are followed by signs of organ system dysfunction, including agitation, hypotension, dysrhythmias, seizures, and coma.

What specific laboratory abnormalities are associated with SMFA poisoning?

1. High anion gap metabolic acidosis
2. Elevated lactate
3. Hypokalemia and hypocalcemia may be present.

Describe the treatment of SMFA poisoning.

Treatment is primarily supportive.

Is there an antidote for SMFA poisoning?

Both ethanol and glycerol monoacetate have been studied as possible treatments. These agents supply acetyl-CoA to competitively inhibit the action of SMFA. Neither agent has definitely been shown to improve patient outcome.

STRYCHNINE

What is strychnine?

An alkaloid, occasionally used as a rodenticide, that is extracted from the seeds of the strychnine tree (*Strychnos nux-vomica*). Use has been limited in modern times; however, historically this poison was widely used in medicinal tonics, as a rodenticide, and for criminal poisonings.

How does strychnine cause poisoning?

Glycine receptor antagonism in the spinal cord, resulting in failure of normal inhibitory signals

What are some signs and symptoms of strychnine poisoning?

Painful generalized muscle spasms that may resemble tonic seizures and are often triggered by external stimuli. Early in the poisoning, patients have a normal mental status, although later may develop AMS secondary to the complications of profound rigidity. Consequences of prolonged muscle spasm include rhabdomyolysis, lactic acidosis, myoglobinuria, and renal failure.

Name the bacterial illness that may be confused with strychnine poisoning.

Tetanus (tetanospasmin)

What is opisthotonus?

Extreme arching of the back that occurs as a result of back muscle spasms. This finding can be seen in both tetanus and strychnine poisoning.

What is "risus sardonicus"?

The grimace produced as a result of contracted facial muscles. This is also seen in both tetanus and strychnine poisoning.

How long after ingestion do symptoms occur?

15–60 min post-ingestion

How does strychnine poisoning occur?

1. Ingestion – accidental, suicidal, homicidal
2. Recently, there are reports of strychnine poisoning occurring as a result of contaminated street drugs.

How can strychnine poisoning be detected?

Blood, urine, and gastric aspirate levels are available but are not likely helpful in the acute setting.

What other laboratory values are useful in strychnine poisoning?	Electrolytes, CPK, and renal function tests to monitor for acidosis, rhabdomyolysis, and renal failure.
How does death occur from strychnine poisoning?	Hypoxia, following generalized muscle spasm with respiratory muscle dysfunction
Is there a specific antidote for strychnine poisoning?	No. Treatment is aimed at relieving muscle spasm. Initially, this consists of benzodiazepines and opioids. For severe symptoms, muscle paralysis with a nondepolarizing agent may be necessary. Hyperthermia from profound muscle hyperactivity may be treated with misting or cooling blankets.

VACOR (PNU)

What is another name for Vacor?	N-3-pyridylmethyl-N'-p-nitrophenyl urea (PNU). Vacor contains 2% PNU. It is also known as pyrimil.
What does it look like?	Yellow-green powder, may resemble corn meal
What are the 2 main clinical conditions that occur with Vacor poisoning?	1. DM (insulin-dependent) 2. Autonomic dysfunction
How does Vacor cause DM?	1. Disrupts nicotinamide metabolism, causing abnormalities in pentose phosphate and, therefore, interfering with RNA metabolism and resulting in destruction of pancreatic islet beta cells (responsible for insulin secretion) 2. Substitutes for nicotinamide in NAD and NADPH, interfering with oxidoreductase reactions
How do patients present after Vacor poisoning?	Within hours of ingestion, patients can present with DKA, peripheral neuropathy, and autonomic neuropathy. The autonomic neuropathy can cause severe orthostatic hypotension, impotence, ↓ sweating, urinary retention, constipation,

and dysphagia. Transient hypoglycemia is possible before hyperglycemia and is due to insulin release from damaged pancreatic cells.

Is Vacor available?

Was withdrawn by the manufacturer in 1979; however, occasional poisonings are still reported

What are common symptoms in patients with Vacor overdose?

Similar to those commonly recognized in DKA, including nausea, vomiting, blurred vision, polyuria, thirst, abdominal pain, generalized weakness and chills

What are common findings on examination of the peripheral nervous system in the patient with Vacor poisoning?

1. Hyporeflexia
2. ↓ vibration and light touch sensation in the extremities
3. Paresthesias
4. Fine tremor

Do patients recover after Vacor poisoning?

Fatalities have occurred secondary to DKA, GI perforation, and dysrhythmias. If a patient survives, they will likely be left with insulin-dependent DM and treatment-resistant orthostatic hypotension.

Is there an antidote to Vacor?

Possibly. Niacinamide (vitamin B_3) has been used; however, a parenteral form of niacinamide is no longer available and now must be substituted with niacin. This is less effective and can cause vasodilation and impaired glucose tolerance, both of which exacerbate the effects of Vacor poisoning. Early administration is essential for clinical benefit.

Why is Vacor poisoning important?

It is a mechanism for the biological induction of insulin-dependent DM, and exposure closely mimics the natural disease.

OTHER

What is red squill?

A plant (*Urginea maritime*) that contains cardiac glycosides (scilliroside) in the bulb

How does red squill kill rodents?

Causes cardiac glycoside poisoning, resulting in pulmonary edema

What is different about rats and humans that contributes to the selective toxicity of red squill in rodents?

Humans vomit upon ingesting the toxin due to its potent emetic effect; rats are unable to do so.

Thallium is used as a rodenticide in countries outside the United States. What are common symptoms of significant thallium poisoning?

Painful peripheral neuropathy and alopecia

In the past, arsenic was commonly used as a rodenticide in the United States. What are 4 mechanisms by which arsenic causes poisoning?

1. Pentavalent arsenic can substitute for phosphorus during glycolysis, forming an unstable intermediate at a critical ATP-generating step.
2. Binds to sulfhydryl groups, inhibiting numerous enzymes (e.g., succinate dehydrogenase, a key enzyme in the citric acid cycle)
3. Production of reactive oxygen species, causing direct injury to a variety of tissues
4. Interference with gene expression, cell signal transduction, and apoptosis

A patient presents with garlic odor, oral burns, phosphorescent (luminous in the dark) "smoking" feces, and vomiting following the ingestion of a rodenticide. What agent has caused the toxicity?

Yellow (or white) phosphorus

Is red phosphorous poisonous?

No

What is the clinical presentation after white phosphorus poisoning?

Classically described in 3 stages:
<u>Stage 1</u> – oral burns, nausea, vomiting, abdominal pain, and possibly diarrhea

occur within minutes to hours post-ingestion. CV collapse or dysrhythmias may occur.

Stage 2 – apparent recovery during this period of systemic absorption

Stage 3 – multi-system organ failure after several days

What are 2 metal phosphides that are used as rodenticides?

1. Zinc phosphide
2. Aluminum phosphide

What does zinc phosphide smell like?

Decaying fish

Zinc phosphide is used as a rodenticide. Is it the zinc or the phosphide that is responsible for the toxicity?

Phosphide (P^{3-}) becomes phosphine (PH_3) upon exposure to moisture or stomach acid and is responsible for the toxic effects. The zinc does not contribute to its toxicity.

How does phosphine cause toxicity?

Phosphine may block cytochrome c oxidase of the electron transport chain. It also causes free radical generation and resultant lipid peroxidation.

What are some common clinical manifestations of phosphide poisoning?

1. GI – profuse vomiting and abdominal pain within 10–30 min
2. Respiratory – cough, excessive sputum production, tachypnea, pulmonary edema
3. CV – palpitations, tachycardia, hypotension, QRS interval prolongation, dysrhythmias (i.e., atrial fibrillation, VT, VF)
4. Endocrine – metabolic acidosis
5. CNS – seizures, coma

Is there an antidote for metal phosphide poisoning?

No. Therapy is supportive. Administering sodium bicarbonate to decrease gastric acidity and lessen phosphine production has been considered but is of unproven benefit.

What is tetramine?

A rodenticide, also called tetramethylene disulfotetramine. It is an odorless, tasteless powder that dissolves easily in water. It has been banned worldwide, but poisoning continues to be reported in China, Hong Kong, and the United States.

What is its mechanism of toxicity?

Noncompetitive $GABA_A$ receptor antagonism → blocks Cl^- influx → cells are more prone to depolarization

How can patients be exposed to tetramine?

Inhalation and ingestion

What clinical manifestations does it cause?

Onset – 10 to 30 min post-ingestion
Mild poisoning – nausea, vomiting, abdominal pain, lethargy, headache, weakness
Severe poisoning – refractory seizures, coma, and death within hours

What is the treatment for tetramine poisoning?

1. Decontaminate patients by removing clothes and cleaning them with soap and water.
2. Activated charcoal may be given if the patient has a well-protected airway.
3. Treat seizures aggressively with benzodiazepines, barbiturates, and pyridoxine.
4. Hemoperfusion or hemofiltration may be effective.

Chapter 7   Chemical Agents of Terrorism

BOTULINUM TOXIN

What is botulinum?

Any one of eight serologically distinct, heat-labile exotoxin heterodimer proteins (labeled A, B, C1, C2, D, E, F, G), of which only A, B, E, and (rarely) F cause illness in humans

What produces botulinum?

The anaerobic, spore-forming, gram-positive bacillus *Clostridium botulinum*

What are the modes of transmission that may be utilized by terrorists / criminals?

Ingestion, inhalation, parenteral

What is the LD_{50} of botulinum toxin?

.001 microgram per kilogram

Is there an antidote to botulinum?

Yes, a trivalent (A, B, E) antitoxin from the CDC and a heptavalent antitoxin from the U.S. Army. Contact the CDC or local state health department to arrange antidote delivery and assist with confirmatory testing.

What is the onset time for an acute botulinum poisoning?

Highly variable—symptoms may appear as early as 2 hrs post-ingestion, with most patients developing symptoms between 10–72 hrs. In some cases, signs and symptoms may not be noticed for up to 8 days. The delay and variability can make identifying a source difficult.

What is the mechanism of toxicity of botulinum?

Toxin is endocytosed by the nerve → light chain of botulin proteolytically cleaves various SNARE proteins → prevents synaptic vesicle fusion with the presynaptic nerve terminus → nerve cannot release ACh, thereby interrupting neurotransmission

What symptoms occur with acute botulinum poisoning?

Presenting symptoms follow a stereotypical pattern of descending weakness:
1. Cranial nerve dysfunction manifested as dysphagia, diplopia, and dysarthria
2. On exam, ptosis, gaze paralysis, and facial palsy are most often noted.
3. Inhibition of muscarinic cholinergic function can cause dry mouth, mydriasis, and constipation.
4. It progresses as a descending motor paralysis affecting the upper limbs, then the lower limbs.
5. In severe cases, the intercostals and diaphragm are affected, possibly necessitating mechanical ventilation.
6. Ingested botulinum may also cause GI symptoms, including nausea, vomiting, constipation, and less commonly, diarrhea that typically precedes neurological symptoms.

How does inhalational botulism present?

In a similar fashion to food-borne botulism. The time-course for inhalational botulism is poorly understood, due to the small number of cases; however, the onset is believed to occur in about 3 days.

What might lead you to suspect that there has been an intentional release of botulinum toxin?

There are several clues that should raise suspicion:
1. A large number of patients
2. Multiple clusters without an identifiable source
3. Groups of patients who share a common geographic connection
4. Outbreaks involving the rare types C, D, E, F, or G

What role does botulinum toxin play in biological warfare?

Botulin oxidizes rapidly upon atmospheric exposure, rendering it harmless. Poisoned air is considered breathable in roughly 1 day. There are no documented warfare uses in history; however, it is the most toxic naturally occurring protein in the world, and there is concern that it could be used as an agent of terror.

How is acute poisoning with botulinum toxin treated?

1. Supportive care, with attention to airway protection and ventilatory support
2. Botulinum antitoxin is the definitive treatment. This will be empiric, based on clinical suspicion, as no rapid confirmatory tests will be readily available. Consider antitoxin administration in any patient with a clinical presentation suspicious for botulism, particularly when a group of 2 or more presents with suggestive symptoms.

INCAPACITATING AGENTS

What is an incapacitating agent?

An agent that transiently impairs an individual in a non-lethal manner by disrupting the CNS and/or PNS

What are some common classes of incapacitating agents?

Anticholinergic agents, ultra-potent opioids, aerosolized benzodiazepines

What anticholinergic agent is an incapacitating agent?

3-quinuclidinyl benzilate (QNB or BZ)

What are ultra-potent opioids?

Typically fentanyl derivatives (e.g., carfentanil, remifentanil) designed to incapacitate through sedation

How are these agents typically used?

Exposure occurs through inhalation after these agents are aerosolized. Clinical effects are those of the opioid toxidrome, including miosis and CNS and respiratory depression.

What is the onset of action of ultra-potent opioids?

Rapid, generally within minutes

During what hostage situation were ultra-potent fentanyl derivatives likely used to subdue captors?

The Moscow Theater, Russia 2002

What are the effects of aerosolized benzodiazepines?	These agents produce the sedative-hypnotic toxidrome. Symptoms include CNS depression with possible respiratory depression after large exposures. While data is limited, effects are expected to be produced rapidly after inhalational exposure.
What prevalent hallucinogen has been studied for use as an incapacitating agent?	LSD, a potent hallucinogen in the ergotamine family that is active in μg quantities. It may be absorbed by ingestion, transdermally, or through mucous membranes. Effects typically begin within 1 hr and may last up to 8 to 12 hrs.

INCENDIARY AGENTS

What are incendiary agents?	Compounds used, primarily by the military, to burn / destroy supplies, equipment, ordnance, and structures
What are the main types of incendiary agents?	Thermite, magnesium, white phosphorus, and gelled hydrocarbons (e.g., napalm) are the most common types.
What is thermite, and what are some of the characteristic injuries it causes?	Mixture of powdered aluminum and iron oxide. Upon ignition, it burns at >2500°C (4500°F). Molten particles of iron may lodge in the skin, causing deep tissue burns.
What is a typical injury from a magnesium burn?	Magnesium burns at >2000°C (4200°F). Deeply embedded magnesium fragments may produce magnesium dihydroxide and localized hydrogen gas, resulting in tissue necrosis.
What are some important chemical characteristics of white phosphorus?	It may spontaneously ignite upon exposure to air. Oxygen must be excluded from the agent (i.e., with water or a wet cloth) in order to stop the burning.
How does ingested white phosphorus result in toxicity?	White phosphorus is a metabolic poison, disrupting electron transport. A large exposure to embedded particles may result in systemic toxicity.

Describe the treatment of white phosphorus burns.

Patients with retained particles on skin or clothing should have those areas covered with water prior to mechanical debridement. Treatment should otherwise follow standard burn therapy.

What is napalm, and what secondary exposure should be considered in patients with napalm burns?

Napalm is a gelled form of gasoline which is more stable and burns longer than normal gasoline. Burning napalm gives off CO, so this secondary exposure must be considered in patients with napalm burns.

What other considerations should be observed in patients exposed to incendiary agents?

Blunt or penetrating trauma may be present, as these agents are typically deployed with explosives.

What type of dressing should you avoid using on a white phosphorus burn?

Oily or greasy dressings. The element is lipid-soluble and can penetrate the tissues.

IRRITANTS

What are irritant gases?

Gases that cause irritation to the respiratory tract. Effects may be immediate or delayed depending on the water solubility of the gas.

What 2 broad categorizations are used for irritant gases?

1. Highly water soluble (e.g., chlorine, sulfur dioxide, ammonia)
2. Poorly water soluble (e.g., nitrogen dioxide, ozone, phosgene)

What are the effects of highly soluble irritant gases?

Because they are highly water soluble, they cause immediate airway irritation upon contact with moist tissue.

What are the effects of poorly soluble irritant gases?

Effects on the pulmonary mucosa take time to develop due to the low water solubility of these gases. Delayed onset pulmonary edema is often seen. Exposure to these gases is typically prolonged, as there is no initial irritation to warn of their presence.

What is the typical presentation of a patient exposed to a highly soluble irritant gas?

Irritation of nose, throat, eyes, and skin, manifesting as oropharyngeal burning, cough, and dyspnea

Describe the mechanism of irritant gas toxicity.

Generate caustic substances and free radicals on contact with airway mucosa

Describe the treatment of irritant gas exposure.

1. Removal from the source with dermal decontamination, if necessary.
2. Oxygen, nebulized bronchodilators, and airway support, as needed.
3. Nebulized sodium bicarbonate may be beneficial after chlorine gas exposure.
4. Observe for delayed sequelae following exposure to gases of low water solubility.

What are lacrimating agents?

Lacrimators (tear gas) are primarily used for riot control and self-protection. They produce irritation of the eyes, skin, and airway.

Name some different types of tear gas.

Chloroacetophenone (CN, aka "mace"), chlorobenzalmalononitrile (CS), and capsaicin, also known as pepper spray. Rarely, CS and CN may cause bronchospasm, pulmonary edema, and skin vesication.

What are the general effects of lacrimators?

Eye and airway irritation, lacrimation, blepharospasm

Describe the treatment for lacrimator exposure.

Removal from exposure, followed by skin and eye irrigation

NERVE AGENTS

What are nerve agents?

Organophosphate (OP) chemical weapons

What is the mechanism of action of nerve agents?

AChE inhibition. Covalent bonding to a serine hydroxyl residue on the active site of the AChE prevents ACh hydrolysis, resulting in accumulation of ACh in the synapse and an exaggeration of the typical action mediated by the postjunctional structure (e.g., neuron, gland, myocyte). This causes excessive cholinergic stimulation.

What are the G-series nerve agents?

Tabun (GA), sarin (GB), soman (GD), cyclosarin (GF)

What are the V-series nerve agents?

VE, VG, VM, VX

What are the physical properties of G- and V-series nerve agents?

The term nerve gas is misleading; nerve agents are in fact liquids at room temperature and must be aerosolized or evaporated to be used effectively as an inhalation agent. The vapors are heavier than air and, therefore, will remain close to the ground and settle in low-lying areas. They have different degrees of volatility. For example, sarin evaporates as readily as water, while VX evaporates 1,500 times more slowly.

What makes the V-series nerve agents so dangerous?

They are persistent agents, resistant to degradation and removal (even by surfactants), so toxic concentrations can remain for weeks to months, long after their initial release.

What are the physical properties of G-series and V-series nerve agents?

Volatile liquids at room temperature, varying from colorless to brown and from odorless to fruity-smelling

What are the Novichok nerve agents?

Stable and safe-to-handle binary solid versions of nerve agents that were developed in the Soviet Union and Russia between 1970 and 2000.

What are the routes of exposure to nerve agents?

Inhalation and dermal

What is the LD$_{50}$ of GB?

Inhalation – 75–100 mg/min/m^3
Dermal – 1700 mg

What is the onset of action for an acute nerve agent exposure?

Inhalation – seconds to minutes (dose dependent)
Dermal – 20 to 30 min after large exposures, otherwise may be delayed up to 18 hrs

What are the signs and symptoms of an acute nerve agent exposure, along with the mnemonic used to remember the cholinergic signs and symptoms of OP poisoning?

DUMBELS
Defecation
Urination
Miosis
Bronchorrhea / **B**ronchospasm / **B**radycardia
Emesis
Lacrimation
Salivation

Does this list include all the possible effects of nerve agent poisoning?

No, it only includes muscarinic effects. The excess cholinergic stimulation will also stimulate nicotinic receptors, causing effects at the motor end plate (e.g., fasciculations, weakness, paralysis) and ganglia (e.g., tachycardia, HTN).

List the target organs of nerve agent exposure and the associated clinical effects.

CNS – agitation, AMS, seizures, coma
Eyes – miosis, lacrimation
Mouth – salivation
Lungs – ↑ bronchial secretions, bronchospasm
CV – tachycardia / bradycardia, QT interval prolongation
GI – diarrhea, emesis, ↑ motility
GU – urinary incontinence
Sweat glands – diaphoresis
Adrenals – ↑ catecholamines
Neuromuscular junction – fasciculations, weakness, paralysis

What is the most reliable physical exam finding for volatilized nerve agent poisoning?

Miosis

How is the presentation of an inhalational exposure different from that of a dermal exposure?

Inhalational – onset within seconds to minutes. With a small vapor exposure, miosis, rhinorrhea, and slight bronchospasm will be seen. This will progress to marked dyspnea with obvious secretions as the exposure continues. Those with large exposures will progress to AMS, generalized fasciculations, seizures, paralysis, and apnea.

Dermal – exposure to liquid nerve agents may have delayed effects (dose dependent). Contact with the skin will cause localized sweating and possibly fasciculations of the underlying muscles. Later, patients will experience nausea, vomiting, diarrhea, generalized sweating, and fatigue. With larger exposures, progression to AMS, seizures, generalized fasciculations, ↑ secretions, paralysis, and apnea will occur. Unlike vapor exposure, a dermal exposure will delay the development of miosis. The delayed presentation and lack of miosis can make the diagnosis of a nerve agent exposure difficult.

What is the mechanism of seizures from OP/nerve agent exposure?

Within the first 5 min, seizures appear to be due to cholinergic overstimulation, and atropine can abort or prevent seizures. After 5 min, other changes are noted, including a decrease in brain norepinephrine, an increased glutaminergic response, and the activation of NMDA receptors. At this point, both atropine and benzodiazepines are needed.

Why might seizure activity be missed in an OP/nerve agent-poisoned patient?

The nicotinic effects can progress from fasciculations to flaccid paralysis, resulting in nonconvulsive seizures. Any comatose patient who experiences this type of exposure should be treated with benzodiazepines, as well as atropine, with emergent EEG monitoring.

Is there an antidote for an acute nerve agent poisoning?

Yes. Atropine and related anticholinergic drugs will antagonize excess cholinergic transmission and compete with ACh. Pralidoxime chloride (2-PAM) serves to reactivate AChE and restore normal cholinergic function. These must be given immediately in order to be effective.

How does pralidoxime (2-PAM) work?

Nerve agents form a covalent bond with the active site of AChE, preventing breakdown of ACh. 2-PAM is attracted to the active site of AChE, and its nucleophilic oxime moiety will attack the phosphate atom of the nerve agent. This will displace it from the active site, reactivating the enzyme.

What is "aging"?

"Aging" occurs when the nerve agent forms an irreversible covalent bond with the AChE enzyme after losing an alkyl side chain, rendering the enzyme permanently inactive. This can take from <1 hr to several days, depending on the particular agent. Pralidoxime will have no effect on an aged AChE complex.

Why is it important to prevent aging?

Once aging occurs, the patient will not regain vital functions, such as muscle strength or respiratory drive, until new enzyme is synthesized. This may take weeks to months

How fast does aging occur after nerve agent poisoning?

Depends on the agent. For example, soman rapidly and permanently disables AChE in 2 to 6 min, whereas sarin and VX age more slowly, with aging half-lives of 5 hrs and 48 hrs, respectively.

What lab test can confirm nerve agent exposure?

Measurement of the activity of erythrocyte AChE and plasma pseudocholinesterase. Results are usually not available quickly enough to affect clinical decisions and are used only to confirm the diagnosis.

What is the treatment for nerve agent poisoning?

1. Removal from exposure source and removal of clothing (avoid secondary exposure of healthcare workers)
2. Copious dermal irrigation with soap and water for liquid exposure
3. Protect the patient's airway, if necessary (use a non-depolarizing paralytic for RSI)
4. Atropine titrated to the drying of pulmonary secretions and resolution of bronchospasm
5. 2-PAM: 1–2 g IV over 10 min, repeated in 1 to 2 hrs. Alternatively, a bolus of 30 mg/kg, followed by an infusion of 8 mg/kg/hr, is advocated by the WHO.
6. Benzodiazepines to prevent and treat seizures

What is a Mark I kit?

A set of auto-injectors which deliver 2 mg of atropine and 600 mg of 2-PAM. There is also a separate auto-injector that will deliver 10 mg of diazepam.

How is it used?

The auto-injectors are designed to deliver medication through protective clothing. For patients with significant poisoning, immediate administration of three Mark I kits is recommended (1,800 mg of 2-PAM). The diazepam auto-injector should also be used for anyone with significant symptoms. If an IV has been established, it is preferable to use this route.

How much atropine is usually needed to treat nerve agent poisoning?

Typical total dose required ranges from 5–20 mg; however, similar to OP insecticide poisonings, there are reports of larger doses (up to 200 mg) of atropine having been used to treat nerve agent casualties

Is tachycardia a contraindication to atropine use in an acute OP exposure?

No. The tachycardia may actually improve due to decreased activation of preganglionic nicotinic sympathetic nerve terminals, decreased release of norepinephrine from the adrenal glands, and alleviation of dyspnea and hypoxia.

What is the goal of atropine therapy?

Drying of pulmonary secretions (reflected by improved oxygenation) and relief of bronchospasm (reflected by ease of breathing/ventilation). Atropine will likely not improve miosis or skeletal muscle paralysis; therefore, reversal of these effects is not a therapeutic endpoint. Attempting to reverse these findings with atropine can result in anticholinergic toxicity.

What is the prognosis of a weapons-grade, acute nerve agent poisoning?

Without rapid antidote treatment, death will occur within minutes.

Just how potent is VX?

Extremely potent. A droplet of VX <20% of the size of the Lincoln Memorial on the back of a penny has the potential to kill the average human within 30 min if placed on unbroken skin.

PHOSGENE

What is phosgene?

Also called carbonyl chloride, it is a colorless gas or liquid at <8°C (46°F) that smells like "freshly mown hay" or "green corn."

Where is phosgene used?

In the production of dyes, resins, pharmaceuticals, and pesticides. It was used as a gaseous warfare agent during WWI, where it was responsible for 80% of poison gas fatalities.

Why was phosgene so effective?

It is heavier than air and, therefore, will settle and accumulate in low-lying areas such as trenches. Also, because of its low water-solubility, it is not as irritating to the upper airways as some irritant gases. This will allow victims to remain in a contaminated area for a prolonged period, increasing exposure.

What is the most common method of phosgene exposure?

Phosgene gas may be produced when chlorinated organic compounds (e.g., freon, household solvents, paint removers, dry-cleaning fluids) are heated. Occupational exposure can occur when welding metals are cleaned with these agents.

What is the mechanism of toxicity of phosgene?

Pulmonary irritation, causing a chemical pneumonitis with inflammation of the small airways and alveoli. Leakage of serum into the alveolar spaces may eventually lead to noncardiogenic pulmonary edema.

What are the symptoms of phosgene exposure?

At high concentrations, it can cause immediate-onset symptoms of eye irritation, cough, reflex hypoventilation, and apnea. Delayed-onset symptoms are due to inflammation of the bronchial and alveolar structures and development of pulmonary edema. This is characterized by progressive dyspnea, potentially leading to respiratory failure.

What must be remembered about the time-to-onset of pulmonary edema in phosgene exposure (and other poorly water-soluble irritants)?

May take up to 12 to 24 hrs to develop; therefore, patients with a suspected phosgene exposure must be observed for 24 hrs

Does the characteristic odor afford adequate warning?

No. The odor threshold is too high to afford adequate warning properties. Also, phosgene can cause olfactory fatigue.

Does significant immediate irritation portend a bad outcome?

No. The degree of delayed toxicity depends on the concentration and duration of exposure; therefore, lack of immediate irritation may in fact be more dangerous, as the victim may not leave the contaminated area.

What can be used to predict outcome?

The latency period until the development of pulmonary edema. Shorter latency = greater exposure and poorer prognosis

What part(s) of the airway are most affected by phosgene inhalation?

Lower respiratory tract and lung parenchyma

What is the treatment for phosgene poisoning?

1. Removal from environment (including contaminated clothing)
2. Wash contaminated skin, and flush eyes if there is ocular exposure.
3. Supportive care. Have low threshold for endotracheal intubation and PPV. Use as large an endotracheal tube as possible, as frequent suctioning may be required.
4. Nebulized beta 2-adrenergic agonists can reduce bronchospasm.

Is there an antidote for phosgene exposure?

No, although administration of steroids is recommended.

3-QUINUCLIDINYL BENZILATE

What is 3-quinuclidinyl benzilate (QNB)?

Odorless, nonirritating anticholinergic psychomimetic classified as a schedule 2 military hallucinogenic incapacitating agent (NATO code = BZ)

Why is QNB considered an incapacitating agent?

QNB is a potent anticholinergic agent that produces delirium at low doses.

What is the mechanism of toxicity of QNB?

Systemic competitive inhibition of ACh at postsynaptic and postjunctional muscarinic receptor sites

What are the routes of exposure to QNB?

1. Inhalation (particulate aerosol)
2. Percutaneous absorption (particulate immersion)

What is the onset time of an acute QNB exposure?

1 to 4 hrs, usually with peak effects at 8 hrs

What are the symptoms of an acute QNB exposure?

Synonymous with an anticholinergic response—dry mucous membranes, mydriasis, tachycardia, urinary retention, flushing, delirium

What is the reported duration of effect of QNB?

Symptoms may not resolve for 2 to 4 days.

Are any laboratory tests helpful for diagnosis?

No

Is there an antidote to QNB?

Physostigmine can be used to reverse anticholinergic symptoms; however, repeat doses may be necessary due to QNB's extended half-life in comparison to physostigmine.

What are the treatment recommendations for an acute QNB exposure?

1. Supportive care is the primary treatment.
2. Decontamination for dermal exposures
3. Benzodiazepines for agitation
4. Physostigmine may be used to reverse anticholinergic symptoms.

What is "Agent 15"?

An anticholinergic glycolate incapacitating agent possessed by the Iraqi military during the Gulf War. It was found to be similar (or possibly identical) to QNB.

RICIN

What is ricin?

A toxalbumin found in castor beans (*Ricinus communis*). When purified, it is a white, water-soluble powder.

How is ricin's heterodimeric structure important to its function?

It has a B chain that allows for cellular entry by binding to galactose-containing receptors on the cell membrane, and an A chain that causes toxicity.

What is the mechanism of toxicity of ricin?

Ricin's A chain inhibits protein synthesis by depurinating an adenine base of the 60S ribosomal subunit. This prevents binding of elongation factor 2 (EF2) and subsequently stops protein translation by RNA polymerase.

By what routes can ricin cause toxicity?

Ingestion, inhalation, parenteral

What limits ricin's oral toxicity?

Poor GI absorption. This is especially true of whole castor beans. Ricin is found within the seed coat and the bean must be chewed to release significant toxin.

How toxic is ricin after an oral ingestion?

Estimated lethal oral dose = 1–20 mg/kg (~8 castor beans)

What are the symptoms associated with acute oral ricin poisoning?

Primarily GI (i.e., vomiting, diarrhea, abdominal pain, oropharyngeal irritation). Patients can have electrolyte abnormalities or develop shock due to dehydration or GI hemorrhage. Multisystem organ failure with hemolysis, renal failure, LFT abnormalities, and AMS can occur.

What is the average onset of action for acute ricin poisoning?

4 to 6 hrs. Presentation beyond 10 hrs post-ingestion is unlikely.

What is the prognosis of oral ricin poisoning?

<5% mortality

How toxic is ricin after parenteral exposure?

Far more toxic than with oral exposure. In mice, the LD_{50} is ~5–10 μg/kg.

What is the presentation after parenteral exposure?

After a delay of up to 12 hrs, the patient will present with nonspecific symptoms, including fever, malaise, headache, nausea, or abdominal pain. There may be inflammation or erythema at the injection site. The patient can develop laboratory abnormalities such as elevated WBC, transaminases, amylase, CPK, and creatinine. Death secondary to multisystem organ failure can occur.

How does an inhalation exposure present?

4 to 8 hrs post-exposure, patients can present with fever, cough, nausea, arthralgias, chest tightness, shortness of

breath, and pulmonary edema. Fatalities are due to respiratory failure. Symptom onset may be delayed for 24 hrs.

How long can ricin poisoning symptoms persist?

If death has not occurred in 3 to 5 days, the patient will often recover; however, full recovery may take weeks.

How do you treat a patient after ricin exposure?

1. Removal from exposure (including clothing) with soap and water decontamination before entry into a healthcare facility. Use PPE if entering a potentially contaminated environment.
2. For oral exposures, activated charcoal should be given.
3. Supportive care with aggressive IV fluid administration and electrolyte repletion. Dialysis is ineffective.
4. Pulmonary edema may require intubation and PPV.

For how long should a patient be observed following an exposure?

<u>Oral exposure:</u> if asymptomatic for 12 hrs, patient may be discharged with instructions to return immediately for any respiratory symptoms
<u>Dermal exposure:</u> observe for 12 hrs, as absorption may occur through compromised skin
Symptomatic patients must be admitted and observed for development of hypovolemia, hemolysis/anemia, renal failure, or hepatotoxicity.

Is there an antidote for ricin?

No; however, the U.S. military has developed a vaccine.

What is ricin's role in biological warfare?

It is listed as a schedule 1 controlled substance and given the military symbol W. Although considered relatively inefficacious due to its rapid atmospheric oxidation (~3 hrs), it is easily obtained and has no antidote.

Has ricin been used as an agent of biological warfare in the past?

1. WWI – United States investigated as a bullet coating
2. WWII – United States investigated as a cluster bomb component
3. Georgi Markov – Bulgarian dissenter, was assassinated in 1978 with injection of encapsulated ricin
4. Terrorist groups – Ansar al-Islam and Al Qaeda have tested weaponized ricin since 2000

What other toxalbumin-producing bean is similar to castor beans?

Jequirity beans (*Abrus precatorius*) are used ornamentally and as rosary beads. Abrin is the specific toxalbumin found in this plant and has properties similar to ricin (reportedly more potent).

TRICHOTHECENE MYCOTOXINS

What are trichothecene mycotoxins?

A group of toxins produced as byproducts of fungal metabolism. T-2 is a specific trichothecene that is regarded as the most toxic of this group. While T-2 acts primarily as a vesicant, it may also exert systemic effects.

Can T-2 mycotoxin be used as a chemical warfare agent?

Yes. "Yellow rain" incidents occurring in Southeast Asia in the 1970s have been controversially linked with T-2 mycotoxin. During these exposures, T-2 toxin was allegedly dispersed by aircraft.

What are the routes of T-2 mycotoxin exposure?

Inhalation, ingestion, dermal

What was the route of alleged T-2 mycotoxin exposure that occurred in past nonmilitary outbreaks?

Ingestion. Multiple natural outbreaks of GI illness related to T-2 have been reported throughout the world. Typically, these outbreaks are related to consumption of moldy wheat or corn that laid unharvested over the winter and was collected the following spring.

What is the mechanism of toxicity of T-2 mycotoxin?

T-2 binds the 60S subunit of eukaryotic ribosomes and obstructs peptidyl transferase activity, thereby interrupting the RNA translation process. This results in the blockade of RNA, protein, and DNA synthesis.

Which tissues are most affected by systemic T-2 mycotoxin poisoning?

Rapidly dividing cells (e.g., GI epithelium, bone marrow)

What are the signs and symptoms of T-2 mycotoxin exposure?

<u>Dermal/ocular exposure</u> – skin and eye irritation, erythema and blistering, possibly progressing to tissue necrosis
<u>Inhalation</u> – oropharyngeal irritation, rhinorrhea, epistaxis, dyspnea, cough, blood-tinged sputum
<u>Inhalation/ingestion</u> – nausea, vomiting, abdominal cramps, diarrhea. GI bleeding is likely, and delayed leukopenia may develop.

Can T-2 mycotoxin exposure be fatal?

Yes, within minutes to days, depending on dose and route

Is there an antidote for T-2 mycotoxin?

No

What is the primary treatment for T-2 mycotoxin ingestion?

Decontamination and supportive care. Granulocyte colony stimulating factor (G-CSF) may be of benefit to treat neutropenia.

VESICANTS

What is a vesicant?

Blister agent characterized for its use in chemical warfare

What are the different types of vesicants (military designations in parentheses)?

1. Sulfur mustards (H, HD, HT, HL)
2. Nitrogen mustards (HN-1, HN-2, HN-3)
3. Lewisite (L)
4. Phosgene (CG)

What is a mustard agent?

Sulfur mustard is an alkylating chemical that was originally used as a weapon in WWI. It is a liquid at room temperature but may readily vaporize in warm environmental conditions. Sulfur mustard agent may be weaponized as a liquid or aerosol. Distilled mustards are usually clear, odorless hydrophobic liquids at room temperature. Impurities or mustard mixtures typically develop a pale yellow/amber to brown color (i.e., look like mustard) and a mustard, garlic, or horseradish smell. Nitrogen mustards are newer agents that have been used for medical purposes, but not in weapon form.

Describe the mechanism of mustard toxicity.

Mustard is an alkylating agent, causing damage to DNA and cellular proteins. After topical exposure, damage occurs to the dermal-epidermal junction, causing vesicle/bullae formation and skin sloughing. Secondary to the alkylation of DNA, systemic manifestations may include bone marrow suppression.

What is Lewisite?

An organic arsenical compound developed for use as a vesicating weapon. Pure Lewisite is a clear, odorless, oily liquid; however, impure Lewisite can turn completely black and faintly smells of geraniums.

What is the chemical mechanism of Lewisite toxicity?

Largely unknown; however, toxicity appears to result from the depletion of glutathione and from the interaction of arsenic with sulfhydryl groups

Is phosgene a vesicant?

While it may cause intense skin irritation, it does not result in skin vesiculation; therefore, it is not a true vesicant.

What are the primary sites of vesicant action?

Eyes, skin, and respiratory tract

How are vesicants able to produce systemic symptoms?	Ingestion, inhalation, dermal absorption. They are lipophilic, and are thus readily (and rapidly) absorbed through epithelia.
What is the onset of action for a vesicant exposure?	Depends on specific compound and route: <u>Mustard</u> – usually 2 to 48 hrs after contact exposure, with gradual escalation in severity <u>Lewisite</u> – immediate
How do acute vesicant exposures typically present?	With severe irritation and decomposition of exposed tissues: <u>Skin</u> – erythema, dermatitis, edema, extreme vesiculation <u>Ocular</u> – conjunctivitis, edema, corneal degradation, photosensitivity, blindness Mucous membranes – mucous hypersecretion, laryngitis, bronchitis, hemorrhage <u>Respiratory</u> – dyspnea, pulmonary edema GI – nausea, vomiting, diarrhea
What are Lewisite-specific symptoms in an acute exposure?	"Lewisite-shock" – hypotension secondary to capillary damage and subsequent third spacing of fluids
What are the sub-acute and chronic risks of vesicant exposure?	Infection, COPD, hepatic/renal dysfunction, bone marrow suppression, immune dysfunction (mustards), carcinogenesis
What treatment is recommended for an acute vesicant exposure?	1. Rapid decontamination 2. Neutralization if available 3. Supportive care
Are antidotes to vesicants available?	1. Mustards – povidone-iodine may help to neutralize 2. Lewisite – British anti-Lewisite (BAL) chelates Lewisite, forming a stable 5-membered ring
What is the mortality rate for acute vesicant exposure?	<5% mortality reported in WWI; however, large surface area (>50%) concentrated contact exposures can be fatal

Are any vesicants used therapeutically?	1. Mustard gas (HD) for psoriasis (discontinued) 2. HN-1 for wart removal (discontinued) 3. Mustine (HN-2) and a variety of non-weaponized nitrogen mustards for cancer chemotherapy

VOMITING AGENTS

What emetics are used as chemical warfare agents?	1. Diphenylchloroarsine (DA or Clark I) 2. Diphenylcyanoarsine (DC or Clark II) 3. Diphenylamine(chloro)arsine (DM, or adamsite)
What are other names for this group of agents?	Sneezing gases, harassing agents, human repellants
How are these agents used as weapons?	1. Non-lethal riot control 2. Emesis induces removal of PPE to enhance exposure to other chemical agents
How are these agents typically deployed?	As smoke or droplet aerosols
When aerosolized, how does adamsite gas look and smell?	Odorless, yellow-green vapor
Historically, when have these agents been employed for warfare?	1. Used by Germany during WWI 2. Stockpiled by Japan in WWII
What are the routes of exposure?	Inhalation, ingestion, dermal
When do clinical symptoms manifest after exposure?	After several minutes
How might this latency affect the toxicity of these agents?	Patients are initially unaware of the exposure and fail to leave the environment before significant absorption occurs.
What are the signs and symptoms of acute exposure?	Initially, mucosal irritation with rhinorrhea, tearing, and coughing. This is followed by nausea, vomiting, diarrhea, abdominal pain, and headache.

Can these agents be lethal?	Rarely. Death can occur with significant exposures, particularly in enclosed spaces.
What is the treatment for toxic exposures to vomiting agents?	Decontamination and supportive care

OTHER

When considering exposure to chemical weapons, what other exposures must one also consider?	Biologic weapons
What are some examples of biologic weapons?	1. Anthrax spores (*Bacillus anthracis*) 2. Plague (*Yersinia pestis*) 3. Tularemia (*Franciscella tularensis*) 4. Small pox (*Variola*) 5. Hemorrhagic fever viruses (e.g., Ebola, Marburg)
What are some similarities between chemical and biologic weapons?	1. Typically vaporized/aerosolized for dissemination 2. Dissemination is weather-dependent. 3. PPE is required when handling.
What are some differences between chemical and biologic weapons?	Biologic agents: 1. Are usually slower-acting, tasteless, and odorless, and are thus harder to identify early 2. Can mimic endemic diseases (e.g., plague still found in United States, inhalation exposure to anthrax during flu season) 3. Decontamination less important because of delayed presentation 4. Isolation usually more important to stop spread
What is another name for anthrax?	"Wool-sorter's disease" because wool workers often contracted the cutaneous form of anthrax via spores from the sheep's wool.

What are the types of anthrax exposures?

1. Inhalational anthrax
2. Cutaneous anthrax
3. Gastrointestinal anthrax

What are the signs and symptoms of inhalational anthrax?

Initial fever, malaise, fatigue, cough, and mild chest pain, progressing to respiratory distress and even hemorrhagic mediastinitis, sepsis, and meningitis

What is the classic cutaneous manifestation of dermal exposure to anthrax?

Black eschar with surrounding edema after inoculation through compromised skin

What clinical syndrome occurs after exposure to aerosolized plague?

Pneumonic plague, occurring 2 to 3 days after inhalation; patient experiences fever with cough / hemoptysis and sepsis, progressing to respiratory distress and CV collapse.

What is bubonic plague?

Vector-borne endemic plague that occurs after exposure to infected fleas and is characterized by buboes (painful adenopathy) with fever and fatigue

What precautions must be employed when a patient is suspected of having plague?

Respiratory isolation with droplet precautions (highly contagious)

What are the characteristics of the skin lesions that develop with smallpox?

Macules which elevate to form papules, vesicles, and pustules

Where are the lesions most prominent?

Extremities and face, may also see oral lesions

What are the extradermal manifestations of smallpox?

Fever, malaise, nausea, vomiting, myalgias

What is aflatoxin?

Mycotoxins produced predominately by *Aspergillus* spp. The Iraqi military was known to possess weaponized aflatoxin during the first Gulf War. Aflatoxins are of lower potency than trichothecene mycotoxins but may cause both acute and chronic disease.

Chapter 8   Natural Toxins

AMPHIBIANS

What are amphibians?

Vertebrate ectothermic (cold-blooded) animals that live part of their life in the water and part on land. This taxonomic class includes frogs, newts, salamanders, and caecelians (worm-like creatures).

What are some poisonous amphibians?

1. Poison dart frogs (*Phyllobates* genus)
2. *Atelopid* frogs
3. Western newts (*Taricha* genus)
4. Red-spotted newt (*Notophthalmus viridescens*)
5. *Bufo* toads – cane toad (*Bufo marinus*); Colorado River toad (*Bufo alvarius*), also called the Sonoran Desert toad

What are toxic components of *Bufo* toad venom?

1. Bufotenine – a tryptamine produced in the parotid gland of the toad; has been speculated to cause hallucinations (unlikely, as it does not cross the blood-brain barrier)
2. Bufodienolide – cardioactive steroids that will inhibit Na-K-ATPase
3. 5-methoxydimethyl tryptamine – secreted by *Bufo alvarius* and is a potent hallucinogen

How can a *Bufo* toad poisoning occur?

Licking/eating the toad. Also, consuming products containing toad venom may cause poisoning. Inhaling or smoking the venom of *Bufo alvarius* can cause hallucinations.

What laboratory drug assay may be abnormal in *Bufo* toad poisoning?

Detectable digoxin level, as the bufodienolide cross-reacts with the digoxin immunoassay

How can *Bufo* toad poisoning be treated?	Digoxin Fab fragments have been successfully used in treating overdoses in patients with bufodienolide poisoning presenting with elevated digoxin levels.
What is the most toxic dart frog?	Golden poison dart frog (*Phyllobates terribilis*), found along the Saija River of Colombia
Where do "dart frogs" get their name?	South American Indians were historically known for rubbing their blowgun darts on the backs of these frogs to make poisonous darts.
What is one of the main toxic substances found in poison dart frogs?	Batrachotoxins, which bind with high affinity to voltage-gated sodium channels and maintain them in an open state → irreversible depolarization → paralysis and cardiac dysrhythmias
What toxin is found in *Atelopid* frogs, western newts, and red-spotted newts?	All produce a toxin identical to tetrodotoxin, which is most commonly associated with pufferfish. When referring to newts, tetrodotoxin is often called tarichatoxin, from the genus *Taricha* to which these animals belong.
What is the mechanism of action of tetrodotoxin?	Blocks neuronal voltage-gated sodium channels → blocks transmission by preventing sodium flux. This is the opposite mechanism of batrachotoxins from the poison dart frog.

ARTHROPODS

BLACK WIDOW SPIDERS

Where (geographically) are black widows (*Latrodectus mactans*) found?	*Latrodectus* species are found in temperate and tropical regions of the world. In the United States, they are found throughout the lower 48 states and Hawaii.
What types of environments does the black widow prefer?	Dark, secluded places (e.g., woodpiles, barns, beneath stones)

What are the distinguishing features of the female black widow?

The female is shiny, black, and 8–10 mm with a red hourglass mark on the ventral surface of its rounded abdomen. Females have large fangs capable of penetrating human skin, unlike the male spiders.

What are the characteristics of a black widow bite?

1. "Bull's eye-like" erythematous region surrounding puncture marks (fades within 12 hrs)
2. Often painless locally since the venom lacks human cytotoxic properties

What is the major toxic component of black widow venom?

Alpha-latrotoxin

What is the mechanism of toxicity of alpha-latrotoxin?

Alpha-latrotoxin $\rightarrow$ presynaptic neuronal Ca^{2+} influx $\rightarrow$ exocytosis of neurotransmitters (including ACh, norepinephrine and dopamine) $\rightarrow$ muscle spasm and sympathomimetic toxidrome

What are the signs and symptoms of systemic toxicity?

Initial signs may be minimal with little or no pain at the bite site. Mild erythema and localized swelling may then be noticed around the bite. As symptoms progress, pain develops from the bite site proximally, along with HTN and tachycardia. Nausea and vomiting may be present. Lower extremity bites often result in intense abdominal pain, whereas upper extremity bites often result in severe chest pain, both of which may resemble surgical or other pathologic processes.

What is lactrodectism?

The general syndrome of pain and catecholamine surge that develops following envenomation

What are the subcategories of lactrodectism?

1. *Hypertoxic myopathic syndrome* – an extreme manifestation of envenomation with severe muscle cramping and weakness accompanied by acute chest or abdominal pain

2. *Facies latrodectismica* – sweating, facial grimace/contortion that may accompany some envenomations
3. *Pavor mortis* – fear of death some patients feel after envenomation

What are the life-threatening complications of the black widow spider bite?

Respiratory distress, severe HTN, CV collapse

What are the treatments of the black widow spider bite?

Commonly, analgesics (i.e., opioids) and muscle relaxants (i.e., benzodiazepines) are adequate to control pain. In severe cases, *Lactrodectus* antivenom may be utilized.

Which groups of individuals may particularly benefit from antivenom therapy?

Young children, the elderly, and those with comorbidities

From what animal is the currently approved (in the U.S.) antivenom derived?

Horses. Consequently, there is a high incidence of anaphylaxis to the antivenom. It should be used cautiously and in a setting with rapid access to the medications and supplies needed to treat anaphylaxis.

BROWN RECLUSE SPIDERS

Where are brown recluse spiders (*Loxosceles reclusa*) found?

In the Mississippi valley region of the U.S., primarily in the southern states, but may extend up to parts of Illinois and Iowa. Other *Loxosceles* species inhabit the southwestern U.S.

What environment does the brown recluse prefer?

Dry, secluded, warm areas (e.g., woodpiles, basements, attics). They dislike areas of activity (i.e., they are "reclusive").

What are the distinguishing features of the female brown recluse?

Brown to grey in color, medium size (6–20 mm) with a dark brown violin-shaped marking on the dorsal side of cephalothorax, and legs 5× the length of the body. Similar to the black widow, the female is larger and considered more dangerous than the male.

Describe a distinguishing feature of the brown recluse eye structure.

Loxosceles species have three sets of eyes arranged in pairs (six total). Most other species of spiders have eight eyes.

When do brown recluse bites most often occur?

When the spider is threatened, mainly during April–October

What is the major toxic component of brown recluse venom?

Sphingomyelinase D

What is the mechanism of toxicity of sphingomyelinase D?

Venom components, including sphingomyelinase D, have both hemolytic and cytotoxic properties. This may result in local tissue thrombosis, ischemia, and necrosis.

What are the cutaneous effects of the brown recluse bite?

Initially, the bite may be painful, but some do go unnoticed. Over a few hours, pain is followed by central blanching and surrounding erythema. A vesicle or bulla may develop in the central area followed by progressive ulceration and necrosis. Erythema and necrosis typically follow a gravitational pattern as the venom spreads throughout the tissue. Symptoms vary with the amount of venom injected; therefore, many bites have few sequelae. Bites tend to be more severe over areas of adipose tissue.

What is systemic loxoscelism?

Syndrome of nausea, vomiting, fever, weakness, rhabdomyolysis, and possibly DIC that has been sporadically described after brown recluse envenomation. Evidence defining the etiology and mechanism of this disease is limited.

What are the cutaneous treatments of the brown recluse spider bite?

1. General wound care including cool compress application
2. Tetanus prophylaxis
3. Extremity immobilization and serial exams
4. Antimicrobial agents for secondary infection

What are the systemic treatments of the brown recluse spider bite?

Analgesics and supportive care

Are there any antidotes for brown recluse envenomation?

No. Historical use of wound excision, dapsone, and even electric shock therapy have not been definitively proven to change outcomes.

SCORPIONS

There are multiple types of scorpions that are indigenous to the U.S. Members of which genus are most dangerous to humans?

Stings from the *Centruroides exilicauda* (the bark scorpion) are the most medically significant, as their venom contains a potentially lethal neurotoxin.

What are the signs and symptoms of a sting from other indigenous scorpions?

Local pain and inflammation

What states have the highest incidence of scorpion envenomation?

Arizona and parts of California, New Mexico, Texas, and Nevada

How many cases of lethal scorpion envenomations have been reported?

Accurate data is sparse and unreliable; however, in the U.S., only one death attributed to the *Centruroides* scorpion has been reported since 1964.

What are the signs and symptoms of a sting by the *Centruroides exilicauda* scorpion?

Pain and swelling at the site of the sting followed by local paresthesias are the most commonly encountered. A number of sympathetic and parasympathetic nervous system manifestations can occur, including vomiting, diarrhea, hypersalivation, sweating, tachydysrhythmias, significant HTN, and wheezing. Muscular weakness, via both peripheral and cranial innervation, may be seen.

How are *Centruroides* envenomations graded?

Grade I – local pain/paresthesias
Grade II – remote pain/paresthesias
Grade III – cranial/autonomic nerve dysfunction *or* skeletal muscle involvement

Grade IV – combined cranial/autonomic nerve dysfunction *and* skeletal muscle involvement

Is there antivenom that can be used in *Centruroides exilicauda* envenomations?

Yes. There are several antibody-derived antivenoms, but their use is controversial, as most envenomations may be adequately managed with supportive care alone. Antivenom may be indicated in grade III or IV envenomations.

What are the physiologic effects of the venom from a *Centruroides* scorpion?

Several individual toxins cause peripheral neuronal sodium channel opening, causing repetitive neuron stimulation. Symptoms may involve both the autonomic (e.g., HTN, tachycardia, salivation) and the somatic nervous systems (e.g., fasciculations, ataxia).

If a scorpion collector is stung, are there other concerns?

Knowing the particular species of scorpion is critical. Exotic scorpions (especially from Africa) can be far more dangerous and have greater health consequences.

TICKS

What causes tick paralysis?

A neurotoxin in the salivary glands of female ticks that is released during feeding

Name 2 tick species that cause tick paralysis in the U.S.

1. *Dermacentor andersoni* (western United States)
2. *Dermacentor variabilis* (southeastern United States)

What symptoms characterize tick paralysis?

Acute, ascending paralysis, beginning with lower extremity weakness and progressing to respiratory failure and death. It can also present with ataxia. Patients can have sensory complaints. Exam will reveal diminished or absent reflexes.

How is tick paralysis treated?

Removing the tick will cause resolution of symptoms within 24 hrs; therefore, a thorough body search (i.e., hair, axillae, perineum, ear canals) is mandatory if this disease is suspected.

What syndrome does tick paralysis mimic, and how can the two be distinguished?

Guillain-Barre syndrome (GBS). They can be distinguished by the finding of normal CSF analysis in tick paralysis (GBS will cause ↑ CSF protein).

How does a tick attach to its host?

Using its chelicerae, the tick creates a hole into the host's epidermis into which it inserts the hypostome. This structure anchors the tick while it feeds. A salivary anticoagulant promotes the free flow of host blood.

For which disease agents do ticks serve as vectors?

Bacteria, viruses, rickettsiae, protozoans

What is the proper way to remove a tick?

With forceps or tweezers, grasp the tick near the head (close to the host skin) and pull the tick straight off (do not twist). Other methods of removal may cause the tick to regurgitate into the wound → ↑ risk of disease transmission.

What is the disease agent that causes Lyme disease?

Borrelia burgdorferi (spirochete)

Which tick species are vectors for Lyme disease?

Ixodes scapularis (eastern U.S.), *I. pacificus* (western U.S.), *I. ricinus* (Europe), *I. persulcatus* (Europe, Asia), *I. ovatus* (Asia), *I. moschiferi* (Asia)

How long must a tick remain attached to transmit Lyme disease?

≥36 hrs

What symptoms are associated with early Lyme disease?

1. Early localized (stage 1) – 7 to 10 days after bite, manifests as erythema migrans ("bull's-eye" rash) in ~75% of patients. This macular dermatitis starts out as a small, painless, circular macule or papule and expands slowly over days to weeks, usually with some central clearing and flu-like symptoms.

2. Early disseminated (stage 2) – weeks to months after the initial infection with fatigue, fever, lymphadenopathy, secondary annular lesions, transient arthralgias, Lyme carditis (conduction abnormalities including AV block), meningitis, Bell's palsy, and radiculopathies

What signs and symptoms are associated with late Lyme disease?

<u>Rheumatologic</u> – severe pain/swelling of the large joints, especially the knees
<u>CNS</u> – encephalopathy

How is Lyme disease diagnosed?

Clinical presentation is key; <50% recall a tick bite. It can be confirmed with titers, but interpretation of the results is complex.

What is the treatment for Lyme disease?

Antibiotics such as amoxicillin, azithromycin, cefuroxime, clarithromycin, doxycycline, and tetracycline are typically used to treat early Lyme disease and are usually taken for 2 to 3 wks. Dose and duration of treatment vary depending on severity. Late Lyme disease with neurological symptoms is treated with IV antibiotics, such as ceftriaxone.

What is the disease agent that causes Rocky Mountain Spotted Fever (RMSF)?

Rickettsia rickettsii

Which tick species are vectors for RMSF?

1. *Dermacentor variabilis* (American dog tick) in the eastern U.S.
2. *Dermacentor andersoni* (Rocky Mountain wood tick) in the western U.S.

What is the classic triad of symptoms associated with RMSF?

1. High fever
2. Rash (2 to 4 days after fever; starts on palms, soles, wrists, and ankles, then spreads centripetally to torso)
3. History of tick bite

What are the other symptoms associated with RMSF?

Severe headache, malaise, chills, myalgias, abdominal pain, nausea, vomiting, diarrhea

Describe the progression of the rash.

Initially a blanching macular rash that develops into a petechial rash

How is RMSF treated?

Tetracycline antibiotics, particularly doxycycline. Chloramphenicol is an alternative for use in pregnant women.

What happens if RMSF goes untreated?

Mortality up to 30%. With appropriate treatment, the mortality rate drops to ~4%.

What is the agent that causes tularemia?

Francisella tularensis – a gram-negative coccobacillus

Which tick species are vectors for tularemia?

1. *Dermacentor andersoni* (Rocky Mountain wood tick) in the western U.S.
2. *Amblyomma americanum* (lone star tick) in the eastern U.S.
3. *Dermacentor variabilis* (American dog tick) in the eastern U.S.
4. *Ixodes ricinus* in Europe

Are ticks the only means of transmitting tularemia?

No. >50% are transmitted by ticks, but it may also be carried in food and water and by other arthropods (e.g., biting flies).

What signs and symptoms are seen with tularemia?

Multiple diverse syndromes are associated with tularemia, but the typical presentation includes abrupt onset of fever, headache, fatigue, and vomiting. A patient not demonstrating an ↑ HR in response to fever is a characteristic finding.

How is tularemia treated?

Antibiotics, such as streptomycin, gentamicin, and tetracycline

What disease agent causes babesiosis?

Protozoans – *Babesia microti* and *Babesia divergens*

Which tick species are vectors for babesiosis?

I. scapularis (U.S.) and *I. ricinus* (Europe)

What signs and symptoms are associated with babesiosis?

Malaria-like symptoms for days to months – fever, chills, fatigue, headache, nausea, vomiting, AMS, DIC, hypotension, respiratory distress, hemolytic anemia

How is babesiosis treated?

Quinine sulfate plus clindamycin

What disease agent causes ehrlichiosis?

1. *Ehrlichia chaffeensis* causes human monocytic ehrlichiosis (HME)
2. *E. phagocytophila* causes human granulocytic ehrlichiosis (HGE)

These are small, gram-negative coccobacilli belonging to the family *Rickettsiaceae*.

What is the difference between HME and HGE?

<u>HME</u> – affects mononuclear phagocytes, found mostly in southern and south-central U.S.
<u>HGE</u> – affects granulocytes, found in upper midwestern and northeastern U.S.

Which tick species transmit ehrlichiosis?

Amblyomma americanum (HME) and *Ixodes scapularis* (HGE)

What signs and symptoms are associated with HME and HGE?

Similar presentations – fever, headache, myalgias, pancytopenia, elevated hepatic transaminases. HME is typically less severe and has a lower mortality rate.

How is ehrlichiosis treated?

Tetracycline antibiotics, such as doxycycline. Rifampin is an alternative for tetracycline-allergic patients.

What disease agent causes tick-borne encephalitis (TBE)?

Tick-borne encephalitis virus (TBEV), a member of the family *Flaviviridae*

What tick species transmit TBE?

Ixodes ricinus (western and central Europe) and *Ixodes persulcatus* (central and eastern Europe)

What signs and symptoms are associated with TBE?

1. Incubation period – 7 to 14 days
2. Viremic phase – 2 to 4 days, flu-like symptoms
3. Remission – up to 8 days

4. Neurogenic phase – only 20% to 30% of patients, meningitis-like presentation (i.e., fever, headache, nuchal rigidity), encephalitis-like presentation (i.e., confusion, drowsiness, sensory disturbances, partial paralysis), or a combination of these

How is TBE treated?

Supportive care. A TBE vaccine exists and is routinely used in Europe.

Is TBE seen in the U.S.?

Powassan encephalitis (POW) is a rare form of TBE seen in the northeastern U.S. and parts of Canada. It is transmitted by *Ixodes cookie* and manifests as severe fever, headache, nuchal rigidity, nausea, vomiting, and fatigue, progressing to confusion, seizures, respiratory distress, and paralysis.

What disease agent causes Colorado tick fever (CTF)?

Colorado tick fever virus (CTFV), a member of the family *Reoviridae*, genus *Coltivirus*

What tick species transmits CTF?

Dermacentor andersoni (western U.S. and Canada)

What signs and symptoms occur with CTF?

After a 4-day incubation period, sudden fever, chills, headache, retroorbital pain, photophobia, myalgias, malaise, rash, abdominal pain, nausea, and vomiting. The presentation may be biphasic with a symptom-free period in between.

How is CTF treated?

Supportive care

What disease agent causes tick-borne relapsing fever (TBRF)?

Borrelia recurrentis (spirochete)

What tick species transmit TBRF?

Soft ticks of the genus *Ornithodoros* (Asia, Africa, Middle East, and North and South America)

What signs and symptoms are associated with TBRF?	Recurrent episodes of high fever along with headache, myalgias, malaise, photophobia, abdominal pain, nausea, vomiting, rash, and confusion. Episodes typically last <1 wk and are separated by 4 to 14 days between relapses.
How is TBRF treated?	Doxycycline or erythromycin
What reaction can occur during treatment of TBRF?	Jarisch-Herxheimer reaction. This includes fever, rigors, headache, diaphoresis, and hypotension.

OTHER

What are the significant species of stinging hymenoptera?	Bees, wasps, and ants
What differentiates the sting of the honeybee from other bees and wasps?	The honeybee stinger characteristically detaches in human flesh.
What is the greatest danger of the honeybee sting?	Allergic reaction to allergens (proteins) in the venom
Should the stinger of a honeybee be removed immediately?	Yes. This prevents additional venom injection.
How does a bee sting result in a fatality?	Respiratory dysfunction and/or anaphylaxis
Why is an Africanized honeybee (AHB) attack more likely to result in a greater number of stings?	1. Heightened defensive reaction (will attack a person within 10 m of the colony) 2. Respond in larger numbers 3. Are more persistent in following a person (up to hundreds of meters from the nest)
If a patient is allergic to the sting of a honeybee, are they also allergic to the stings of other hymenoptera?	Not necessarily. The allergic reaction to bees is very species-specific.

What is the mechanism of toxicity of the *Vespid* wasp venom?	Causes pain by directly affecting neurons or by releasing pain-inducing compounds
What is the protein in wasp venom that causes the release of histamine from mast cells?	Peptides called mastoparans
Which stinging ants are of medical significance?	Red fire ants and harvester ants
What is significant about the red fire ant sting?	Red fire ants respond to disturbance with vigorous mass stinging
What is the active chemical in fire ant venom?	Alkaloids. These are cytotoxic, resulting in skin necrosis, and they inhibit the Na-K-ATPase of muscle cell membranes, resulting in a postsynaptic neuromuscular blockade.
How does a fire ant sting progress?	Initial burning sting, followed by a wheal (10 mm) with pruritus and edema; 4 hrs later, sterile vesicles form, and by 24 hrs, they turn into necrotic pustules.
Can fire ant bites cause significant morbidity or mortality?	Yes. Systemic symptoms (and even fatalities) have been reported when immobile victims (e.g., infants, frail elderly) have suffered massive numbers of stings.
Which spider's bite mimics the dermonecrotic lesion of the *Loxosceles reclusa* (brown recluse) and lives in the Pacific Northwest?	Hobo spider (*Tegenaria agrestis*)
Which spider's body color can change from yellow to greenish, pink, or tan depending on its last meal?	Yellow sac spider (Family *Clubionidae*), whose bites are usually self-limited

The bite of which webless, aggressive, South American spider (often found around banana plants) is neurotoxic and can manifest with immediate pain, salivation, priapism, bradycardia, hypotension, and occasional death?

The armed (or banana) spider (*Phoneutria*). Note that in North America there is a large yellow spider, called the banana spider, that is relatively harmless.

Which spider found in Africa and South America possesses 6 eyes and is considered very poisonous (and there is no antivenom)?

The six-eyed crab spider (*Sicarius*)

What is the result of the six-eyed crab spider bite?

Severe tissue damage (more extensive than that of the brown recluse) and possibly death

Which large, aggressive spider found along the eastern coast of Australia can cause a syndrome of paresthesias, hypersalivation, nausea, vomiting, confusion, dyspnea, profuse sweating, hypotension, and death due to pulmonary edema?

Australian funnel-web spiders (*Atrax* and *Hadronyche*)

What is the mechanism of action of the venom?

Slows closing of voltage-gated sodium channels → repetitive action potentials → excessive release and eventual exhaustion of neurotransmitters

Is there antivenom for the funnel-web spider?

Yes

Do tarantulas have a venomous bite?

Yes. Reported problems are not typically related to the bite, however. The spider's barbed hairs can get stuck in the eyes or nose, causing irritation.

What is Spanish fly?

A purported aphrodisiac made from dried blister beetles. Blister beetles contain cantharidin, which can cause severe oropharyngeal irritation, mucosal erosion, hematemesis, flank pain, hematuria, and renal dysfunction.

What is the blister beetle's primary route of toxicity?

When a beetle is crushed, it releases cantharidin, which will cause vesicle formation on contact with the skin; these are not painful unless ruptured. Ocular exposure will cause conjunctivitis.

BOTULISM

What is botulism?

A disease caused by systemic absorption of botulinum toxin, which includes eight serologically distinct, heat-labile proteins (labeled A, B, C1, C2, D, E, F, G), of which only A, B, E, and (rarely) F cause illness in humans.

What produces botulinum?

The anaerobic, spore-forming gram-positive bacillus, *Clostridium botulinum*

What are the forms of botulism?

1. Infant
2. Food-borne
3. Wound
4. Adult intestinal
5. Inhalational
6. Parenteral/injection

What conditions are hospitable to *C. botulinum*?

An anaerobic, low-sodium, and non-acidic medium. The toxin can be inactivated by heating at 85°C (185°F) for 5 min.

Where do *C. botulinum* contaminations typically occur?

1. Under-processed canned/jarred foods
2. Poorly preserved meat, sausage, fish, shellfish, jerky
3. Vegetables, fruit, olives (less common)

What is the mechanism of toxicity of botulinum toxin?

Toxin is endocytosed by the neuron → light chain of botulin proteolytically cleaves various SNARE proteins → failure of synaptic vesicle fusion at presynaptic nerve terminus → no ACh release → no neurotransmission

What is the onset time for an acute botulin poisoning?

Highly variable – symptoms may appear as early as 2 hrs post ingestion, with most patients developing symptoms between 10 to 72 hrs; however, signs and symptoms may not be noticed for up to 8 days

What symptoms occur with acute botulin poisoning?

The presenting symptoms follow a stereotypical pattern of descending weakness:
1. Cranial nerve dysfunction – dysphagia, diplopia, dysarthria
2. Exam – ptosis, gaze paralysis, and facial palsy are most often noted
3. Inhibition of muscarinic cholinergic function – dry mouth, dilated pupils, constipation
4. Descending motor paralysis affecting the upper limbs, then the lower limbs
5. In severe cases, the intercostals and diaphragm are affected, possibly necessitating mechanical ventilation.
6. Food-borne botulism also may have GI symptoms, including nausea, vomiting, constipation, and diarrhea (less common), that typically precede neurological symptoms.

How does botulin poisoning affect mental status?

Toxin cannot cross the blood-brain barrier and, therefore, only affects the PNS. Mental status should be normal unless respiratory insufficiency has caused hypoxia or hypercarbia. Also, botulin will not cause sensory deficits.

How is acute botulism treated?

1. Supportive care, with attention to airway protection and ventilatory support
2. Botulinum antitoxin. This therapy will be empiric, based on clinical

suspicion, as no confirmatory tests will be readily available.

Why is it important to administer botulinum antitoxin as early as possible?

The paralysis caused by botulinum toxin will persist until neural end plates are regenerated. If a patient's condition progresses to the point of requiring mechanical ventilation, that patient may become ventilator-dependent for several months. For this reason, it is important to recognize botulism and initiate treatment with antitoxin early.

Are antibiotics indicated for food-borne botulism?

No. They have no effect on preformed toxin; however, they may be needed to treat secondary infections.

Which antibiotics should not be used when treating a patient with botulism?

Aminoglycosides and clindamycin may exacerbate neuromuscular blockade.

What causes infant botulism?

Infant botulism is the most common form of botulism. It occurs when *C. botulinum* spores are ingested and germinate in the GI tract. The bacteria then produce toxin, which are absorbed into the body. Adult intestinal botulism is similar to infant botulism. It occurs in adults who have altered GI flora due to antibiotic use, abdominal surgery, achlorhydria, or inflammatory bowel disease.

What is the classic source of infant botulism?

Honey. In actuality, infant botulism is usually contracted by ingesting dust containing *C. botulinum* spores. The soil in southeastern Pennsylvania, Utah, and California has the greatest chance of containing these spores.

How does infant botulism present?

May be subtle. Constipation is often the initial symptom and may precede neurological symptoms by days. This can progress to poor feeding, weak cry, ptosis, weakness, and respiratory insufficiency.

What is wound botulism?

Occurs when *C. botulinum* spores contaminate wounds. They can germinate and produce the toxin, which is then systemically absorbed. Clinical manifestations are similar to food-borne botulism.

How is wound botulism treated?

Same as food-borne botulism; however, administration of antibiotics and drainage and/or debridement of infected tissue must also be performed

What is the LD_{50} of botulinum toxin?

1 ng/kg; therefore, 50–100 ng can be fatal

Is there an antidote to botulism?

Yes, a trivalent (A, B, E) antitoxin from the CDC and a heptavalent antitoxin from the US Army

Is the trivalent antidote available from the CDC used to treat infant botulism?

No. This is, in part, due to the high rate of adverse reactions and fear of sensitizing infants against horses and equine-derived products.

Is there an antidote for infant botulism?

Yes. Recently, a human-derived immune globulin (baby-BIG) has been introduced and should be used to treat infant botulism.

Can the presence of botulism be detected?

Yes. Diagnosis can be confirmed by detecting toxin in the patient's serum, stool, or wound drainage. The suspected food should also be tested. The CDC or local state health department should be contacted to help with testing. They will also provide the antitoxin.

What does an acute botulin poisoning electromyograph (EMG) look like?

First, this should only be done in a stabilized patient.
1. Brief low-voltage compound motor units
2. Low M wave amplitudes
3. Abundant action potentials
Note that up to 15% of affected individuals will have a normal EMG.

What is the prognosis for botulin poisoning?	Variable. With careful attention to respiratory status, recovery is common, although full recovery may take months.
How is botulin A used therapeutically?	1. Strabismus 2. Blepharospasm 3. Spasmodic torticollis 4. Achalasia (investigational)
What adverse reactions can occur following therapeutic botulin A administration?	1. Local dermatitis 2. Ocular edema 3. Photophobia 4. Symptoms consistent with poisoning

ESSENTIAL OILS

What are essential oils?	Polyaromatic hydrocarbons that have been extracted from a single type of plant. The oils are obtained through steam distillation or cold pressing of the desired part (i.e., root, leaves, flowers) of the parent plant.
Why are essential oils so toxic?	The chemicals in essential oils are highly concentrated and, when ingested, are quickly absorbed.
How are essential oils used?	For their aromatic properties and as alternative medicinal remedies
What is pennyroyal oil?	Pennyroyal is derived from the plant *Mentha pulegium* and has been used since antiquity as an abortifacient and insect repellant.
What is the mechanism of pennyroyal toxicity?	<u>Pulegone</u> (primary toxin) – binds to cellular proteins and depletes glutathione, resulting in centrilobular hepatic necrosis <u>Menthofuran</u> (P450 metabolite of pulegone) – inhibits glucose-6-phosphatase → prevents glycogen breakdown → hypoglycemia
Describe the treatment of pennyroyal ingestion.	Primarily supportive with close monitoring for hypoglycemia. *N*-acetylcysteine may be beneficial in repleting glutathione

and decreasing the incidence of liver failure.

How does oil of wintergreen cause toxicity?

Oil of wintergreen contains methyl salicylate. Toxicity is identical to aspirin poisoning, although the oil is more quickly absorbed, which results in a faster onset of symptoms.

How many mL of pure oil of wintergreen is equal to 7 g of aspirin?

5 mL (1 tsp) or ~21 regular strength (325 mg) aspirin tablets

What is the treatment for oil of wintergreen poisoning?

Follows standard salicylate guidelines. Hydration and urine alkalinization are indicated for mild toxicity. Hemodialysis may be needed for severe toxicity.

What other essential oil is known to cause hepatotoxicity?

Clove oil. Ingestion of concentrated clove oil may also result in CNS depression and seizures.

What are the manifestations of camphor toxicity?

Initially, nausea, vomiting, tachycardia, confusion, agitation, and CNS depression. Seizures often develop within 30 min of ingestion. Camphor odor may be evident on the breath.

From what plant is camphor derived?

Cinnamomum camphora tree

Describe the toxic effects of eucalyptus oil.

Primary manifestation is CNS depression/coma. Coma has been reported with ingestion of as little as 5 mL.

What is melaleuca oil?

Also known as tea tree oil, it is found in a variety of cosmetic products. Contact dermatitis and photosensitivity are common after dermal exposure. CNS depression and ataxia are reported after ingestion of concentrated solutions.

FOOD POISONING, BACTERIAL

What is the most potent of the bacterial food poisons?

Botulin

Which bacteria produce preformed toxins in food?	1. *Staphylococcus aureus* 2. *Clostridium perfringens* 3. *Bacillus cereus* 4. *Clostridium botulinum*
What property of preformed toxins makes them difficult to eradicate?	Heat-resistance (i.e., not easily removed; or deactivated by cooking/boiling)
What is the incubation period for bacteria with preformed toxins?	Short – symptom onset within 6 to 12 hrs of consumption
What characterizes staphylococcal food poisoning?	From 1 to 6 hrs post-ingestion, victims develop nausea with profuse vomiting and abdominal cramps. This is usually followed by diarrhea. Fever is rare, and symptoms typically last <12 hrs.
What characterizes food poisoning caused by *C. perfringens*?	From 8 to 16 hrs post-ingestion, patients develop watery diarrhea, abdominal cramping, and vomiting, though vomiting is less frequently encountered. Symptoms last 12 to 24 hrs.
What is unique about *Bacillus cereus* food poisoning?	It causes two distinct clinical syndromes: 1. An "emetic" syndrome caused by a preformed toxin. This results in vomiting and abdominal cramping within 1 to 6 hrs and recovery within 12 hrs. 2. A "diarrhea" syndrome believed to be caused by toxin produced in the gut. This causes diarrhea and abdominal cramping 8 to 16 hrs post-ingestion with recovery by 24 hrs (usually).
What is the classic vehicle for *B. cereus* food poisoning?	Reheated fried rice
Will antibiotics be of benefit for gastroenteritis caused by preformed toxins?	No
Which types of bacteria produce toxins in the gut?	1. *Bacillus cereus* 2. *Campylobacter jejuni*

3. Enterotoxigenic and enterohemorrhagic *Escherichia coli*
4. *Vibrio parahemolyticus*
5. *Clostridium perfringens*

Consumption of which types of bacteria may cause serious systemic poisoning?

1. *Clostridium botulinum*
2. *Listeria monocytogenes*
3. *Escherichia coli* O157:H7
4. *Shigella*

Which types of bacteria, when ingested, may cause an invasive gastroenteritis?

1. *Listeria monocytogenes*
2. *Salmonella*
3. *Vibrio parahemolyticus*
4. *Shigella*
5. *Yersinia enterolytica*
6. *Campylobacter jejuni*
7. Enteroinvasive *Escherichia coli*

What is the etiology of "traveler's diarrhea"?

Enterotoxigenic *Escherichia coli* (ETEC)

Found in milk, raw hot dogs, deli meat, and unpasteurized soft cheeses, which bacteria typically causes a gastroenteritis syndrome but can cause an invasive infection in immunocompromised individuals?

Listeria monocytogenes. This is why pregnant women are advised to avoid cold cuts and soft cheeses.

Which bacteria produces a toxin in food and in the gut, and may be found in meats and gravy?

Clostridium perfringens

What finding on a stool smear may differentiate a bacterial etiology from other causes of food poisoning?

Abundant WBCs

Administration of antibiotics to patients with *E. coli* O157:H7 increases the risk of what condition?

Hemolytic-uremic syndrome (HUS)

What is the most important preventative measure in controlling food-borne illness?	Hand washing

HERBAL PRODUCTS

What is the inherent risk in taking herbal products?	Quality control is relaxed and not regulated by the FDA, resulting in variability in potency and purity.
For what is *Ginkgo biloba* used?	1. Dementia syndromes/memory aid 2. Peripheral vascular disease 3. Tinnitus 4. Vertigo
What toxic effects may result from *Ginkgo biloba* ingestion?	Antiplatelet effects and GI distress
What is the mechanism of action of ephedra?	1. Agonism at alpha 1-, alpha 2-, beta 1-, and beta 2-adrenergic receptors 2. Release of stored catecholamines from presynaptic nerve terminals and inhibition of catecholamine reuptake
For what indications do people take ephedra?	1. Weight loss 2. Enhance athletic performance (boost energy)
What are the toxic effects of ephedra?	Tachycardia, HTN, cardiac dysrhythmias, psychosis, seizures, and possibly CVA. Secondary to these effects, ephedra is currently banned in the U.S.
Which herbal product classically causes photosensitivity?	St. John's Wort. It is also associated with early cataracts.
What are the reported uses of St. John's Wort?	1. Antidepressant (for mild depression) 2. Anti-inflammatory 3. Antimicrobial
How does St. John's Wort induce drug interactions?	It is a CYP3A4 and P-glycoprotein inducer

What drug levels have been reported to be altered by St. John's Wort?

Cyclosporin A, indinavir, nevirapine, midazolam, theophylline, amitriptyline, warfarin, digoxin, oral contraceptives

What hyperthermic, drug-induced syndrome can (theoretically) result from St. John's Wort?

Serotonin syndrome. This may result when St. John's wort is combined with other serotonergic agents.

What herbs have been associated with hepatotoxicity?

Bajiaolian (*Dysosma pleianthum*), black cohosh (*Cimicifuga racemosa*), cascara (*Rhamnus purshiana*), celandine (*Chelidonium majus*), chaparral (*Larrea tridentata*), common comfrey (*Symphytum officinale*), Russian comfrey (*Symphytum uplandicum*), prickly comfrey (*Symphytum asperum*), common germander (*Teucrium chamaedrys*), felty germander (*Teucrium polium*), impila (*Callilepsis laureola*), jin bu huan (*Polygala chinensis*), kava (*Piper methysticum*), ma huang (*Ephedra sinica*), American pennyroyal (*Hedeoma pulegoides*), European pennyroyal (*Mentha pulegium*), skullcap (*Scutellaria lateriflora*), white chameleon (*Atractylis gummifera*)

How does kava kava cause hepatotoxicity?

Mechanism is unknown, but it is thought to arise from contaminants in the manufacturing process. Natural kava, used primarily by Pacific Islanders, has not resulted in hepatotoxicity.

What is the hepatotoxic element in comfrey, and what are its specific effects on the liver?

Pyrrolizidine alkaloids, which can cause veno-occlusive disease of the liver

For what indications is goldenseal used?

1. As an antimicrobial (especially for colds, in combination with echinacea)
2. Fever/inflammation
3. Drug abuse masking agent
4. Gallbladder disease

What are the toxic effects of goldenseal?

Large doses have been associated with nausea, vomiting, CNS depression, hyperreflexia, seizures, paralysis, and respiratory failure.

What electrolyte abnormalities are associated with licorice consumption?

Chronic consumption of licorice root, which contains glycyrrhizic acid, may cause pseudohyperaldosteronism, resulting in hypokalemia and hypernatremia.

What herbal product used for smoking cessation contains a substance similar to nicotine?

Lobelia, which contains lobeline

What dietary supplement was associated with eosinophilia-myalgia syndrome?

Manufactured L-tryptophan. This syndrome of myalgias, arthralgias, and eosinophilia was associated with L-tryptophan produced by a single manufacturer in 1989 and 1990.

How is yohimbine used?

Yohimbine is an alpha 2-adrenergic antagonist derived from the yohimbe tree and is often used as a stimulant and for erectile dysfunction. Adverse effects include tachycardia, HTN, nausea, vomiting, and diaphoresis.

Cantharidin, used as a topical wart remover, has what toxic side effects?

Dermal irritation, GI hemorrhage, delirium, ataxia, renal toxicity

From where is cantharidin obtained?

It is a vesicant produced by blister beetles, most notably the Spanish fly.

What is the biggest danger of chamomile use?

Anaphylaxis in those allergic to the *Asteraceae/Compositae* families (ragweed pollens)

Which herbals increase INR and put patients who take warfarin at risk?

Devil's claw, dong quai, garlic, ginseng, papaya

What are "Chinese patent medicines"?

"Herbal" medicines produced by poorly regulated Chinese pharmaceutical companies. Their popularity has expanded as the worldwide use of alternative medicine has grown. While touted to be herbal, these products have been found to contain a variety of contaminants, including heavy metals, pharmaceutical products (e.g., benzodiazepines, NSAIDs), and other potentially harmful biologic products (e.g., centipede, toad secretions).

What are Ayurvedic medicines?

Traditional Indian remedies that usually contain heavy metals and herbal products. Lead, arsenic, and mercury may be present in large quantities in these products.

MARINE

INGESTED

Name some marine toxins that cause their effects after ingestion.

Scombroid, ciguatera, tetrodotoxin (TTX), paralytic shellfish poisoning (PSP), neurotoxic shellfish poisoning (NSP), amnesic shellfish poisoning (ASP), diarrheal shellfish poisoning (DSP)

Scombroid poisoning typically presents with what signs and symptoms?

Flushing of face and/or neck, sensation of warmth without fever, metallic and/or peppery taste in mouth, burning sensation of mouth and/or throat, nausea, abdominal cramping, diarrhea. Bronchospasm and hypotension are possible.

How soon after ingestion of scombrotoxic fish do symptoms present?

5 to 90 min

How long do symptoms typically last?

12 to 24 hrs

How do humans acquire scombroid poisoning?

Ingestion of poorly refrigerated or poorly preserved dark, or red-muscled, fish (e.g., tuna, mackerel, mahi-mahi, herring, sardine, anchovies)

What is the pathophysiology of scombroid poisoning?

Effects are caused by large amounts of histamine present in these fish, along with other toxins that may potentiate histamine's effect.

Does cooking these fish prevent scombroid poisoning?

No. Histamine is heat-stable and unaffected by cooking.

What is the treatment for scombroid poisoning?

1. Antihistamines – IV H_1 and H_2 blockers (e.g., diphenhydramine and cimetidine, respectively)
2. Bronchodilators (e.g., albuterol) can be helpful for bronchospasm.
3. Severe cases with hypotension and respiratory distress will require aggressive treatment with IV fluids, airway control, and possibly epinephrine.

Ingestion of what types of fish have been implicated in ciguatera poisoning?

Large predatory reef fish, including snapper, grouper, sea bass, barracuda, amberjack, mullet, tuna, and moray eel. Sturgeon have also been implicated.

How is ciguatoxin (CTX) bioaccumulated?

It is produced by the marine dinoflagellate *Gambierdiscus toxicus*, which grow on algae and dead coral and are consumed by herbivorous fish. The toxin is concentrated up the food chain as larger predatory fish consume multiple prey containing CTX.

Onset of symptoms occurs how long after ingestion of these contaminated fish?

Shows significant variability – as rapidly as 15 min, but delays may occur out to 24 hrs. Symptoms usually appear within 4 to 6 hrs following ingestion of contaminated fish.

What are the most common presenting symptoms of ciguatera poisoning?

CNS – seizures, respiratory depression, coma
CV – hypotension. Symptomatic bradycardia has occurred and has been hypothesized to be due to CTX's effects on the muscarinic autonomic nervous system.
GI – nausea, vomiting, diarrhea, abdominal pain
PNS – paresthesias, hot/cold reversal, headache, weakness, vertigo, ataxia, myalgias, pruritus

Hot and cold reversal is often cited as a classic symptom of ciguatera poisoning. What does this actually describe?

Often described as cold objects feeling hot. More accurately, though, contact with cold seems to cause painful tingling, burning discomfort, or an electric shock sensation.

Co-ingestion of what other toxin potentiates these symptoms?

Ethanol. Ingestion of ethanol after recovery can cause a recurrence of symptoms, and, therefore, should be avoided for up to 6 months.

What is the mechanism of action of CTX?

Binds to sodium channels $\rightarrow$ $\uparrow$ Na^+ influx $\rightarrow$ repetitive firing and constant activation. Also, sodium influx may lead to axonal swelling and slowed conduction.

What characteristics make CTX a highly effective human poison?

Stability in hot, cold, and acidic environments. It also does not alter the taste or appearance of the fish.

What are the suggested treatments for CTX poisoning?

1. Administer supportive care with attention to the common presentation of dehydration with potential electrolyte abnormalities secondary to vomiting and diarrhea.
2. Symptomatic bradycardia should be treated with atropine.
3. Pruritus can be treated with antihistamines.
4. Mannitol 1 g/kg over 45 min has been used to treat acute neurological symptoms (although evidence for its effectiveness is questioned)
5. Amitriptyline and gabapentin have been used to lessen residual neurologic symptoms.

Are there any long-term sequelae from CTX poisoning?

Yes. Patients may suffer from intermittent paresthesias, pruritus, and myalgias for months to years after acute poisonings.

Is the ingestion of pufferfish the only cause of tetrodotoxin (TTX) poisoning?

No. TTX is found in many species, including blowfish, xanthid crabs, horseshoe crabs, toadfish, California and Oregon newts, and the blue-ringed octopus.

TTX poisoning presents with what array of symptoms?

1. Paresthesias are common and typically the first symptom to be reported, usually beginning within an hour post-ingestion. Paresthesias initially affect the tongue, lips, and mouth and progress to involve the extremities.
2. GI symptoms may be seen and include nausea, vomiting, and diarrhea (less often).
3. Headache, blurred vision, pleuritic chest pain, dizziness, diaphoresis, hypersalivation, and bronchorrhea have been reported.
4. Dysphagia, aphonia, and other cranial nerve abnormalities are possible.
5. Ascending paralysis progressing to respiratory failure
6. Bradycardia, hypotension, and refractory heart block
7. Death can occur within hours secondary to respiratory muscle paralysis or profound hypotension.

What is the mechanism of action of TTX?

1. Binds to voltage-gated sodium channel site named toxin site 1 → inhibits Na^+ influx → blockade of neurotransmission at central, peripheral, and autonomic sites → poor nerve and muscle function
2. Direct relaxation of vascular smooth muscle → hypotension

What is the treatment for TTX poisoning?

1. Aggressive supportive care, ensuring adequate ventilation.
2. Hypotension should be treated with IV fluids and vasopressors, if necessary.
3. Temporary pacing for refractory heart block may be needed.
4. Activated charcoal and gastric lavage with alkaline solution can be considered early following ingestion, although these treatments are of unproven benefit.

5. Most patients require admission, with care in an ICU setting if they demonstrate significant clinical effects.
6. Long-term sequelae are rare if the patient survives.

Can patients be exposed to TTX by routes other than ingestion?

Yes. The bite of the blue-ringed octopus can cause TTX poisoning.

What are the neurological syndromes caused by shellfish poisoning?

PSP, NSP, ASP (see above)

What is the major toxic component that causes PSP?

Saxitoxin (STX)

What is the primary mechanism of STX?

Similar to TTX, it binds to site 1 on the voltage-gated sodium channel, causing inhibition of sodium influx.

What are the signs and symptoms of PSP, and how is it treated?

Presents in a similar fashion to TTX and should be treated the same way

What agent is responsible for amnestic shellfish poisoning?

Domoic acid

What is the mechanism of action of domoic acid?

Domoic acid is a structural analogue of glutamic acid and kainic acid and, therefore, will act as an excitatory neurotransmitter. Overstimulation of the neurons → excessive Ca^{2+} influx → cell death

What are the clinical manifestations of domoic acid poisoning?

Onset is from 15 min to 38 hrs post-ingestion and can manifest with nausea, vomiting, abdominal cramps, diarrhea, headache, confusion, ophthalmoplegia, purposeless chewing, grimacing, bronchorrhea, hypotension, dysrhythmias, seizures, coma, and death.

What is the prognosis?

Mortality is ~2%. Up to 10% can suffer long-term antegrade memory deficits.

Autopsy results implicate damage to both the hippocampus and the amygdala.

What agent is responsible for NSP?

Brevetoxin

What is the mechanism of action of brevetoxin?

Opens sodium channels, producing similar manifestations to ciguatera poisoning

How does DSP present?

Severe GI symptoms (e.g., nausea, vomiting, abdominal cramps, diarrhea) without neurological symptoms. Onset is typically 30 to 120 min post-ingestion and should be treated supportively.

What is clupeotoxism?

Poisoning from the ingestion of plankton-eating fish (i.e., sardines, herring, anchovies). Although rare, it is widespread in the tropical and subtropical regions. It can cause severe poisoning with a metallic taste, GI distress, paresthesias, paralysis, coma, and possibly death.

What is the treatment?

Supportive care

What is palytoxin?

A toxin originating in soft coral species and occasionally found in the flesh of some crabs and fish

What is the mechanism of action of palytoxin?

Allows influx of cations into smooth, skeletal, and cardiac myocytes, causing muscle contraction

What are the symptoms of palytoxin poisoning?

Severe myalgias, low back pain, chest pain, respiratory distress (asthma-like), hemolysis, and cardiac arrest

What do CTX, PSP, ASP, NSP, and DSP have in common?

The toxins involved in all of these originate in dinoflagellates.

Does there need to be a "red tide" in order for there to be a risk of dinoflagellate-associated shellfish poisonings?

No. Not all outbreaks are associated with toxic algal blooms.

INVERTEBRATES

Venomous marine invertebrates come from which phyla?	1. Porifera (sponges) 2. Annelida (bristleworms) 3. Cnidaria (jellyfish, corals) 4. Mollusca (octopus, cone snails) 5. Echinodermata (starfish, sea urchins)
What jellyfish are commonly implicated in human envenomations?	1. Box jellyfish (especially *Chironex fleckeri* and *Carukia barnesi*) 2. Portuguese man-of-war (*Physalia* spp.) 3. Sea nettles (*Chrysaora* spp.)
How do jellyfish envenomate humans?	With nematocysts – stinging cells that fire a venom-containing, harpoon-like apparatus into the victim
What are the common signs and symptoms of jellyfish envenomation?	Immediate local pain/irritation and urticaria
Describe the general treatment of Cnidaria envenomation.	1. Remove attached tentacles with hand protection or a mechanical device. 2. Vinegar can be applied to inactivate the venom. 3. Cover the affected area with paste of baking soda, sand, or shaving cream, and scrape with a flat-edged object to remove remaining nematocysts. 4. Topical anesthetics may be used for pain relief.
What treatments should be avoided after envenomation?	Avoid washing with fresh water or rubbing the site of envenomation, as either of these actions may result in discharge of the nematocysts.
***Chironex fleckeri* envenomation has caused multiple deaths along the coast of what country?**	Australia
***Chironex fleckeri* venom is believed to cause death by what mechanism?**	Cardiotoxicity

To what jellyfish is there an antivenom?

Chironex fleckeri

What is Irukandji syndrome?

A painful hypertensive syndrome that has been described following stings from the Irukandji jellyfish. The syndrome is characterized by generalized and severe pain, muscle spasm, HTN, tachydysrhythmias, and rarely pulmonary edema.

The venom of which jellyfish causes Irukandji syndrome, and where is it found?

Carukia barnesi, found in the Indo-Pacific region. A similar syndrome has been described following stings of other jellyfish in U.S. waters. The latter is rare.

When should a baking soda slurry be used instead of vinegar to treat a jellyfish envenomation?

When a sea nettle envenomation is suspected (Chesapeake Bay)

What is sea bather's eruption?

A reaction to the venom of jellyfish larvae that causes a pruritic, maculopapular rash

How can sea bather's eruption be avoided?

Remove swimwear and wash with salt water (freshwater causes larvae to sting)

What echinoderms can envenomate humans?

1. Sea urchins
2. Crown-of-thorns seastar
3. Sea cucumbers

What are the signs and symptoms of echinoderm envenomation?

Local pain and swelling, conjunctivitis (from sea cucumber venom), rarely systemic features (i.e., nausea, vomiting, hypotension)

What test can be useful in evaluating echinoderm envenomation?

Plain x-ray to look for embedded spines

How do sponges generally cause injury?

They contain silica or calcium carbonate spicules that embed in the skin, resulting in mild dermatitis. These spicules can usually be removed with adhesive tape.

How should "fire sponge" envenomations be treated?

Copious irrigation and vinegar

Bristleworm stings cause what signs and symptoms?

Local burning, urticaria, erythema

Cone snail venom can cause death by what mechanism?

Respiratory failure due to paralysis. Cone snail venom contains a variety of "cono-toxins" that generally work by blocking neuronal ion channels.

What octopus has been known to envenomate humans?

The Australian blue-ringed octopus (*Hapalochlaena* spp.)

What is the mechanism of the *Hapalochlaena* spp. venom?

Neurotoxin that blocks voltage-sensitive sodium channels

***Hapalochlaena* spp. venom is identical to what other marine toxin?**

Tetrodotoxin

VERTEBRATES

What are three ways marine vertebrates can poison people?

1. Venomous spines – sting rays, venomous fish
2. Venomous fangs – sea snakes
3. Ingestion – ciguatera, scombroid

What is the mechanism of stingray injury?

Both traumatic and venomous. A whip-ping tail movement results in puncture wounds from the serrated spine, at which time venom is introduced into the wound.

Where on the body do most stingrays strike people?

Lower legs. After being stepped on, the tail of the stingray reflexively curls like a scorpion, usually striking the leg.

What is the treatment of a stingray envenomation?

1. Irrigation of the wound with removal of any remaining spines
2. Immersion of the injured area in hot (45°C/113°F) water for 30 to 90 min
3. Additional pain control with opioids and local anesthesia may be necessary.

4. Evaluate with radiography for retained foreign body.
5. Prophylactic antibiotics

Why is hot water used to treat stingray envenomations?

The toxin is heat-labile and degrades at higher temperatures.

Name some other fish that cause painful envenomations.

Scorpionfish, stonefish, weeverfish, catfish

Describe the manifestations of these envenomations.

Extreme pain is the primary symptom. Blanching of the skin around the wound may occur. Systemic symptoms are generally mild but may include HTN, tachycardia, nausea, vomiting, weakness, and vertigo. Wounds should be evaluated for the presence of foreign bodies.

Stonefish are native to which waters?

Tropical waters of the Central Pacific, Indo-Pacific, and East African coastline

How is a stonefish envenomation treated?

Similar to stingray envenomation (i.e., remove foreign material, irrigate, soak in hot water, pain control). An antivenom to stonefish is also available.

Where are venomous sea snakes found?

Tropical waters of the Indian and Pacific Oceans, including Hawaii. They are not found in the Atlantic Ocean.

What are the clinical findings of a sea snake envenomation?

Generalized muscle aches and weakness usually begin 30 min to 4 hrs after envenomation. This may be followed by varying degrees of ascending and bulbar paralysis, depending on the extent of envenomation. Nausea and vomiting will also likely be present.

Describe the mechanism of action of sea snake venom.

Neurotoxins cause paralysis and respiratory failure. Hemotoxins and myotoxins are also present, but to a lesser extent.

What is the treatment of venomous sea snake bites?	1. Light pressure immobilization of the affected limb may be beneficial for field transport. 2. Supportive care, including respiratory support 3. Polyvalent sea snake antivenom is available for multiple species.

MUSHROOMS

COPRINE GROUP

What is the name of the most common coprine-containing mushroom?	*Coprinus atramentarius* (aka "alcohol inky" or "inky cap")
What is the appearance and the habitat of *C. atramentarius*?	<u>Cap</u> – 3 to 7 cm, smooth, ovular, grayish-brown. The cap turns black and liquefies after being picked. <u>Stalk</u> – 4 to 5 cm <u>Spores</u> – black <u>Habitat</u> – along roadsides and in urban areas during the fall months
Coprine toxins cause toxic symptoms when consumed in combination with what substance?	Ethanol
What physiologic enzyme is inhibited by coprine toxin?	Aldehyde dehydrogenase
What pharmacotherapy for alcohol abuse yields symptoms similar to coprine toxin?	Disulfiram
What mushroom produces symptoms identical to *Coprinus* species but has not been shown to contain coprine toxin?	*Clitocybe clavipes* (also known as "club-foot funnel cap")
Describe the appearance of *C. clavipes*.	<u>Cap</u> – 2–6 cm, flat, grayish-brown, with gills extending down to the stalk

Stalk – 1–5 cm with a thickened base
Spores – white

What physical manifestations are associated with coprine toxicity?

Symptoms are the same as those of a disulfiram reaction – nausea, vomiting, flushing, distal paresthesias, tachycardia, possibly hypotension

What is the timing of symptom onset?

30 to 60 min after consumption of ethanol. The toxin can remain systemically active up to 5 days; thus, symptoms can occur with delayed ethanol ingestion.

What is the treatment for coprine toxicity?

1. IV fluids and supportive care
2. Antiemetics
3. Vasopressors for refractory hypotension

CORTINARIUS GROUP

What is the principle toxin responsible for poisoning from *Cortinarius* mushrooms?

Orellanine

Describe the appearance and habitat of the most common orellanine-containing mushroom, *C. orellanus*.

Cap – small, bell-shaped, bright orange-brown
Stalk – yellow stalk
Gills and spores – rust-colored
Habitat – endemic to Europe and Japan, increasingly found in the U.S., most often grow beneath hardwood trees

What is the physiologic mechanism whereby orellanine causes toxicity?

Mechanism is poorly defined, but it is thought to work by inhibition of alkaline phosphatase in the renal tubules → ↓ production of ADP and impaired cellular metabolism

What are the initial clinical manifestations of toxicity?

The symptoms are variable and dose-dependent:
24 to 36 hrs post-ingestion – abdominal pain, nausea, vomiting, thirst

2 days to 2 wks post-ingestion – chills, night sweats, flank pain, polyuria, or oliguria

What is the ultimate outcome for nearly 50% of patients with orellanine toxicity?

Tubulointerstitial nephritis and acute renal failure, occurring 3 to 20 days post-ingestion

What 4 laboratory findings may be helpful in detecting early toxic renal failure?

1. Microscopic hematuria
2. Leukocyturia
3. Elevated BUN
4. Elevated creatinine

What measures are recommended to treat orellanine toxicity?

Supportive care with special attention to renal function, which returns in ~50% to 65% of affected patients

CYCLOPEPTIDE GROUP

What are the 3 subgroups of cyclopeptides?

1. Amatoxin
2. Phallotoxin
3. Virotoxin

Which subgroup is primarily associated with potentially lethal toxicity?

Amatoxins. Phallotoxins may cause GI upset if a large quantity is ingested, while virotoxins are nontoxic to humans.

Can amatoxins be deactivated by proper preparation?

No. They resist heating, drying, and all forms of cooking and are insoluble in water.

What is the name of the most notorious and most lethal of the cyclopeptide mushrooms?

Amanita phalloides (aka the "death cap")

Describe the appearance of *A. phalloides*.

<u>Cap</u> – 4 to 15 cm, convex, white or greenish
<u>Stalk</u> – 5 to 17 cm, thick with a thin ring and a large bulb at its base
<u>Gills</u> – white or green
Spores – white

What is the natural habitat of *A. phalloides*?

Throughout Europe and the coastal U.S., growing from late summer through fall, often around hardwood trees (e.g., oak chestnut, beech, birch, pine). It shares both appearance and distribution with many nontoxic mushrooms.

Through what physiologic mechanism do amatoxins cause toxicity?

Bind and inhibit RNA polymerase II, preventing protein and DNA synthesis and causing cell death. This most profoundly affects tissues of high cellular turnover in the liver, renal tubules, and GI tract.

What is the triad of clinical phases encountered following amatoxin ingestion?

Phase 1 (6 to 24 hrs) – delayed-onset GI distress
Phase 2 (24 to 96 hrs) – apparent clinical recovery but declining hepatic and renal function
Phase 3 (2 to 4 days up to 2 wks) – fulminant hepatic and renal failure

What physical manifestations typify phase 1 of amatoxin poisoning?

Primarily GI – severe abdominal pain, cramping, watery diarrhea and emesis, potentially leading to dehydration and circulatory collapse

What are the most ominous clinical predictors of mortality in phase 3 of amatoxin poisoning?

Hepatic encephalopathy, hypoglycemia, coagulopathy, metabolic acidosis

What is the Meixner test, and how can it detect the presence of amatoxin?

Juice from a mushroom is dripped onto newspaper (must contain lignin) and allowed to dry. HCl is then added. A blue color change within several minutes suggests amatoxin is present.

What toxin can yield a false-positive Meixner test?

Psilocybin

Does activated charcoal have a role in amatoxin exposure?

Possibly. It can be repeated q2–4 hrs for 48 hrs following ingestion.

What are three specific pharmacologic therapies that may provide hepatoprotection from amatoxin poisoning (though supportive studies in humans are still lacking)?

1. Silibinin (milk thistle)
2. *N*-acetylcysteine
3. Penicillin (high-dose)

What other treatments may be effective in treating amatoxin poisoning?

Extracorporeal albumin dialysis or liver transplant for patients with hepatic failure. Treatment is otherwise supportive.

GASTROINTESTINAL IRRITANT GROUP

How many genera of mushrooms are classified as GI irritants?

19 (including hundreds of species)

What is the most commonly ingested GI irritant mushroom in North America?

Chlorophyllum molybdites

Describe the appearance of *C. molybdites*.

<u>Cap</u> – 10 to 40 cm, smooth, round, white, occasionally with brownish warts
<u>Stalk</u> – 5 to 25 cm, white, smooth
<u>Gills</u> – yellow, become green as the mushroom ages
<u>Spores</u> – green

How can toxicity from the majority of GI irritant mushrooms be reduced or prevented?

Adequate preparation – heating/boiling is sufficient for many species

What is the clinical presentation of acute toxicity?

GI symptoms within 30 to 120 min of ingestion – abdominal cramping, watery diarrhea, nausea, emesis. Chills, headaches, and myalgias may also be present.

How long do symptoms typically last?

Commonly 6 to 12 hrs, but the time-course is dose- and species-dependent

What is the primary course of treatment for toxicity?

Supportive care with consideration of other, more toxic mushrooms that may have been co-ingested (especially if onset of symptoms is >2 hrs)

What is the general rule concerning the time-course of symptoms following mushroom ingestion?

Patients with nausea and vomiting within 6 hrs of ingestion typically have a benign course, whereas patients with nausea and vomiting beyond 6 hrs post-ingestion are more likely to have ingested a cyclopetide or other more toxic group of mushrooms; however, one must always consider a mixed-species ingestion.

What other poisonings must be considered for nausea and vomiting following mushroom ingestion?

Pesticide, herbicide, bacterial food poisoning

HALLUCINOGEN GROUP

What is the primary toxin responsible for the psychoactive effects of hallucinogenic mushrooms?

Psilocybin

What is the most common genus of psilocybin-containing mushrooms?

Psilocybe (also, some members of genera *Gymnopilus*, *Panaeolus*, and *Stropharia*)

Describe the common appearance of a *Psilocybe* mushroom.

Cap – 0.5 to 4 cm, brown, smooth, may become slippery or sticky when wet
Stalk – 4 to 15 cm, thin
Spores – dark brown or black

With what drug of abuse does psilocybin share a similar structure and function?

LSD. Both augment serotonergic neuronal activity.

What is the common term for hallucinogenic mushrooms?

"Magic mushrooms"

What ancient civilization is known to have used hallucinogenic mushrooms in religious ceremonies?

The Aztecs

What are the clinical manifestations of psilocybin intoxication?	30 to 60 min post-ingestion – euphoria, paresthesias, tachycardia, mydriasis, visual hallucinations, synesthesia, time distortion. Seizures have been reported with heavy intoxication.
How long do hallucinations typically last?	4 to 6 hrs
What is the primary mode of treatment for toxicity?	Observation and supportive care. Placing patient in a dark room without sensory stimuli may reduce hallucinations.
What pharmacologic therapies are recommended for intoxication?	Benzodiazepines for seizures or agitation

IBOTENIC/MUSCIMOL GROUP

What two species of mushrooms are primarily known to contain ibotenic acid and muscimol toxins?	1. *Amanita muscaria* 2. *Amanita pantherina*
What prominent children's book depicts the *Amanita muscaria* mushroom?	*Alice in Wonderland*
Describe the appearance and habitat of *A. muscarina*.	<u>Cap</u> – 5 to 30 cm, bright orange or red, covered in white warts <u>Stalk</u> – hollow, white, upward-tapering <u>Habitat</u> – often found under hardwood and conifer trees throughout North America, primarily in the western states
Describe the appearance and habitat of *A. pantherina*.	<u>Cap</u> – 5 to 15 cm, reddish-brown that darkens with age, may or may not have warts <u>Stem</u> – white with distinct rings <u>Habitat</u> – found throughout North America
What is the physiologic mechanism of ibotenic acid toxicity?	Ibotenic acid resembles the stimulatory neurotransmitter glutamate and causes hallucinations, myoclonic activity, and possibly seizures.

To what substance is ibotenic acid metabolized?

Muscimol

What is the physiologic mechanism of muscimol toxicity?

Muscimol agonizes GABA receptors, thereby causing CNS depression.

What are the clinical manifestations of toxicity?

Variable and can resemble both the excitatory or inhibitory nature of the toxin. Symptoms include emesis, followed by drowsiness, dizziness, ataxia, and confusion. This may progress to myoclonic jerking, hallucinations, delirium, seizures, or coma.

What is the typical duration of symptoms?

Typically 6 to 8 hrs, but may take up to 48 hrs for full resolution

What pharmacologic therapies are recommended for toxicity?

Benzodiazepines for seizures or severe agitation

What is the primary treatment for toxicity?

Supportive care, as the course is typically self-limiting

MONOMETHYLHYDRAZINES GROUP

What species of mushroom is responsible for monomethylhydrazine toxicity?

Gyromitra species, the most common being *Gyromitra esculenta*. These species contain the toxin gyromitrin (monomethylhydrazine).

What are three common names for *G. esculenta*?

1. "Brain fungi"
2. "Beefsteak mushroom"
3. "False morel"

What is the appearance and the habitat of *G. esculenta*?

<u>Cap</u> – dark, reddish-brown, irregular shape (i.e., folded and resembles a brain)
<u>Stalk</u> – 5 to 15 cm, long, thick, hollow
<u>Habitat</u> – endemic to Eastern Europe and throughout N. America, grows in sandy soil near pine trees during the spring months

For which highly sought-after, edible mushroom is G. esculenta commonly mistaken?

Morchella esculenta (common morel)

What is the physiologic mechanism whereby monomethylhydrazine causes toxicity?

Competitive inhibition of pyridoxine kinase → functional pyridoxine deficiency → ↓ GABA production/availability

What anti-tuberculosis therapy has an adverse reaction profile similar to monomethylhydrazine?

Isoniazid (INH)

In what industry is monomethylhydrazine found?

Aerospace industry. It is a primary component of rocket fuel.

Can toxicity be reduced or prevented by adequate preparation prior to ingestion?

Yes, with sufficient boiling; however, inhaling the hydrazine vapors can also be toxic

Describe the initial clinical presentation of toxicity.

5 to 12 hrs post-ingestion – emesis and diarrhea, followed by fatigue, dizziness, and headache, with potential progression to delirium, seizure, and coma

What late complication may occur from toxicity?

Liver failure (3 to 4 days post-ingestion)

What hematologic manifestation can result from toxicity?

Methemoglobinemia or hemolysis

What are three specific pharmacologic therapies available for toxicity complications?

1. Pyridoxine (vitamin B_6) for delirium and seizures
2. Methylene blue for symptomatic methemoglobinemia or methemoglobin level >30%
3. Glucose for hypoglycemia

MUSCARINE GROUP

What are the primary genera of mushrooms containing sufficient levels of muscarine to produce toxicity?	1. *Clitocybe* 2. *Inocybe* Contrary to its name, *Amanita muscaria* contains very little muscarine.
Describe the appearance and habitat of *Clitocybe* mushrooms.	Cap – 1.5 to 3 cm, flattened, grayish-brown Stalk – 1 to 5 cm, tapered Gills – run down along stalk Habitat – found on lawns and in parks during the summer and fall months
Describe the appearance and habitat of *Inocybe* mushrooms.	<u>Cap</u> – 5 to 6 cm, conical, brown <u>Stalk</u> – 2 to 10 cm, thin, covered in fine white hairs <u>Gills</u> – brown <u>Spores</u> – brown <u>Habitat</u> – found under conifer and hardwood trees during the summer and fall months
What is the physiologic mechanism of toxicity from muscarine?	It is a pro-cholinergic agent, with the primary effect of stimulating acetylcholine-sensitive receptors of the parasympathetic nervous system.
What acronym is helpful for remembering the symptoms associated with toxicity?	DUMBELS **D**efecation **U**rination **M**iosis **B**ronchorrhea/**B**ronchospasm/ **B**radycardia **E**mesis **L**acrimation **S**alivation
How long following toxin ingestion do symptoms typically present?	15 to 45 min
How long do symptoms typically last?	6 to 24 hrs, but this is dose-dependent

Is activated charcoal effective in toxicity?

Yes, if initiated soon after ingestion

List three pharmacologic therapies that may be beneficial in muscarine toxicity.

1. Atropine for severe cholinergic symptoms. Respiratory symptoms, such as bronchospasm and bronchorrhea, should guide therapy.
2. Albuterol for bronchospasm
3. Benzodiazepines for agitation or seizures

MYCOTOXINS

What are mycotoxins?

Mycotoxins are chemicals produced by filamentous fungi that may impart disease to other organisms. Toxic substances in mushrooms are not considered true mycotoxins.

What is the purpose of mycotoxins?

Mycotoxins are produced by fungal metabolism and generally have little or no use to the organism; however, some have been speculated to provide an evolutionary advantage to the fungi.

How are humans typically exposed to mycotoxins?

Mycotoxins are found in small quantities in many grains, nuts, and seeds. Occasionally, quantities are sufficient to cause acute disease in humans. Examples include outbreaks of hepatitis in India related to aflatoxin, "red mold disease" caused by trichothecene mycotoxins in Japan and Korea, and even an outbreak of possible ergotism that led to the Salem Witch Trials. More recently, mycotoxins have reportedly been used as biologic weapons.

Which are potential bioterrorism weapons?

Trichothecenes (T-2 toxin and vomitoxin), aflatoxins, ochratoxins, ergot alkaloids, and fumonisin are capable of inducing disease in humans and have the most potential to be used as bioweapons.

What are trichothecenes?

A family of >60 compounds produced by several fungi, including *Fusarium*, *Myrothecium*, *Phomopsis*, *Stachybotrys*, *Trichoderma*, and *Trichothecium*. All contain a common 12, 13-epoxytrichothene skeleton. T-2 toxin is regarded as the most toxic of this class and has a reported LD_{50} of ~1 mg/kg.

How was T-2 discovered?

Multiple outbreaks of hemorrhagic GI illness and leukopenia were reported in the Ukraine and in Orenburg, Russia in the 1930s and 1940s. In 1940, Soviet scientists coined the term "stachybotryotoxicosis" to describe the acute syndrome of sore throat, bloody nasal discharge, dyspnea, cough, and fever due to *Stachybotrys* mycotoxins. These outbreaks resulted in the isolation of T-2 toxin in 1968.

To what does the term "yellow rain" refer?

The "yellow rain" attacks occurred in Southeast Asia in the late 1970s. Reportedly, a sticky yellow substance was aerosolized by aircraft and bombs among the Hmong tribes in Laos and Cambodia. When falling on trees and dwellings, it had the sound of rain. While speculated to be T-2 toxin, debate exists as to the true identity of yellow rain.

What are the routes of T-2 exposure?

Inhalation, ingestion, dermal. This makes the toxin a highly effective bioweapon due to its multiple portals of entry.

How can T-2 be delivered as a biological warfare agent?

The toxins are extremely stable proteins resistant to heat, autoclaving, hypochlorite, and ultraviolet light. They can be delivered as dusts, droplets, or aerosols from various dispersal systems and exploding munitions.

What are the signs and symptoms of T-2 exposure?

Skin itching/irritation, vesicles, nausea, vomiting, diarrhea, upper airway irritation, and GI hemorrhage

What is the management of T-2 toxicity?

1. Supportive care, removal from the source of exposure, and decontamination
2. Dexamethasone has improved survival times in animal studies
3. Granulocyte colony-stimulating factor (G-CSF) may be beneficial for bone marrow suppression.

Are there any helpful laboratory studies?

None will be diagnostic:
1. CBC – useful in evaluating blood loss due to GI hemorrhage and to monitor for bone marrow suppression
2. Electrolytes and organ function tests (i.e., LFTs, RFTs) should be monitored as markers of the degree of toxicity.

What are aflatoxins?

Naturally occurring mycotoxins produced by many species of *Aspergillus*. Aflatoxin B1 is considered the most potent natural carcinogen known.

Where are aflatoxins found?

Crops frequently affected are cereals, oilseeds, and tree nuts. They can also be found in the milk of animals that have ingested contaminated feed.

Can aflatoxins be used as bioweapons?

Yes. Iraq was known to have weaponized alfatoxins before the first Gulf War.

What are the physical effects of exposure?

High-level exposure produces acute hepatic necrosis and cirrhosis. Chronic subclinical exposure leads to an elevated risk of liver cancer (IARC Group 1).

Is there any other associated disease that increases the risks of chronic aflatoxin exposure?

Concurrent infection with hepatitis B virus (HBV) during aflatoxin exposure increases the risk of hepatocellular carcinoma.

How does ochratoxin cause disease?

Nephrotoxicity. Its mechanism of action appears to be inhibition of protein synthesis and induction of oxidation in the renal tubules.

Does ochratoxin cause acute toxicity?

No. Ochratoxin appears to cause disease only after chronic ingestion. Signs and symptoms are those of progressive renal failure.

How do ergot alkaloids cause toxicity?

Ergot alkaloids possess an indole ring structure and alpha-adrenergic agonist properties. These features can result in hallucinations and peripheral vasoconstriction.

What is gangrenous ergotism?

Peripheral vascular insufficiency caused by the vasoconstrictive effects of ergots results in limb pain, numbness, and possibly progression to dry gangrene and limb loss.

By what name was ergotism known in the Middle Ages?

St. Anthony's fire

From which fungus is ergot derived?

Claviceps purpurea

What is convulsive ergotism?

Seizures, muscle spasms, paresthesias, mania, and psychosis that occur as a result of the toxin. GI effects (i.e., nausea, vomiting, diarrhea) precede CNS effects. Hallucinations may occur and are similar to those produced by LSD.

What is the treatment for ergot poisoning?

1. Remove the source of exposure.
2. Benzodiazepines for seizures
3. Sodium nitroprusside or phentolamine may be used for treatment of vasoconstriction.

PLANTS

ANTICHOLINERGIC

Name the prototypical anticholinergic plant.

Atropa belladonna (aka "deadly nightshade")

List other plants known to contain anticholinergic alkaloids.

1. *Datura stramonium* (jimsonweed)
2. *Mandragora officinarum* (European mandrake)

3. *Hyosyamus niger* (henbane)
4. *Brugmansia arborea* (angel's trumpet)
5. *Atropa belladonna* (deadly nightshade)

What is the primary toxin in anticholinergic plants?

Atropine, may contain hyoscyamine and scopolamine

Describe the pathophysiology of atropine poisoning.

Competitive inhibition of postsynaptic muscarinic receptors

How many milligrams of atropine are contained in each jimsonweed seed?

~0.1 mg

Which plant was responsible for poisoning British troops at Jamestown during the American Revolutionary War?

Datura stramonium, aka "Jamestown weed" or jimsonweed

Recite the mnemonic used to remember anticholinergic signs and symptoms.

"Dry as a bone, red as a beet, mad as a hatter, blind as a bat, hot as a hare, full as a flask"

List signs and symptoms characteristic of the anticholinergic toxidrome.

Dry mucous membranes, dry and flushed skin, psychosis/delirium, mydriasis, hyperthermia, loss of bowel sounds, urinary retention, tachycardia

Why are anticholinergic plants often abused?

They have the ability to produce hallucinations.

How long may symptoms last following ingestion of an anticholinergic plant?

May last for days, depending on species and part of the plant ingested

List basic treatment principles.

1. Supportive care with consideration of activated charcoal
2. Benzodiazepines for agitation
3. Consider physostigmine for therapeutic or diagnostic purposes.

What is the half-life of physostigmine?

~1 hr; therefore, anticholinergic symptoms are likely to recur

CARDIAC GLYCOSIDES

What plants are known to contain cardiac glycosides?	1. Oleander (*Nerium oleander*) 2. Yellow oleander (*Thevetia peruviana*) 3. Foxglove (*Digitalis purpurea*) 4. Lily of the valley (*Convallaria majalis*) 5. Red squill (*Urginea maritime*)
How do cardiac glycosides exert their toxic effects on a cellular level?	Natural cardiac glycosides (e.g., ouabain, oleandrin, scilliroside, thevetin) resemble the medication digoxin. Inhibition of Na-K-ATPase $\rightarrow \uparrow$ intracellular Ca^{2+} (via sodium-calcium exchange) and $\uparrow$ extracellular K^+.
What effects do cardiac glycosides have on myocardial tissues?	1. Positive inotropy 2. Negative AV nodal dromotropy 3. Generation of myocardial irritability
How might an acute overdose of cardiac glycosides present?	Nausea, vomiting, bradycardia (or tachycardia), AMS, blurred/discolored vision (yellow-green halos around objects), headache, fatigue
What is the most common ECG manifestation of cardiac glycoside toxicity?	PVCs
What are the other possible ECG manifestations?	Tachydysrhythmias with AV block are typical, but almost any dysrhythmia may occur; exceptions to this are atrial fibrillation or flutter with rapid ventricular response. Pathognomonic rhythms include biventricular tachycardia and paroxysmal atrial tachycardia with AV block.
What doses of cardiac glycosides are considered toxic?	As little as a few seeds or a few leaves may be enough to cause severe toxicity. Patients may also become symptomatic after inhalation of smoke from these plants.
What laboratory tests are particularly useful for evaluation?	Potassium level and ECG

What electrolyte abnormality is a marker of toxicity?	Hyperkalemia
Are digoxin levels useful for evaluation?	Cardiac glycosides often cross-react with serum digoxin levels; therefore, they are useful as a marker of exposure but are not predictive of toxicity or outcome.
List the basic principles of treatment.	1. Supportive care with consideration of activated charcoal 2. Treatment of hyperkalemia 3. Digoxin immune Fab for select cases
List the indications for digoxin immune Fab.	1. Hyperkalemia (K^+ >5.0 mEq/L) 2. New AV block 3. Dysrhythmias
Should standard digoxin immune Fab formulas apply for treatment of plant-induced cardiac glycoside toxicity?	No. These formulas will underestimate the total dose necessary.
Which cardiac glycoside-containing plant is a major cause of intentional self-poisoning in underdeveloped countries, such as Sri Lanka?	Yellow oleander (*Thevetia peruviana*)

CYANOGENIC GLYCOSIDES

What are some common plant sources of cyanide toxicity?	Cassava root (*Manihot esculenta*), hydrangea (*Hydrangea* spp.), bitter almonds (*Prunus* spp.), peach pits (*Prunus* spp.), apricot pits (*Prunus* spp.), apple seeds (*Malus* spp.)
What are the 2 most prevalent cyanogenic glycosides?	1. Amygdalin 2. Linamarin
Name the amygdalin-containing product that was historically promoted for cancer treatment.	Laetrile

What is the pathophysiology of poisoning from cyanogenic glycosides?

Hydrolysis of cyanogenic glycosides → release of hydrogen cyanide → cytochrome oxidase a_3 inhibition → blockade of electron transport and oxygen utilization

What are the symptoms of acute cyanide toxicity?

Headache, dizziness, nausea, vomiting, abdominal pain, and anxiety minutes to hours post-ingestion. In severe cases, this may be followed by confusion, hypotension, seizures, coma, and death.

What are the signs of acute cyanide toxicity?

High anion-gap metabolic acidosis, ↑ lactic acid, ↑ venous oxygen saturation

What is the reported characteristic odor associated with cyanide toxicity?

"Bitter almond" odor on breath or vomitus

Describe the manifestations of chronic cyanogenic glycoside exposure.

Signs of upper motor neuron toxicity, (e.g., spasticity, hyperreflexia), visual disturbances, and hypothyroidism

By what names is this disease known?

Konzo or tropical spastic paraparesis

How is acute cyanide toxicity treated?

1. Supportive care with consideration of activated charcoal
2. Patients with symptom progression and those with acidosis should receive a cyanide antidote.

What cyanide antidotes are available for treatment?

1. Traditional cyanide antidote kit – amyl and sodium nitrite (induce methemoglobinemia to bind cyanide), thiosulfate (provides sulfur for conversion of cyanide to thiocyanate)
2. Hydroxocobalamin (preferred) – alternative treatment used in Europe and recently approved by the FDA for use in the United States. It binds cyanide to form cyanocobalamin (vitamin B_{12}).

DERMATITIS-PRODUCING

What plants most commonly cause allergic contact dermatitis?	Poison ivy, poison oak, and poison sumac (in that order). These members of the genus *Toxicodendron* exceed all other causes combined.
Where are poison ivy, poison oak, and poison sumac found?	In the U.S. Poison ivy is found primarily east of the Rockies, poison oak to the west of the Rockies, and poison sumac in marshy areas of the southeast.
What are other plants associated with allergic contact dermatitis?	Ginkgo tree, mango tree and fruit, and cashew tree and nuts. Mango and cashew are in the same plant family as poison ivy (*Anacardiaceae*).
What is the toxic compound released by these plants, and what type of response do they elicit?	An oleoresin called urushiol causes a type IV hypersensitivity response. In severe cases, a type I response with anaphylaxis may be seen.
How long after exposure is the dermatitis seen?	Usually within 1 to 2 days in a previously sensitized person and within 10 days in an individual without prior exposure. Symptom onset in <5 min may occur in the rare case of anaphylaxis.
What are the physical findings?	<u>Mild</u> – linear, erythematous and pruritic lesions with small papules and vesicles <u>Severe</u> – diffuse erythema and edema, severe pruritus/pain, bullae Respiratory symptoms (i.e., cough, dyspnea, oropharyngeal swelling) may occur following aerosol exposure from burning plants.
What percentage of people are susceptible?	50% to 70% react to exposure, though this is dose-dependent. 10% to 15% are extremely sensitive.
How is allergic contact dermatitis treated?	1. Immediate washing with soap and water 2. Topical preparations (e.g., domeboro, calamine, oatmeal baths, Burrow

solution) may help alleviate mild to moderate symptoms.
3. PO antihistamines for pruritus
4. Topical steroids are acceptable for mild symptoms; severe symptoms warrant oral steroids tapered over a 2-wk period.

What type of response is elicited by exposure to stinging nettle (*Urtica dioica*)?

Rapid response to direct toxin injection (i.e., histamine, ACh, serotonin) from the plant when disturbed. The histamine is responsible for skin irritation, while the ACh causes a burning sensation.

Where is stinging nettle found?

Northern Europe, Asia, and North America

Do plants cause other forms of dermatitis?

Yes. Plants can cause irritant dermatitis by both immune and nonimmune-mediated mechanisms.

What are some plants that cause nonimmune-mediated irritant dermatitis?

Wolfsbane (*Aconitum napellus*), Christmas rose (*Helleborus niger*), buttercup (*Ranunculus* spp.), meadow rue (*Thalictrum foliosum*)

What is the mechanism of toxicity of these plants?

These plants contain toxins that pass through the dermis and cause direct release of histamine from mast cells.

Name some plants that cause immune-mediated irritant dermatitis.

Tulips (*Tulipa* spp.), mustard (*Brassica* and *Sinapis* spp.), rapeseed (*Brassica* spp.), garlic (*Allium sativum*)

What is the mechanism of this type of dermatitis?

Transdermally absorbed toxins from these plants produce a type I hypersensitivity reaction.

What is the most common toxin involved in phytophototoxic reactions?

Furocoumarins

What is a phytophototoxic reaction?

Certain ingested or dermally absorbed plant toxins may cause sensitivity to UV rays, resulting in severe sunburn symptoms in sun-exposed areas. Chronic hyperpigmentation of the involved skin may occur after the exposure.

Name some common plants that may cause phytophototoxic reactions.	Celery (*Apium graveolens dulce*), carrot (*Daucus carota*), parsley (*Petroselinum crispum*), parsnip (*Pastinaca sativa*), Queen Anne's lace (*Ammi majus*), grapefruit (*Citrus paradissi*), lemon (*Citrus limon*), lime (*Citrus aurantifolia*)

GASTROINTESTINAL IRRITANTS

What are some plants that are commonly reported to cause GI irritation as their sole toxic effect?	1. Pokeweed (*Phytolacca americana*) 2. Hollybush (*Ilex aquifolium*) 3. English ivy (*Hedera helix*) 4. Wisteria (*Wisteria* spp.) 5. Poinsettia (*Euphorbia* spp.)
Are these the only plants that cause GI upset?	No. Many poisonous plants are irritating to the GI tract, but these plants solely produce GI symptoms.
What is the general mechanism of GI irritants?	Many of these plants contain saponin glycosides, which cause direct GI irritation.
What specific laboratory abnormality may be found after pokeweed exposure?	Mitogens in pokeweed stimulate leukocyte proliferation and may cause significant leukocytosis. This finding may be present 2 to 4 days following ingestion or exposure through compromised skin and may last for weeks.
What are the general symptoms of GI irritant toxicity?	Nausea, vomiting, abdominal pain, diarrhea
When do symptoms of GI irritant poisoning typically arise?	Generally within 2 to 4 hrs of ingestion, but onset is dose-dependent
Can pokeweed be eaten without harmful effects?	Yes, but only after the toxin (phytolaccotoxin) is properly boiled out (parboiled)

How much mistletoe can be consumed without toxic effect?

As few as 3 mistletoe berries can cause significant GI upset.

What symptoms accompany holly toxicity?

Nausea, vomiting, diarrhea. Death has been reported from aspiration of berries.

How should GI irritant toxicity be managed?

Supportive care with consideration of activated charcoal if within 2 hrs of ingestion. Fluid and electrolyte abnormalities may be sufficient to warrant hospital admission.

NICOTINICS

What are some common plant sources of nicotine toxicity?

All plants in the genus *Nicotiana* (tobacco), including *Nicotiana rustica* (Indian or Aztec tobacco), *Nicotiana tabacum* (common tobacco) and *Nicotiana glauca* (tree tobacco)

What other alkaloids are similar to nicotine?

Coniine, lobeline, sparteine, arecoline, cytosine, *N*-methylcytisine

What plants contain nicotine-like alkaloids?

Broom (sparteine), blue cohosh (*N*-methylcytisine), golden chain (cytisine), hemlock (coniine)

What herbal substance is often used to treat nicotine addiction?

Lobeline, a nicotine receptor agonist from the species *Lobelia inflata*

What famous philosopher was put to death by coniine poisoning?

Socrates, from the poison hemlock plant (*Conium maculatum*)

What are the signs and symptoms of nicotine poisoning?

GI symptoms (i.e., nausea, vomiting, diarrhea), followed by headache, diaphoresis, tachycardia, muscle fasciculations, hyperthermia, progressing to seizures, respiratory depression, bradycardia, paralysis, and death.

Describe the symptomatic progression of nicotine poisoning.

Stimulatory symptoms (sympathetic) appear to dominate initially and are then followed by muscarinic effects.

Describe the pathophysiology of nicotine poisoning.

Nicotine results in stimulation of the sympathetic and parasympathetic post-ganglionic neurons along with stimulation of the motor end plate.

What is green tobacco illness?

Nicotinic symptoms due to transdermal nicotine absorption into the systemic circulation in tobacco workers following repetitive exposure to moist, green tobacco leaves

How is nicotine poisoning treated?

1. Supportive care
2. Atropine may be given for bronchorrhea, bronchoconstriction, or bradycardia.
3. Benzodiazepines should be given for seizures.

What is the LD$_{50}$ of nicotine?

Adult – 40 to 60 mg (~1 mg/kg body weight)
Child – amount in one cigarette (or three cigarette butts), when ingested, is enough to make a child severely ill

OXALATES

What are the two types of oxalates found in plants?

Soluble and insoluble

What plants most commonly cause toxicity due to insoluble calcium oxalate?

Philodendron spp., *Caladium* spp., *Dieffenbachia* spp. (dumb cane), *Spathiphyllum* spp. (peace lily), *Arisaema* spp. (jack-in-the-pulpit)

What is the pathophysiology of insoluble oxalate toxicity?

Calcium oxalate crystals are contained in needle-like bundles called raphides. When the leaves are broken or chewed, mechanical stimulation of these raphides causes discharge of the oxalate needles. These needles cause irritation of the oral mucosa, lips, and tongue, as well as the skin and conjunctivae, resulting in local pain and edema.

What population is most susceptible to insoluble oxalate exposure?

Children <5 yrs who inquisitively ingest houseplants; however, others also have been exposed (e.g., foragers)

What treatment modalities are available for oxalate exposure?

1. As most cases are self-limited, analgesics are often sufficient.
2. Remove plant material from the mouth, and assess the airway in oral exposures.
3. Irrigate eyes and skin for these exposures.
4. Monitor for airway compromise due to edema.

What are soluble oxalates?

Oxalic acid is found in rhubarb leaves (*Rheum officinale*), sorrel (*Rumex* spp.), and starfruit (*Averrhoa carambola*), among others.

How do soluble oxalates cause toxicity?

Chelation of calcium and other divalent cations. Hypocalcemia may result in weakness, hyperreflexia, tetany, dysrhythmias, and seizures. Formation of calcium oxalate crystals in the renal tubules may result in renal failure. Rarely, calcium oxalate crystals may form in other organs (e.g., brain, spinal cord), resulting in AMS, paralysis, or other systemic toxicity.

What ECG findings may be present with soluble oxalate toxicity?

QTc prolongation (due to hypocalcemia)

What is the treatment of soluble oxalate toxicity?

IV calcium should be given for dysrhythmias, tetany, and seizures. Adequate urine output should be maintained with IV fluids.

SODIUM CHANNEL OPENERS

What role do sodium channels play in cells?

Control Na^+ influx through the cell's plasma membrane in response to action potentials

What plants contain substances that cause toxicity by opening (activating) sodium channels?

1. *Veratrum viride* (false hellebore), *Veratrum album* (white hellebore), *Veratrum californicum* (skunk cabbage), and some plants from genus *Zigadenus* (e.g., death camus) contain veratrum alkaloids.
2. *Rhododendron* spp., *Kalmia angustifolia* (sheep laurel), and *Kalmia latifolia* (mountain laurel) contain grayanotoxins.
3. *Aconitum* spp. (e.g., wolfsbane, monkshood) contain aconitine.

How do they enter the body?

Primarily by ingestion, although there can be absorption through mucous membranes (e.g., sneezing powder made from white hellebore)

By what mechanism do these toxins affect the sodium channels?

Bind to and open voltage-gated sodium channels $\rightarrow$ $\uparrow$ Na^+ influx

What clinical effects occur with poisoning by these plants?

Vomiting, diarrhea, abdominal pain, paresthesias, diaphoresis, blurred vision, hypotension, syncope, convulsions. Cardiotoxic effects may develop and include sinus bradycardia, nodal rhythms, and complete AV block with hypotension. Other conduction abnormalities, such as a transient Wolff-Parkinson-White pattern, have been observed.

Are any antidotes available for the sodium channel openers?

No. Treatment is primarily supportive. Hypotension and bradycardia can be treated with IV fluids and atropine. Activated charcoal can be considered if the patient presents soon after ingestion.

Sodium channel opener toxicity mimics the effects of what other toxin?

Cardiac glycosides. Both $\uparrow$ intracellular Na^+ $\rightarrow$ $\uparrow$ automaticity and $\uparrow$ vagal tone.

What laboratory value will help distinguish poisoning with a sodium channel opener from poisoning with a cardiac glycoside?

Potassium. Sodium channel openers do not affect the Na-K-ATPase and, therefore, will not cause hyperkalemia.

What is mad honey poisoning?

Toxicity resulting from the ingestion of honey produced by bees primarily using nectar from grayanotoxin-containing *Rhododendron* spp.

What genus of poisonous plants is mistaken for edible leeks (*Allium tricoccum*)?

Veratrum

Why might someone ingest death camases (*Zigadenus* spp.)?

Its bulb resembles that of an onion.

SOLANINE

What plants are common sources of solanine toxicity?

Most members of the genus *Solanum* contain solanine to varying degrees. The toxin is most concentrated in unripe fruits, sprouts, stalks, and stems.

Name some common solanine-containing plants.

1. *Solanum nigrum* (black nightshade)
2. *S. tuberosum* (common potato)
3. *S. melongena* (eggplant)
4. *S. pseudocapsicum* (Jerusalem cherry)
5. *Lycopersicon esculentum* (tomato)

Does cooking these plants alter their toxicity?

Baking, boiling, and microwaving appear to only minimally lower the levels of solanine. Deep frying at 170°C (338°F) is known to degrade solanine and substantially lower levels.

What are the signs and symptoms of solanine toxicity?

Nausea, vomiting, diarrhea, abdominal cramps, and hyperthermia are the predominant symptoms. In severe cases, hallucinations, delirium, cardiac dysrhythmias, seizures, and coma have been reported.

What is the typical time-course of symptoms?	Onset is 2 to 24 hrs post-ingestion, and duration is up to several days but depends on the amount and parts of the plant ingested.
Describe the mechanism of solanine toxicity.	Solanine inhibits cholinesterase in vitro, which is speculated to cause the majority of toxic effects. In addition, the solanine structure resembles that of cardiac glycosides, and it appears to alter cell membrane sodium transport, both of which may be mechanisms of cardiotoxicity.
What is the treatment for solanine poisoning?	Supportive care
What novel depicts an Alaskan adventurer whose demise may have been hastened by the effects of solanine poisoning?	*Into the Wild* by Jon Krakauer

TOXALBUMINS

What plants contain toxalbumins?	*Ricinus communis, Abrus precatorius, Jatropha curcas*
What toxalbumin is listed as Schedule 1 under the Chemical Weapons Convention?	Ricin
What toxalbumin was found enclosed in letters sent through the U.S. mail on multiple occasions?	Ricin
What are the plant sources of ricin and abrin?	Castor beans (ricin) and jequirity beans (abrin)
Where are the castor bean plant (*Ricinus communis*) and the jequirity bean plant (*Abrus precatorius*) found?	<u>Castor bean plant</u> – native to east Africa, although now grows in many tropical and warm regions, including the southern U.S. <u>Jequirity bean plant</u> – primarily in Southeast Asia, has spread to some subtropical regions, including Florida

What is the most common use of jequirity beans?

Ornamental purposes (e.g., rosary beads, maracas). They are known as "rosary peas."

Describe the structure and toxic mechanism of the toxalbumins.

They consist of an A and a B subunit. The B subunit allows for cellular entry by binding to galactose-containing receptors on the cell membrane, while the A subunit causes toxicity. The A subunit depurinates an adenine base of the 60S ribosomal subunit. This prevents binding of elongation factor 2 (EF2) and subsequently stops protein translation by RNA polymerase.

What are the signs and symptoms of toxalbumin exposure?

The clinical effects depend on the route and amount of exposure, with parenteral and inhalational exposure being most potent. The most frequent presentation after oral exposure is oropharyngeal irritation and GI distress, with abdominal pain, nausea, vomiting, and diarrhea. With more severe poisonings, symptoms can progress to dehydration, shock, GI hemorrhage, hemolysis, and renal or hepatic injury. If symptoms are severe, delirium, seizures, coma, and death may ensue.

What is the time course for symptom development?

After ingestion of ricin, symptoms will usually be evident within 4 to 6 hrs, although this may be delayed for up to 10 hrs. The symptom progression can take 4 to 36 hrs to fully manifest.

How is toxalbumin exposure treated?

Supportive care focusing on adequate hydration. If a patient presents early after ingestion, activated charcoal should be given.

Is swallowing a whole castor or jequirity bean dangerous?

No. The toxin is found primarily within the seed coat, and the bean must be chewed to break the hard outer shell and release the toxalbumin.

OTHER

Betel nut (*Areca catechu*) is a commonly chewed plant in the Indian, Asian, and Pacific cultures. What are the symptoms of intoxication?	Hallucinations and cholinergic symptoms – sweating, salivation, hyperthermia
What is the primary toxin in betel nuts?	Arecoline, a cholinergic agent that also has weak nicotinic effects
What is the potential long-term health effect of betel nut chewing?	Oral cancers
Tea made from which "medicinal" plant may contain pyrrolizidine alkaloids?	Comfrey
Pyrrolizidine alkaloid poisonings affect what organ in the body?	Chronic exposures cause veno-occlusive hepatic disease, and acute poisoning results in hepatic necrosis.
What is the mechanism of pyrrolizidine alkaloid toxicity?	These agents are metabolized to reactive pyrrole species by the P450 system. Chronic exposure results in intimal proliferation in the hepatic vasculature, sinusoidal congestion, and veno-occlusive disease. Acute toxicity appears to be mediated through oxidative stress.
Plants of the *Strychnos* genus contain what two potent toxins?	Strychnine (seeds – *Strychnos nux-vomica*) and curare (bark – *Strychnos* spp.)
Acute poisoning by the strychnine toxin causes what symptoms?	Muscle spasms and rigidity with preserved mental status
By what mechanism does strychnine act?	Antagonizes glycine receptors in the spinal cord and brainstem

Toxic ingestion of the curare toxin causes paralysis by what mechanism?

Competitive acetylcholine antagonism at the nicotinic receptors in the neuromuscular junction. It has been used to derive nondepolarizing neuromuscular blockers.

Glycyrrhizin found in licorice root causes what disorder in humans?

Pseudohyperaldosteronism, resulting in hypokalemia and hypertension, along with sodium and water retention

By what mechanism does glycyrrhizin act?

Inhibits 11-beta-hydroxysteroid dehydrogenase, which is the enzyme necessary for conversion of cortisol to cortisone, resulting in elevated cortisol levels

Morning glory and peyote cactus are consumed by humans because they have what properties?

Hallucinogenic properties secondary to direct serotonin effects

Name two common plants that contain colchicine.

1. *Colchicum autumnale* (Autumn crocus)
2. *Gloriosa superba* (Meadow saffron)

What other plant toxins acts similarly to colchicine?

Podophyllin and vinca alkaloids

What species of plants contain podophyllin?

Podophyllum spp. (the American mandrake, or mayapple, and the wild mandrake)

What is the mechanism of colchicine, podophyllin, and vinca alkaloid toxicity?

They inhibit cellular division by blocking microtubule formation

What are the symptoms of colchicine, podophylline, and vinca alkaloid poisoning?

Nausea, vomiting, diarrhea, bradycardia, hypotension, alopecia, bone marrow suppression, and progression to multisystem organ failure. Vinca alkaloid and podophyllin ingestions may also result in peripheral neuropathy.

Name the toxin that is the most common cause of plant-related deaths in the U.S.

Cicutoxin, from the water hemlock (*Cicuta maculata*)

Cicutoxin poisoning produces what signs and symptoms?

Nausea, vomiting, diaphoresis, bradycardia, hypotension, ↑ bronchial secretions, seizures that may progress to status epilepticus

What should be the approach for treatment of the cicutoxic patient?

1. Aggressive supportive care and immediate gastric lavage
2. Benzodiazepines for seizures
3. Atropine for ↑ secretions
4. Consider hemodialysis

Karwinskia toxin, found in buckthorn, wild cherry, and coyotillo, causes what symptomatology?

Ascending symmetric motor neuropathy, similar to Guillain-Barre Syndrome (GBS)

How does the _Karwinskia_ toxic neuropathy differ from GBS?

Cerebral spinal fluid is normal in _Karwinskia_ toxicity, as opposed to GBS, which has ↑ proteins in the CSF.

What is the treatment for _Karwinskia_ toxic neuropathy?

Supportive therapy. Recovery is generally slow.

Esculoside is the toxin found in horse chestnut and may cause which symptoms?

Vomiting, diarrhea, muscle twitching, weakness, incoordination, mydriasis, paralysis, stupor

What is capsaicin?

The active ingredient in peppers and pepper spray

How does capsaicin work?

It induces release of substance P from sensory nerve terminals

REPTILES

SNAKES

Elapidae

What are the major species of Elapidae and where are they found?

The family Elapidae consists of coral snakes found in the U.S., as well as cobras, mambas, and kraits found in Africa, Asia, Australia, and the Pacific Ocean regions.

What are the three genera of the Elapidae family found in the U.S.?

Micrurus fulvius fulvius (Eastern coral snake), *Micruroides euryxanthus* (Sonoran coral snake), *Micrurus fulvius tenere* (Texas coral snake)

What physical characteristics do coral snakes display?

1. Small, round head with no pits and a black snout
2. Round pupils
3. Short fangs (1–3 mm) attached to maxillae
4. Bright bands of black and red separated by yellow rings
5. Often confused with Scarlet King Snake, which has yellow and red bands separated by black rings

What is the old folk rhyme that is used to identify coral snakes?

"Red on yellow, kill a fellow, red on black, venom lack."

What are the local characteristics of a coral snake bite?

1. Snake exhibits "chewing" mechanism on extremity or digit, but absence of cytotoxins leaves little localized injury.
2. Minimal edema
3. Minor pain immediately following bite

How do Elapid venoms exert their effect?

Through neurotoxins that interfere with neuronal transmission at the neuromuscular junction to provoke an often delayed onset of neurologic symptoms

What are the signs and symptoms of systemic toxicity resulting from Elapid envenomation?

General malaise, weakness, paresthesias, slurred speech, diplopia, dysphagia, stridor, respiratory arrest, total body paralysis (up to 3 to 5 days)

What is the life-threatening complication from Elapid envenomation?

Respiratory arrest

What are the treatments for Elapid envenomation?

1. Limb immobilization with loose compression dressing may be beneficial for field transport.

2. Aggressive airway management at first indication of paralysis
3. Following coral snake bite, *Micrurus fulvius* antivenom is indicated if patient reports any indication of a legitimate bite, despite presence of signs or symptoms
4. All symptomatic patients should receive antivenom
5. Antivenom for exotic species may be available from zoos. Local poison centers may be helpful in obtaining antivenom.
6. Supportive care, monitor for hypersensitivity to antivenom

Viperidae

What 2 subfamilies of snakes does the Viperidae family contain?

1. Crotalinae – pit vipers
2. Viperinae – vipers without pits

Which is most commonly found in the United States?

Crotalinae

What are the three genera that comprise the Crotalinae subfamily?

Crotalus (large rattlesnakes), *Sistrurus* (massasauguas and pigmy rattlesnakes), *Agkistrodon* (copperheads and cottonmouths)

Where are Crotalinae found?

Approximately 25 species reside in the U.S. and are mostly confined to the southeast, southwest, and the Appalachian mountain regions.

What physical characteristics do Crotalinae display?

1. Triangular heads
2. Elliptical pupils
3. Paired, hollow fangs that can contract into roof of mouth and can grow up to 2–4 cm in length
4. "Pits" (heat sensing organs) located between the eye and the nostril
5. A single row of sub-caudal scales

6. Copperheads have distinct reddish-brown heads with hourglass patterns on body
7. Cottonmouths have a unique white-colored buccal mucosa

When do the Crotalinae most often strike?

Usually when startled or provoked, with a striking range of half the body length. Most bites occur between May and October, as the snakes hibernate during the colder months.

What are the primary features of crotaline envenomation?

As these venoms are primarily digestive enzymes, local tissue necrosis and coagulopathy are the predominant findings.

What are the local characteristics of a crotaline bite?

1. Puncture wounds, which can be single or multiple and involve localized pain. Serosanguinous drainage may occur from the wounds.
2. Localized edema and ecchymosis typically beginning 15 to 30 min after the bite and may progress throughout entire limb in 6 to 8 hrs, dependent upon amount of venom injected
3. Hemorrhagic blistering may occur within 24 to 36 hrs after bite
4. Localized tissue necrosis may occur several days after bite

Do all bites result in envenomation?

No. Up to 20% of bites do not result in envenomation; these are referred to as "dry bites."

What are the major toxic components of crotalind venom?

Collagenase, hyaluronidase, lecithin, and divalent metal ions such as zinc, copper, and magnesium, ribonuclease and deoxyribonuclease, acetylcholinesterase, phospholipase, protease

What are the 3 distinct hematologic effects of crotalid venom?

1. Benign defibrination
2. Isolated thrombocytopenia
3. DIC = like syndrome

Which U.S. rattlesnake carries a neurotoxic venom?

Crotalus scutulatus (Mojave rattlesnake) – Mojave toxin A

What are the neurotoxic effects of rattlesnake venom?

Blockade of ACh at the neuromuscular junction, causing paresthesias, fasciculations, cranial nerve paresis, respiratory arrest

What are the signs and symptoms of systemic toxicity as caused by crotaline envenomation?

Pain at site of puncture, metallic taste in mouth, generalized weakness, confusion, progressive edema, abdominal pain, nausea and vomiting, dyspnea, tachycardia, hypotension

What are the life-threatening complications arising from a severe envenomation?

Anaphylaxis, cardiac/pulmonary/cerebral edema, ARDS, shock, DIC, multi-organ system failure

What laboratory tests may be helpful?

CBC, electrolytes, PT/PTT, INR, fibrinogen, BUN, blood glucose, UA, electrolytes

What treatments should be avoided in the prehospital care of an envenomation?

Suction, ice, warmth, constriction bands, incision, excision, charcoal poultices

What are the treatments for envenomation?

1. Immobilize the limb
2. In moderate to severe envenomation, crotaline polyvalent immune Fab antivenom (CroFab) is indicated and should be administered as early as possible. Monitor for hypersensitivity reaction to antivenom.
3. Antivenom for exotic species may be available from zoos. Local poison centers may be helpful in obtaining antivenom.
4. Provide supportive care.
5. FFP and platelets as indicated by significant bleeding
6. Local wound care
7. Observation for at least 4 hrs in suspected "dry bites"

OTHER

What are the two species of venomous lizards?	1. Gila monster (*Heloderma suspectum*) 2. Mexican beaded lizard (*Heloderma horridum*)
Where is the Gila monster found?	The U.S. southwest and northern Mexico
Where is the Mexican beaded lizard found?	Mexico
Of what is the venom composed?	Similar to the venom produced by rattlesnakes, including serotonin, phospholipase A_2, kallikrein-like bradykinin-releasing substances, and gilatoxin
Describe venom production and release.	Venom is produced in glands in the lower jaw and is secreted into the saliva when the animal is agitated. Envenomation occurs when the animal bites the victim, attaching itself and performing a chewing motion. Venom is introduced into the wound through grooves in the loosely attached teeth. Accidental envenomations are extremely rare.
What systemic signs and symptoms may occur?	Common signs include nausea, vomiting, diaphoresis, and dizziness. Rarely, hypotension, tachycardia, respiratory distress, nonspecific T-wave changes or conduction delays on ECG, and hemorrhage (due to abnormal hemostasis) may occur.
What local signs and symptoms may occur?	Severe pain, edema, lymphangitis, vasospasm, hemorrhage, cyanosis, necrosis (rare)
What complication of a lizard bite may lead to a more severe envenomation?	These lizards are notorious for being difficult to remove once attached.

What are the risk factors for systemic involvement?

Long bite time (most important), extremes of age, comorbid illness. Prior exposures may result in anaphylaxis.

What initial wound care is advised?

1. Irrigate/clean thoroughly
2. Direct pressure to control bleeding
3. Dress and splint affected extremities to limit movement.
4. Elevate affected extremity to minimize edema and pain.
5. DO NOT USE suction devices, tourniquets, pressure immobilization devices, or ice, as they may result in additional tissue damage.

What treatments are advised in the systemically symptomatic patient?

1. Supportive care
2. Opiate analgesia (often for days to weeks)
3. Wound exploration with plain x-ray to help identify retained teeth
4. Update tetanus. Prophylactic antibiotics are not typically necessary.

What laboratory studies should be ordered?

CBC, BMP, coags, UA. May see leukocytosis and thrombocytopenia (rare). If infection is suspected (rare), wound cultures should be obtained.

What wound care instructions should the patient receive at discharge?

1. Clean wound with soap and water daily.
2. Flush wound with hydrogen peroxide.
3. Apply topical antiseptic.
4. Redress wound in clean dressings.

Which lizard's saliva stimulates insulin secretion in hyperglycemia and is used in some diabetic medications?

Gila monster – it contains an incretin analog, promoting insulin secretion.

What other species of lizard might be considered "toxic"?

The komodo dragon (*Varanus komodoensis*) does not have a true venom, but contains over 50 types of bacteria in its saliva that cause infection and sepsis following a bite.

TETANUS

Which toxin-producing anaerobe is responsible for causing the neurologic disorder tetanus?

Clostridium tetani

What are the four clinical patterns associated with tetanus?

1. Local
2. Cephalic
3. General
4. Neonatal

How many cases of tetanus occur in the U.S. annually?

There were an average of 43 cases per year from 1998–2000. The prevalence is much higher in developing nations due to poor vaccination rates, poor sanitation, and improper wound care.

How does *Clostridium tetani* cause tetanus?

Spores from *C. tetani* are ubiquitous in the environment. They can enter the body through any break in the integument. Once in the body they transform into a vegetative bacterium that produces tetanospasmin (aka "tetanus toxin"), which travels to alpha motor neuron synapses in the spinal cord and brainstem via retrograde axonal transport. Once there, it blocks muscle relaxation by blocking the release of the presynaptic inhibitory neurotransmitters GABA and glycine, resulting in tonic muscular contractions and intense muscle spasms due to disinhibition of spinal cord reflex arcs.

What conditions must be present to allow *C. tetani* to cause disease?

The spores germinate under anaerobic conditions. Trauma usually introduces *C. tetani* spores, with chronic skin ulcers, gangrene, and parenteral drug abuse also being causes. Co-infection with other bacteria, presence of a foreign body, necrotizing tissue, crushed tissue, and localized ischemia may all contribute to infection.

What is the incubation period for *C. tetani*?

1 day to 2 months, but averages 7 days. This is partially dependent on wound location in relation to the CNS (tetanospasmin must travel centripetally).

What is the relationship between incubation period length and disease severity?

The longer the incubation period, the milder the clinical symptoms

What is the most common form of tetanus, and what is the most common presenting symptom?

Generalized tetanus, with trismus ("lockjaw") and *risus sardonicus* (from ↑ tone in the orbicularis oris) often appearing first. Initial complaints are often neck stiffness, sore throat, or difficulty opening the mouth.

How does generalized tetanus progress?

1. Other muscle groups, beginning with the neck muscles and progressing to involve the trunk and extremities, develop rigidity and spasms. This can result in opisthotonus (extreme arching of the back and neck).
2. Uncontrolled spasms in response to even minor external stimuli which can resemble convulsions. These can be severe enough to cause fractures or tendon avulsions.
3. Laryngospasm can cause asphyxiation, and chest wall rigidity can also cause respiratory compromise.
4. Autonomic hyperactivity, manifesting as irritability, tachycardia, dysrhythmias, HTN, hyperthermia, and bronchorrhea
5. Mentation is typically preserved.

Why does tetanus cause these autonomic symptoms?

Tetanoplasmin also disinhibits sympathetic reflexes at the spinal level, which may result in autonomic dysfunction.

How long do symptoms last?

Symptoms can progress for up to 2 wks, after which autonomic disturbances and spasm resolve in ~2 wks. Rigidity may last an additional 6 wks.

What toxicologic causes should be considered when evaluating a patient for tetanus?

1. Strychnine
2. Dystonia

What is localized tetanus?

Occurs when the rigidity and pain stay localized to the site of the inoculation. This has a better prognosis if it remains localized.

What is cephalic tetanus?

A pattern of tetanus that results from a head wound or from chronic otitis media. It presents with cranial nerve palsies and may progress to generalized tetanus.

What is the most common cause of neonatal tetanus?

Failure to use aseptic technique while cleaning the necrotic umbilical stump of neonates born to poorly immunized mothers

When does neonatal tetanus usually manifest itself?

First 14 days of life. It usually begins with weakness, poor feeding, and irritability and progresses to rigidity and spasms. Prognosis is extremely poor, with a mortality rate of up to 90%.

What serum test may indicate a reduced likelihood of tetanus?

Serum antibody level >0.01 IU/mL, as this suggests immunity

What are the major goals in the treatment of tetanus?

1. Supportive care – ensure an intact airway and adequate ventilation. Be prepared to intubate.
2. Stop toxin production – wound care and antibiotics
3. Neutralize unbound toxin – IM human tetanus immune globulin
4. Control muscle spasms – initially administer benzodiazepines, NMB may be necessary to control spasms/allow adequate ventilation
5. IV $MgSO_4$ can inhibit neurotransmitter release, helping to control muscle spasms and autonomic hyperactivity.
6. Labetalol may be considered for refractory HTN.

What is the traditional drug of choice against _C. tetani_?	Penicillin G
Why is penicillin not an ideal choice to treat tetanus?	It can function as a GABA antagonist and worsen symptoms. Metronidazole is the antibiotic of choice.
How frequently should tetanus toxoid immunizations be administered?	Immunization series in childhood with boosters q10 yrs
What are the two general types of immunization?	1. Active – administration of an antigen to stimulate immunologic defenses against a repeat exposure 2. Passive – administration of preformed antibodies to neutralize circulating antigen
Which types of immunization are tetanus toxoid and tetanus immune globulin?	Tetanus toxoid is a form of active immunization, while tetanus immune globulin is a form of passive immunization.
Does tetanus immune globulin neutralize bound tetanospasmin?	No. The immune globulin only neutralizes unbound toxin.
Is the tetanus immune globulin effective in neutralizing unbound toxin in the brain?	No. It does not penetrate the blood-brain barrier.
What should be administered if a patient needs tetanus immune globulin but has had a previous serum sickness reaction to equine-derived products?	Human tetanus immune globulin
In what types of wounds should one consider tetanus prophylaxis?	It should be considered in all wounds in which the dermal barrier has been breached.

How does the management of tetanus in the elderly differ from that in younger patients?

Tetanus immune globulin may need to be administered more frequently to elderly patients with tetanus due to declining antibody titers with age.

What should one do if a patient presents with a clean, minor wound and does not know if he has received a primary series of three doses of tetanus toxoid?

Give tetanus toxoid. Administration of tetanus toxoid is indicated in all wounds without a known record of a primary series of three doses of toxoid.

A patient presents with a high-risk (i.e., puncture, contaminated, or with crush injury) wound and states that she last received a tetanus booster 7 years ago. What should be done?

Give tetanus toxoid. Administration of tetanus toxoid is indicated for all serious wounds if it has been >5 yrs since the last booster and for all minor wounds if it has been >10 yrs.

A patient presents with a high-risk wound and states that he has not received the primary series of tetanus toxoid. What do you do?

Administer tetanus immune globulin prophylactically to provide passive immunity, and initiate the series of tetanus toxoid administration.

Can tetanus toxoid be given during pregnancy?

Yes. Tetanus toxoid is FDA category C (indeterminate) and may be used in pregnancy.

Chapter 9   Therapies

ACETYLCYSTEINE (*N*-ACETYLCYSTEINE, NAC)

What is *N*-acetylcysteine (NAC)?

An amino acid derivative with known efficacy in cases of APAP overdose

What is the mechanism of action of NAC in APAP overdose?

1. It is a precursor to glutathione and binds to the APAP P450 metabolite NAPQI, preventing its hepatotoxic effects and facilitating its renal excretion.
2. May also bind NAPQI directly and reduce it back to APAP
3. Binds to NO to form *S*-nitrosothiol, whose vasodilatory effects can improve brain, cardiac and renal perfusion
4. Acts as a free radical scavenger

When should NAC be started after a toxic ingestion?

Within 8 hrs of ingestion to prevent hepatic damage. If the patient presents soon after ingestion, it is acceptable to wait for a 4-hr APAP level. If close to or beyond 8 hrs post-ingestion, NAC should be started upon arrival while APAP and transaminase levels are pending.

How may NAC be administered?

PO, IV

What are the benefits of the IV preparation?

1. Better patient tolerability and compliance
2. Can easily be given to lethargic/intubated patients
3. Requires less overall nursing time
4. May decrease length of hospital stay

What is the standard NAC dosing for acute, uncomplicated APAP toxicity?

PO – loading dose of 140 mg/kg (diluted to 5% in flavored beverage to make more palatable), then 70 mg/kg q4 hrs for total of 18 doses

IV – three steps:

1. Loading dose of 150 mg/kg, diluted in 200 mL D5W, given over 15 min
2. Second dose of 50 mg/kg, diluted in 500 mL D5W, given over 4 hrs
3. Third dose of 100 mg/kg, diluted in 1 L D5W, given over 16 hrs

In uncomplicated cases of APAP overdose, for how long should NAC therapy be given?

Generally, APAP levels must be undetectable, the patient should have minimal to no symptoms of APAP poisoning (i.e., nausea, vomiting, abdominal pain), and the parameters of liver damage (i.e., transaminases, INR) should be normal or significantly improved from peak levels.

What complications are associated with NAC therapy?

PO – unpleasant taste, nausea, vomiting, urticaria (rare)

IV – anaphylactoid reaction (i.e., flushing, rash, hypotension), which is rate-dependent

Are there contraindications to using NAC therapy in pregnancy or in children?

1. Pregnancy category B. The risk of APAP toxicity is far more dangerous to mother and fetus than the risk of an anaphylactoid reaction.
2. Young children may have difficulty with excess free water when giving the standard adult IV solution; in this instance, a final NAC concentration of 40 mg/mL should be used.
3. Neonates (preterm and full-term) have been safely treated with the IV preparations; however, necrotizing enterocolitis has been seen with oral solutions.

For what other toxic ingestions may NAC be of theoretical benefit?

1. *Amanita* mushroom
2. Pennyroyal
3. Clove oil, chloroform, carbon tetrachloride, and valproic acid-induced hepatotoxicity

ANTIVENOM

BLACK WIDOW

What is the effect of black widow (*Latrodectus mactans*) antivenom?

Significantly shortens course and decreases severity of symptoms, speeds recovery

From what animal is the current U.S. antivenom derived?

Horses (equine)

How is the antivenom produced?

Horses are hyperimmunized with *Latrodectus mactans* venom. Serum is then removed, and antibodies (along with residual proteins) are extracted.

What is the biggest concern when giving black widow antivenom?

Anaphylaxis and serum sickness. Caregivers should always be prepared for anaphylaxis and have IV fluids, epinephrine, diphenhydramine, and intubation equipment at the bedside prior to administering the antivenom.

What are indications for antivenom administration?

1. Systemic symptoms, including pain and HTN, refractory to muscle relaxants and analgesics
2. Pregnant patients with concern for uterine contractions
3. Vulnerable patients, including children and the elderly, should lower one's threshold for giving antivenom.

Are there any contraindications to antivenom therapy?

Known hypersensitivity to horse serum or black widow antivenom

How should the antivenom be administered?

1. In a setting with full resuscitation capabilities, by slow IV drip over 15 to 30 min
2. Reconstitute lyophilized vial, and swirl for up to 30 min (do not shake), then dilute in saline to total volume of 50 mL.

How many vials are used? Typically 1, but more may be used based on symptoms, not weight.

Are other black widow antivenoms available? Antivenoms are made in South Africa, Australia, and Mexico but are not currently available in the U.S.

SCORPION

How many species of scorpion found in the U.S. are systemically poisonous? 1, the bark scorpion (*Centruroides exilicauda*)

Where is the bark scorpion found? Southwestern U.S. and northern Mexico

Is there an antidote? Yes. In the U.S., an antivenom was developed by the Arizona State University Antivenom Production Laboratory for use only in Arizona but was never approved by the FDA and is no longer in production, so supplies are limited. Scorpion antivenom is also manufactured in Mexico for various *Centruroides* species but is currently unavailable in the U.S.

From what animal is the U.S. antivenom produced? The antivenom is made from the serum of goats who have been hyperimmunized with bark scorpion venom.

What is the mechanism of action of the antivenom? Immunoglobulins in the antivenom bind directly to the scorpion venom.

What are the indications for giving scorpion antivenom? Scorpion antivenom may be used for severe symptoms, including grade 3 and 4 envenomations. Vulnerable populations, including children and the elderly, are more likely to benefit from antivenom.

What is the concern with using the antivenom? Anaphylaxis and serum sickness. Caregivers should always be prepared for anaphylaxis and have IV fluids, epinephrine, diphenhydramine, and intubation equipment at the bedside prior to administering the antivenom.

Are there any contraindications to scorpion antivenom therapy?	Known hypersensitivity to goat serum or scorpion antivenom
What should be done before administering the antivenom?	Skin test for hypersensitivity, although a negative skin test does not exclude an anaphylactic reaction.

SNAKE

What antivenoms are available for crotaline envenomation in the U.S.?	1. Crotalidae polyvalent antivenom (Wyeth-Ayerst) 2. Crotalidae polyvalent immune Fab (CroFab)
From what animals are these antivenoms derived?	1. Wyeth-Ayerst – horses (equine) 2. CroFab – sheep (ovine)
What is the benefit of a Fab fragment?	It lacks the immunogenic F_c fragment and is, therefore, much less likely to result in anaphylaxis or serum sickness.
How are Fab fragments made?	After sheep are immunized to 4 North American snake species (*Crotalus adamanteus, Crotalus atrox, Crotalus scutulatus,* and *Agkistrodon piscivorus*), the IgG is cleaved with papain to isolate the Fab portion from the immunoglobulin.
What are the indications for crotalidae polyvalent immune Fab therapy?	Persistent proximal progression of swelling or significant systemic symptoms (e.g., tachycardia, hypotension, coagulopathy, thrombocytopenia)
What is the standard dosing of crotalidae polyvalent immune Fab?	1. Initial dose is 4 to 6 vials (based on symptom severity) 2. If systemic symptoms and proximal progression are not controlled after initial treatment, an additional 2 vials may be given up to three times. 3. After achieving control, 2 vials should be given q6 hrs × 3 doses.

What are the potential adverse effects of crotalidae polyvalent immune Fab administration?

Anaphylactoid reactions, febrile reactions, serum sickness. True anaphylaxis is rare.

Are there any contraindications to giving crotalidae polyvalent immune Fab?

Relative contraindications include hypersensitivity to sheep serum, papayas, or papain.

What are the adverse effects of crotalidae polyvalent antivenom (Wyeth)?

High incidence of allergic reaction/anaphylaxis (25%) and even higher rate of serum sickness (50%)

Are there any contraindications to crotalidae polyvalent antivenom therapy?

Known hypersensitivity to horse serum or crotalidae polyvalent antivenom

What is the standard dosing of crotalidae polyvalent antivenom?

Typically, 3 to 5 vials initially. An additional 3 to 5 vials can be given, based on severity.

What antivenom is available for Elapidae envenomation?

The only elapid native to the U.S. is the coral snake. An equine-derived antivenom is available for this species; however, this antivenom is no longer in production, and supplies are expected to become limited.

What are the indications for coral snake antivenom therapy?

Any neurologic symptoms related to Eastern or Texas coral snake envenomation

What are common side effects of coral snake antivenom?

Similar to those of crotalidae polyvalent antivenom, including high rates of allergic/anaphylactic reactions and serum sickness

What additional treatment measures should be considered when administering antivenom?

Be prepared for anaphylactic reactions by having fluids, epinephrine, diphenhydramine, and intubation equipment at the bedside.

Are antivenoms available for exotic snakes?	Yes. In the U.S., many are available through zoos, depending on the species involved. Dosing instructions vary greatly. Indications for antivenom administration are similar to those of U.S. snakes and depend on the type of toxin involved (i.e., neurotoxin vs. tissue toxin). Caregivers should always anticipate anaphylactic reactions.
What is not taken into account when dosing any snake antivenom?	The patient's weight

ATROPINE AND GLYCOPYRROLATE

What is the physiologic mechanism of action of both atropine and glycopyrrolate?	Competitive inhibition of ACh binding at muscarinic receptors
How do the effects of atropine and glycopyrrolate differ?	Atropine has central and peripheral effects, while glycopyrrolate does not cross the blood-brain barrier and, therefore, acts only peripherally.
What are the toxicologic indications for atropine therapy?	1. Treatment of respiratory and GI symptoms due to poisoning with AChE inhibitors (e.g., organo-phosphates, carbamates) 2. Treatment of respiratory and GI symptoms due to poisoning with muscarinic agents (e.g., pilocarpine, methacholine, muscarinic mushroom poisoning) 3. Treatment of drug-induced bradycardia secondary to increased parasympathetic tone or AV nodal conduction abnormalities
What is the dosing of atropine in organophosphorus compound and carbamate poisonings?	<u>Adults</u> – 1 to 2 mg IV initially <u>Children</u> – 0.02 mg/kg IV (minimum 0.1 mg) <u>Both</u> – double dose if no improvement after 3 to 5 min. OP and carbamate poisonings may require very large doses

(10–100 mg over a few hours) to achieve appropriate atropinization.

What is the typical dose of atropine for drug-induced bradycardia?

<u>Adults</u> – 0.5 to 1 mg IV
<u>Children</u> – 0.02 mg/kg (maintain dose within 0.1 to 1 mg)

What are the primary dosing endpoints when treating organophosphorus compound and carbamate poisonings?

Respiratory symptoms (i.e., bronchorrhea and bronchoconstriction) should guide treatment, with the endpoint of therapy being drying of secretions, ease of ventilation, and clear lung fields on exam.

In organophosphorus and carbamate poisonings, does tachycardia preclude atropine therapy?

No. Tachycardia may be a response to hypoxia and may improve once respiratory symptoms improve.

What are the potential side effects of atropine therapy?

Anticholinergic toxidrome

Are there any contraindications to treating with atropine or glycopyrrolate?

Pre-existing anticholinergic toxidrome, urinary retention, acute angle closure glaucoma. History of cardiac disease is a relative contraindication as these patients may not tolerate a faster heart rate; however, if a marked cholinergic syndrome exists, atropine can be administered even if the patient has a history of urinary retention, heart disease, or angle closure glaucoma.

What is the dose of atropine delivered by the military auto-injector (Mark I kit)?

2 mg atropine IM

What other component is included in the Mark I kit?

Pralidoxime 600 mg

BARBITURATES

What is the mechanism of action of barbiturates?

Enhance GABA effects by ↑ duration of $GABA_A$-mediated chloride channel opening → ↑ intracellular Cl^- → membrane hyperpolarization and ↓ neuronal electrical activity

Barbiturates are useful in treating what toxicologic problems?

Generally used as second/third line agents for treating toxin-induced seizures and ethanol withdrawal refractory to benzodiazepines

Which barbiturate is most commonly used when treating seizures and other toxicologic conditions?

Phenobarbital

Barbiturates are more effective than benzodiazepines in animal models for treating or preventing seizures due to what class of agents?

Theophylline

Why might phenobarbital be useful in treating isoniazid-induced seizures?

At high concentrations, barbiturates can directly open the GABA$_A$ chloride channel. For this reason, phenobarbital may be useful in conditions of GABA depletion, where benzodiazepines are ineffective. Rapid administration of pyridoxine is imperative, regardless of the adjunctive therapy used.

Barbiturates may be necessary if seizures develop following administration of what antidote?

Flumazenil. Phenobarbital is the treatment of choice for seizures precipitated by administration of flumazenil.

What are possible adverse effects of barbiturate administration?

Hypotension and respiratory depression

Patients with what condition should not receive barbiturates?

Porphyria

The metabolism of which drug is enhanced by acute phenobarbital use?

None. Induction of hepatic enzymes is seen only with chronic use.

BENZODIAZEPINES

What are some examples of benzodiazepines?

1. Short-acting – triazolam, alprazolam, midazolam
2. Long-acting – lorazepam, clonazepam, diazepam, flurazepam

How are benzodiazepines commonly used for treatment of the toxicologic patient?

1. Seizures
2. Agitation
3. Ethanol/sedative-hypnotic withdrawal
4. Toxin-induced sympathomimetic syndrome
5. Serotonin syndrome
6. Muscle relaxation

How are benzodiazepines administered?

PO, IM, IV

What is the mechanism of action of benzodiazepines?

Bind GABA receptors and increase their frequency of opening in response to endogenous GABA, thereby increasing the inhibitory effect of GABA. Benzodiazepines do not open GABA receptors independently of GABA binding, whereas high-dose barbiturates can.

Why are benzodiazepines considered first-line treatment for toxin-induced seizures?

They target the route of the seizure, which is generally a lack of neuro-inhibitory transmission (GABA).

How do benzodiazepines treat cocaine-induced chest pain?

They blunt the cocaine-induced catecholamine surge and the corresponding HTN, tachycardia, and vasoconstriction.

What is the typical dosing of lorazepam?

<u>Adults</u> – 1 to 2 mg IV/PO/IM initially, then titrate to effect
<u>Children</u> – 0.05 to 0.1 mg/kg initially

Are there any contraindications to benzodiazepines?

Known hypersensitivity to benzodiazepines. Monitor for CNS and respiratory depression.

BENZTROPINE

For what condition is benztropine utilized in toxicology?	Dystonic reactions
What is the mechanism of action of benztropine?	Antagonizes ACh (muscarinic) and histamine receptors
How does benztropine work to treat dystonia?	While the mechanism is not fully known, it appears to help restore the balance between dopaminergic and cholinergic transmission.
What is the dosing for benztropine?	In adults, 1 to 2 mg IV/IM (0.02 mg/kg for children) for dystonic reactions. The PO form is generally given as prophylaxis for recurrence of dystonia (1 to 2 mg q12 hrs). Following a dystonic reaction, PO benztropine should be continued for the following 48 to 72 hrs.
What are the adverse effects of benztropine?	Anticholinergic toxidrome
Are there any contraindications to giving benztropine?	Pre-existing anticholinergic toxidrome, urinary retention, acute angle closure glaucoma. History of cardiac disease is a relative contraindication, as these patients may not tolerate a fast heart rate.

BICARBONATE

When bicarbonate is given IV, with what cation is it usually combined?	Sodium, as sodium bicarbonate ($NaHCO_3$)
Toxicity from what OTC medication is treated with sodium bicarbonate to enhance elimination?	ASA
What electrocardiogram finding(s) associated with drug toxicity is treated with sodium bicarbonate?	QRS prolongation and subsequent dysrhythmias (drug-induced cardiac sodium channel inhibition)

How does sodium bicarbonate treat sodium channel blockade?

Generally, the excess sodium load is thought to competitively overcome sodium channel blockade. Some medications (i.e., CAs) have been shown to bind sodium channels less tightly in an alkalotic environment. This may pertain to other sodium channel blockers as well.

What are the criteria for giving sodium bicarbonate for sodium channel blocker toxicity?

QRS widening >100 msec, dysrhythmias, hypotension

What ECG findings are further suggestive of sodium channel blockade?

QRS widening with RAD in the terminal 40 msec of the QRS, best seen as positive forces ("terminal R wave") at the end of the QRS in lead aVR

How do you administer sodium bicarbonate in sodium channel blocker overdose?

1 to 2 mEq/kg IV bolus initially. Repeated treatment should be based on clinical condition and ECG findings (i.e., widened QRS), with a goal serum pH of 7.45 to 7.55.

How does sodium bicarbonate treat salicylate toxicity?

Salicylate is a weak acid. In the presence of an alkalotic environment, a greater fraction of salicylate becomes ionized. This helps to prevent distribution of salicylate into the tissues, as well as salicylate resorption in the kidneys.

Above what toxic salicylate level is sodium bicarbonate therapy considered?

>40 mg/dL

How is sodium bicarbonate dosed for treatment of salicylate toxicity?

Combine 150 mEq sodium bicarbonate with 1 L of D5W. 40 mEq of potassium chloride should be added per liter once urine is produced, in order to prevent hypokalemia. The rate should be started at twice the maintenance fluid rate.

What potentially lethal complication of sodium bicarbonate therapy must be considered in patients treated for either salicylate or sodium channel blocker toxicity?	Hypokalemia secondary to intracellular shifts and renal elimination of K^+ in exchange for H^+. In the setting of hypokalemia, the kidney preferentially reabsorbs K^+ in exchange for H^+. This prevents effective urinary alkalinization. Serum K^+ levels should be checked frequently during therapy.
For which irritant gas exposure may nebulized sodium bicarbonate be an effective therapy?	Chlorine gas. Bicarbonate helps to neutralize the formed hydrochloric acid. The large surface area of the lungs is thought to dissipate heat and prevent thermal injury.
How should sodium bicarbonate be dosed in chlorine gas exposure?	For symptomatic patients, 1 mL of sodium bicarbonate (7.5% or 8.4% solution) can be added to 3 mL of sterile water and nebulized.
Are there any contraindications to bicarbonate therapy?	Care should be taken in patients with renal failure, CHF, volume overload, hypernatremia, or preexisting alkalemia.

BOTULINUM ANTITOXIN

What is contained in botulinum antitoxin?	Antibodies to botulin types A, B, and E
In what animal is the antitoxin made?	Horse; therefore, patients receive equine-derived serum
What is the action of botulinum antitoxin?	Binds circulating toxin, halting disease *progression*. It has no action on toxin bound to nerve terminals; therefore, it *does not reverse* the disease. As a result, early administration is important to limit disability.
Where can physicians obtain antitoxin?	1. Local/state health departments 2. The Centers for Disease Control and Prevention
What is the dose and route of administration?	1 vial diluted in saline (10 mL), infused IV over 30 to 60 min

What is the indication for antitoxin administration?

High clinical suspicion of botulism poisoning. Do not delay treatment waiting for confirmatory lab results.

What is the incidence of allergic reaction to antitoxin?

Historically reported as 9%, so be well-prepared to address anaphylactic reactions. Skin testing has previously been recommended prior to administration of the antitoxin; however, this may not predict an allergic reaction, as one study showed 50% of those with an acute reaction had a negative skin test. The rate of serious adverse reactions has been only ~1% since the recommended dose was reduced to 1 vial. As a result of these points, treatment of severe exposures should not be delayed to perform skin testing.

Which patients should not routinely receive antitoxin?

The equine-derived antitoxin is not recommended to treat infant botulism. This is not only because of the high rate of adverse reactions, but also due to the fear of lifelong sensitization of infants to horses and equine-derived products.

Is there an antitoxin available for children?

A human-derived immune globulin (baby-BIG) is available and should be used to treat infant botulism. Currently, this antidote is only available from the California State Health Department.

Is there an antitoxin effective against type F botulism?

Yes. The US army possesses an antitoxin against all 7 (A–G) serotypes of botulism

BROMOCRIPTINE

For what indications has bromocriptine been advocated in the toxicologic patient?

1. Neuroleptic malignant syndrome (NMS)
2. Cocaine withdrawal (controversial)

What is the mechanism of action of bromocriptine?

1. Dopamine receptor agonism (hypothalamus and neostriatum)
2. Mild alpha-adrenergic receptor antagonism

How is bromocriptine administered?	PO, with poor bioavailability (6%). This may limit its use in an intubated patient.
What are the adverse effects of bromocriptine?	Common side effects include GI upset (e.g., nausea, vomiting, diarrhea) and transient hypotension with initiation of therapy, with a potential for the development of HTN. Cardiac dysrhythmias, exacerbation of angina, thrombosis (e.g., myocardial infarction), peripheral vasoconstriction, and uterine contractions have also been reported but are rare.
What is the typical dosing of bromocriptine?	2.5 to 10 mg PO q6 to 8 hrs for adults

CALCIUM

What are the clinical indications for use of calcium?	1. Hypotension due to CCB poisoning 2. To reduce pain and extent of injury due to hydrofluoric acid burns 3. Symptomatic hypocalcemia from fluoride, ethylene glycol, oxalate, or IV citrate toxicity 4. Hyperkalemia with ECG changes or cardiac symptoms 5. Hypermagnesemia
When is calcium gluconate indicated over calcium chloride?	1. When administering through a peripheral IV, as calcium chloride can cause significant extravasation injury 2. For topical application and intra-arterial or local injection following exposure to hydrofluoric acid
How is calcium dosed when treating a CCB overdose?	Recommendations vary. A reasonable strategy would be an initial bolus of 0.6 mL/kg of 10% calcium gluconate or 0.2 mL/kg of 10% calcium chloride infused over 5 to 10 min. Additional calcium can be given based on the clinical response. Repeated boluses or an infusion are both acceptable.

Is calcium useful in beta-blocker overdose?

Yes. Although more commonly used in CCB overdoses, calcium has been shown to increase inotropy in animal studies and case reports of beta-blocker overdose.

What is the mechanism of action of calcium?

A rise in intracellular Ca^{2+} is necessary for appropriate excitation-contraction coupling. Both CCBs and beta blockers blunt the rise in intracellular Ca^{2+} in response to depolarization. In theory, increasing the amount of extracellular Ca^{2+} can overcome competitive blockade, and/or increase Ca^{2+} entry through unaffected channels and, thus, improve inotropy.

What are some adverse effects of IV calcium administration?

Rapid administration can cause bradycardia and hypotension. Large doses can cause weakness, nausea, somnolence, and syncope. Extravasation can cause significant local tissue necrosis.

What has been theorized as an important interaction of calcium and digoxin toxicity?

Calcium administration was theorized to exacerbate the increase in intracellular Ca^{2+} caused by digoxin, thereby potentially increasing the risk of dysrhythmias or cardiac arrest caused by impaired relaxation of the myocytes. Animal studies, however, have not demonstrated this effect.

How could a patient with a mixed CCB and digoxin overdose be treated?

Administer digoxin immune Fab followed by calcium.

How is calcium utilized in treating hydrofluoric acid exposure?

1. First-line treatment involves making a 2.5% calcium gluconate gel for topical application. Mix 3.5 g of powdered calcium gluconate in 150 mL of water-soluble lubricant.
2. If pain is not relieved, calcium gluconate may be administered intra-arterially or IM.
3. Ocular exposures may be treated with 1% calcium gluconate eye drops.

4. Systemic hypocalcemia, manifested by cardiac dysrhythmias or tetany, must be treated with IV calcium.

Is calcium advocated for treating black widow spider bites?

IV calcium has been advocated in the past to alleviate pain and muscle spasm associated with black widow envenomations; however, evidence for its effectiveness is lacking, and its use is currently not recommended.

CALCIUM DISODIUM ETHYLENEDIAMINE-TETRAACETIC ACID (CaNa$_2$EDTA)

What is CaNa$_2$EDTA?

A water-soluble chelating agent for enhanced elimination of toxic metals

How does CaNa$_2$EDTA eliminate toxic metals?

Divalent metals displace calcium, forming a water-soluble complex that is excreted renally.

With which metals does CaNa$_2$EDTA interact?

Lead (primary target of therapy), zinc, iron, manganese, copper

What is the primary toxicologic use of CaNa$_2$EDTA?

Chelation of lead in patients with marked toxicity

Can CaNa$_2$EDTA alone be used as a treatment for lead encephalopathy?

No. CaNa$_2$EDTA does not cross the blood-brain barrier. It may mobilize body lead stores that then redistribute to the brain, worsening encephalopathy. When used for lead encephalopathy, CaNa$_2$EDTA must be preceded by BAL.

How is CaNa$_2$EDTA administered?

IV, IM

How is CaNa$_2$EDTA typically dosed for lead encephalopathy?

<u>Adults</u> – 2 to 4 g IV over 24 hrs
<u>Children</u> – 1000 to 1500 mg/m^2 IV over 24 hrs
<u>Both</u> – infusion should not start until 4 hrs following dose of BAL

How is CaNa$_2$EDTA metabolized?

Excreted unchanged

What are contraindications to CaNa₂EDTA administration?	1. Renal insufficiency, especially anuria 2. Hepatitis
What are the effects of CaNa₂EDTA?	Chelation of other essential metals (especially zinc), nephrotoxicity, dehydration, muscle weakness, and cramps
Can *disodium* EDTA be used to chelate lead?	No! *Disodium EDTA* primarily chelates Ca^+, which may result in QT prolongation, dysrhythmias, seizures, and death.

L-CARNITINE

What is L-carnitine, and what does it do?	1. Amino acid derivative 2. Assists in bringing long-chain fatty acids into mitochondria 3. Assists in bringing short-/medium-chain fatty acids out of mitochondria
How does valproic acid induce carnitine deficiency?	Carnitine is necessary for valproic acid metabolism. While the mechanism of carnitine depletion is not fully known, one mechanism appears to be the combination of valproic acid with carnitine to form valproylcarnitine, which is excreted in the urine.
How is L-carnitine used for valproic acid toxicity?	1. Treatment of valproic acid-induced hyperammonemia, especially in patients with AMS/encephalopathy 2. Treatment of valproic acid-induced hepatitis 3. Prophylactic therapy for prevention of valproic acid-induced hyperammonemia (theoretical) 4. Acute valproic acid overdose with high (>450 mg/L) valproic acid levels (theoretical)
How does L-carnitine work as an effective therapy?	1. Supplies the carnitine necessary for metabolism of valproic acid 2. Allows for metabolism of long-chain fatty acids 3. ↓ endogenous ammonia concentrations

What is the recommended dose of L-carnitine to treat valproic acid-induced encephalopathy or hepatotoxicity?	100 mg/kg IV q8 hrs
What is the route of intake of L-carnitine?	IV, PO (commercial PO preparation is acetyl-L-carnitine)
What are the side effects of L-carnitine use?	Primarily GI – nausea, vomiting, diarrhea, abdominal cramps. Patients may also develop a "fishy" body odor.

CHARCOAL (ACTIVATED)

How do you "activate" charcoal?	Heating charcoal in the presence of steam puts holes in the charcoal, increasing its surface area.
Activated charcoal (AC) works by using what chemical property?	Adsorption of toxins onto the surface of the charcoal
One gram of AC has how much surface area?	400 m^2 (a tennis court covers 260 m^2)
What is the standard initial dose of AC for the treatment of toxic ingestions?	1 g/kg, optimally in a 10:1 ratio of AC to xenobiotic
Why should you not give charcoal to a patient who is confused or somnolent?	Risk of aspiration. Aspirated charcoal causes severe lung injury. Numerous deaths have been reported. Intubated patients may receive charcoal via NG tube.
What medication is often co-administered with AC, and why?	Sorbitol, in order to promote passage of the charcoal through the GI tract
Following what type of poisoning is charcoal absolutely contraindicated?	Caustics
What is the position of the American Academy of Clinical Toxicology on AC?	The AACT's 2005 position paper states, "activated charcoal should not be administered routinely in the management of

poisoned patients. There is no evidence that the administration of activated charcoal improves clinical outcome." Guidelines from other societies vary, with most recommending charcoal in the first hour in patients at low risk for aspiration.

Can activated charcoal be given by prehospital care providers without physician contact?

Yes. Although prehospital protocols vary, most prehospital providers may give activated charcoal without physician contact to patients with suspected recent ingestions; however, definitive proof does not exist to demonstrate that this changes outcome.

For how long after an ingestion is it helpful to give AC?

Generally, within the first hour

For which toxic ingestions may multidose activated charcoal be beneficial?

Theophylline, caffeine, salicylate, phenobarbital, carbamazepine, phenytoin, and sustained-release products

Multidose activated charcoal is recommended for the treatment of what highly toxic mushroom for which there is no known antidote?

Amanita phalloides ("death cap"). This may be helpful in clearing the toxin because enterohepatic circulation occurs.

If you give multidose activated charcoal, do you give sorbitol with each dose?

No. Sorbitol is not given multiple times because of the risk of electrolyte abnormalities.

What are the risks of multidose AC?

As with a single dose, aspiration is a risk. Additionally, multidose charcoal increases the risk of bowel obstruction and electrolyte abnormalities (e.g., hypernatremia, hypermagnesemia).

CYPROHEPTADINE

What was the first use of cyproheptadine?

As an antihistamine to treat allergy symptoms and urticaria

For what toxicologic syndrome can treatment with cyproheptadine be considered?

Serotonin syndrome

Why might cyproheptadine be effective in treating serotonin syndrome?

It is an antagonist at $5HT_{1a}$ and $5HT_{2a}$ receptors. Overstimulation of these receptors causes serotonin syndrome, and cyproheptadine has proven beneficial in animal models and human case reports.

What is the classic triad of serotonin syndrome?

1. AMS
2. Autonomic instability (e.g., hyperthermia, tachycardia)
3. Neuromuscular dysfunction

What are the limitations of using cyproheptadine to treat serotonin syndrome?

1. Only available PO – limits usefulness in patients with profound symptoms
2. Can cause sedation – may be beneficial but clouds the clinical picture
3. Anticholinergic properties preclude its use if there is any suspicion of anticholinergic toxicity.
4. Effectiveness has not been proven in rigorous clinical experiments; therefore, supportive care, benzodiazepines, and active cooling are the cornerstones of treatment for serotonin syndrome.

What dose of cyproheptadine should be given to treat serotonin syndrome?

Dosing has been inconsistent among case reports. A reasonable regimen is 4 to 8 mg q6 hrs with/without a loading dose of 12 mg. Avoid administering >32 mg over 24 hrs.

Cyproheptadine can be considered in the treatment of what other toxicologic issue?

Ergot-induced vasospasm

What other agents have $5HT_2$ blocking effects and have been considered for the treatment of serotonin syndrome?

Chlorpromazine and olanzapine

CYANIDE ANTIDOTE PACKAGE

What three medications are contained in the cyanide antidote kit?

1. Amyl nitrite
2. Sodium nitrite
3. Sodium thiosulfate

How are the medications packaged?

Sodium thiosulfate and sodium nitrite are IV preparations. Amyl nitrite is in the form of pearls for inhalation. Each kit contains enough medication to treat two adults.

What is the adult dose for each medication?

Amyl nitrite – pearls are crushed and inhaled or administered through bag-valve-mask. They are administered intermittently, and a new pearl should be used q 3 min.
Sodium nitrite – 300 mg IV (packaged in 10 mL)
Sodium thiosulfate – 12.5 g IV (packaged in 50 mL)

How are these medications dosed in children?

Sodium nitrite – use caution due to risk of excessive methemoglobinemia. Ideally, doses are calculated using weight and Hgb level. When Hgb is normal, 10 mg/kg is recommended. If Hgb is unknown, 6 mg/kg is reasonable, as this will be safe even with significant anemia.
Sodium thiosulfate – 1.65 mL/kg of 25% solution IV over 10 min

Do all three medications need to be administered?

No. Amyl nitrite is included for those patients without IV access. If sodium nitrite can be administered IV, there is no need to give amyl nitrite via inhalation.

What is the mechanism of action of the amyl and sodium nitrite?

Nitrites induce methemoglobinemia; methemoglobin has a higher affinity for cyanide than does normal Hgb. Methemoglobin will draw both bound and unbound cyanide away from cytochrome a_3, allowing it to return to its primary role in the production of ATP.

What is the mechanism of action of sodium thiosulfate?

Thiosulfate donates a sulfur moiety to hepatic rhodanese, which catalyzes the metabolism of cyanide. The availability of sulfur is typically the rate-limiting step in the conversion of cyanide to its less toxic metabolite, thiocyanate.

What are the potential side effects of nitrite administration?

Hypotension is the most significant side effect (secondary to the vasodilatory effects of nitrites). Also, methemoglobinemia lowers the oxygen-carrying capacity. This is especially concerning when treating cyanide-poisoned patients with presumed carbon monoxide exposure, as occurs in smoke inhalation victims.

What patient population can have adverse effects after sodium thiosulfate administration?

Renal failure. Thiocyanate can accumulate and have toxic effects, including abdominal pain, vomiting, rash, hypertertension, and CNS dysfunction. If symptoms are severe enough, thiocyanate may be dialyzed.

What additional therapy should always be administered to patients with a potential cyanide exposure?

Although antidotal therapy is extremely important, supportive care, including 100% oxygen, hemodynamic support, and correction of acidosis, is vital.

What are the indications for treatment with the cyanide antidote kit?

Any patient clinically suspected of having cyanide toxicity. This should be considered in any patient with sudden loss of consciousness and any combination of seizures or hemodynamic instability without a definitive cause. There are several laboratory clues for cyanide poisoning, including metabolic acidosis (lactic acidosis) and a narrowing of the oxygen saturation between an arterial and a mixed venous blood sample; however, therapeutic action may be needed before the results of these diagnostic tests are available.

How is the use of the cyanide antidote kit different for a victim of smoke inhalation?

It is often recommended that one forgo administration of the nitrite component in smoke inhalation victims, at least until a carboxyhemoglobin level is determined.

DANTROLENE

Name two conditions or diagnoses for which dantrolene is most commonly used as a therapeutic agent.	1. Malignant hyperthermia (MH) 2. NMS
For what other conditions has dantrolene been used (with some anecdotal evidence)?	1. Serotonin syndrome refractory to traditional therapy 2. Severe hyperthermia/heatstroke with associated muscular rigidity
What is the rationale for using dantrolene?	Dantrolene "uncouples" skeletal muscle contraction from nerve impulses. It can, therefore, be used to relieve muscular rigidity and subsequent hypermetabolic/hyperthermic states.
What is the mechanism of action of dantrolene?	Binds ryanodine receptor (RYR-1) $\rightarrow \downarrow Ca^{2+}$ release from sarcoplasmic reticulum $\rightarrow$ limits actin-myosin interaction $\rightarrow \downarrow$ skeletal muscle tone
What is the dose of dantrolene?	2 to 3 mg/kg IV q15 min, titrated to effect (max 10 mg/kg). Generally, a maintenance dose of 1 to 2 mg/kg IV/PO q6 hrs is needed for 2 to 3 days to prevent recurrence.
What are the most common side effects?	Nausea and vomiting following PO administration. Weakness is expected to occur, which may lead to respiratory depression. Sedation, confusion, and photosensitivity have also been reported.
Does dantrolene cause myocardial suppression or affect smooth muscles?	No. These muscle types contain the RYR-2 ryanodine receptor, which is not affected by dantrolene.

DEFEROXAMINE

For what clinical indication is deferoxamine primarily used?	Iron poisoning

From what is deferoxamine derived?

Culture of *Streptomyces pilosus*

At what iron level should you initiate treatment with deferoxamine?

There is no absolute level. The decision to treat with deferoxamine must be made on clinical grounds and should not be delayed to wait for a serum level; however, a level >500 mg/dL is generally accepted as a critical threshold to warrant treatment.

What are the clinical indications for deferoxamine treatment?

Persistent emesis and/or diarrhea, metabolic acidosis, shock, AMS (i.e., lethargy, coma), and/or an x-ray positive for multiple pills

What is the mechanism of action of deferoxamine?

Forms octahedral complexes with loosely bound/unbound Fe^{3+} to form a water-soluble complex, ferrioxamine, which is eliminated in the urine

How should it be administered?

Start at 15 mg/kg/hr IV over 6 hrs (max 1 g/hr), then reevaluate need for further therapy

What is the most common adverse effect?

Deferoxamine-induced hypotension may occur, especially with rapid infusion. Adequate hydration must be assured before infusion is initiated.

What is the risk of prolonged infusion?

Infusions administered >24 hrs may cause acute lung injury, according to case reports.

What are the contraindications to deferoxamine?

1. Primary hemochromatosis
2. Documented hypersensitivity to deferoxamine
3. Severe renal disease (unless the patient is undergoing dialysis)

For which infections are iron-overloaded patients at higher risk after deferoxamine treatment?

1. *Yersinia enterocolitica*
2. *Zygomycetes*
3. *Aeromonas hydrophila*

What are the major drug interactions with deferoxamine?	1. Prochlorperazine – may cause coma or AMS 2. Vitamin C – may lead to cardiac dysfunction
What color does the urine turn following deferoxamine administration in iron-toxic patients?	May turn pink ("vin rosé") due to ferrioxamine
For what other metal toxicity is deferoxamine used?	Aluminum

DIALYSIS

What are the characteristics of a toxin that is amenable to removal from blood by dialysis?	1. Low protein-binding 2. Low volume of distribution (<1 L/kg) 3. Water-solubility 4. Low molecular weight (<500 Daltons)
What toxins are readily removed from blood by dialysis?	SMEL IT **S**alicylates **M**ethanol/metformin **E**thylene glycol **L**ithium **I**sopropanol (usually indicated only in severe cases) **T**heophylline
What factors are considered when deciding whether to initiate dialysis for treatment of overdose?	1. Is the toxin readily removed by dialysis? 2. Does the toxin, in the amount ingested, have significant toxicity? 3. Serum toxin level (varies by toxin) 4. Clinical status 5. Acid-base status 6. Availability of resources and appropriate vascular access 7. Can other methods be used to treat the poisoning (antidotes)? 8. Is the normal means of elimination impaired (renal failure)?
Is dialysis effective in removing salicylate from blood with a low serum salicylate level?	No. At low (therapeutic) blood levels, salicylates are highly protein-bound. The percentage of unbound salicylate increases as blood levels rise to the point of toxicity.

What additional treatment benefits does hemodialysis provide?	1. Correction of acid-base status 2. Control of fluid status 3. Metabolite removal
What are the possible adverse reactions to dialysis?	1. Hypotension 2. Hypo- or hyperthermia 3. Removal of other therapeutic drugs

DIMERCAPTOPROPANESULFONIC ACID (DMPS)

What is DMPS?	1. Water-soluble chelating agent used in heavy metal poisoning 2. Analog of dimercaprol (British anti-Lewisite or BAL)
For which heavy metal toxicities is DMPS typically used?	Mercury, arsenic, lead
Is DMPS approved for use in the U.S.?	Not currently FDA-approved but is available for use as an investigational drug
What are the possible routes of administration for DMPS?	PO, IV, IM
Why is DMPS potentially more neuroprotective than the common chelator, BAL?	DMPS does not cross the blood-brain barrier and, therefore, does not allow mercury redistribution to the CNS.
How is DMPS excreted?	Primarily renally, but also through the bile
How is DMPS dosed for a severe mercury or arsenic exposure?	<u>IV</u> bolus (sterile water solution) – 3 to 5 mg/kg q4 hrs over 20 min <u>PO</u> (once clinically stable) – 4 to 8 mg/kg q6 hrs
What are the potential adverse effects of DMPS?	1. Urticaria 2. Local irritation 3. Hypotension (rate-related in IV infusions) 4. Erythema multiforme/Stevens-Johnson syndrome (rare) 5. Chelation of other essential metals

What, if any, are the contra-indications to DMPS use?	Known hypersensitivity or severe renal insufficiency

DIETHYLDITHIOCARBAMATE

What are the indications for diethyldithiocarbamate (DDC)?	Treatment of choice for nickel carbonyl poisoning, although still considered an investigational drug. It is not indicated for elemental or inorganic nickel.
How is DDC administered?	PO
What is the mechanism of action of DDC?	Chelation of organic nickel compounds to excretable forms
What intoxicating substance must be avoided with DDC therapy?	Ethanol. DDC may produce a disulfiram reaction, yielding flushing, nausea, vomiting, vertigo, tachycardia, and hypotension.
How is DDC similar to disulfiram?	Disulfiram is metabolized to DDC and produces the same aldehyde dehydrogenase and dopamine hydroxylase inhibition.

DIGOXIN IMMUNE FAB

What are the two preparations of digoxin immune fragments?	Digifab (Protherics) and Digibind (GlaxoSmithKline)
What are the parts of an immunoglobulin (antibody)?	<u>Fc fragment</u> – the fragment "crystallizable" region that binds to receptors on immune cells and complement proteins <u>Fab fragment</u> – the fragment "antigen binding" that binds the specific antigen
How are the digoxin immune fragments prepared?	After sheep are injected with digoxindicarboxymethoxylamine (DDMA), they develop a cross-reactive antibody to digoxin. This is isolated from the serum, and the Fc portion is proteolytically cleaved with papain, leaving the Fab fragments as the primarily component of the preparation.

What patients may have an allergy to digoxin immune fragments?

Those with known allergies to:
1. Sheep proteins
2. Papaya
3. Papain (derived from papaya)

What are the indications for digoxin immune fragments?

1. Potassium >5.0 mEq/L following acute cardiac glycoside ingestion
2. Hemodynamic instability
3. Life-threatening dysrhythmias
4. History of large ingestion (i.e., 10 mg in an adult) or serum level >10 ng/mL 4 to 6 hrs post-ingestion may warrant treatment, regardless of symptoms.

What are the benefits of treatment with digoxin Fab fragments?

Reversal of digitalis-induced dysrhythmias, conduction disturbances, myocardial depression, and hyperkalemia in severely poisoned patients.

What are the sources of cardiac glycoside poisoning?

1. Digoxin
2. Venom of toads from the *Bufo* genus
3. Ingestion of plants containing cardiac glycosides (e.g., oleander, lily of the valley, foxglove)

How does use change in a patient with renal failure?

The digoxin-Fab complex is excreted in the urine; therefore, elimination of the digoxin-Fab complex is delayed in renal failure, and free digoxin levels gradually increase after Fab administration. Rebound cardiac glycoside toxicity is rare but has been reported.

Can dialysis be used to eliminate the digoxin-Fab complexes?

No. Hemodialysis does not enhance elimination of digoxin-Fab complex.

If the digoxin concentration is unknown, how much Digifab should be administered?

If severely poisoned acutely, 5 to 10 vials should be given at a time, with subsequent observation of clinical response. An empiric dose of 2 vials is often sufficient for chronic digoxin poisoning.

How much digoxin will 40 mg (1 vial) of Digifab bind?

0.5 mg digoxin

How do you calculate how much Digifab to administer?

1. Known amount ingested:

$$\text{the number of vials to administer} = \frac{\text{Total digitalis ingested (mg)}}{0.5 \text{ mg}}$$

2. Known serum level in chronic steady state:

$$\text{the number of vials to administer} = \left[\frac{\text{Serum digoxin concentration (ng/mL)} \times \text{patient's body weight (kg)}}{100}\right]$$

How do the doses differ in poisoning with non-digoxin cardiac glycosides?

Higher doses may be required due to lower affinity for the non-digoxin cardiac glycosides.

How should it be administered?

If cardiac arrest is imminent or has occurred, the dose can be given as a bolus; however, it should be infused over 30 min in stable patients.

How quickly does it work?

Patients can have reversal of ventricular dysrhythmias within 2 min, and most patients have settling of toxic dysrhythmias within 30 min of Fab administration. Within 6 hrs, 90% of patients will have completely or partially responded to the medication.

What laboratory test is unreliable after digoxin immune fragment administration?

Serum digoxin concentration. Measured digoxin levels may increase soon after administration of digoxin immune fragments, although the digoxin will not be pharmacologically active because it is largely bound to the immune fragments.

DIMERCAPROL

For what purpose was dimercaprol developed?

Developed by the British as an antidote for Lewisite, an organic arsenical compound used as a vesicating chemical weapon. It is also known as British anti-Lewisite, or BAL.

How is dimercaprol administered for heavy metal chelation?

Deep IM

In what substance is dimercaprol dissolved?	Peanut oil
What are its indications?	1. Treatment of lead encephalopathy as adjunctive therapy with $CaNa_2EDTA$ 2. Severe inorganic arsenic toxicity 3. Inorganic mercury toxicity 4. Gold toxicity
What is the mechanism of action of dimercaprol?	Dimercaprol's sulfhydryl groups chelate heavy metals to form a stable complex capable of renal excretion
What are the contraindications for dimercaprol?	1. Iron, cadmium, selenium, or uranium poisoning, as these metal-dimercaprol complexes are toxic 2. Peanut allergy 3. G6PD deficiency (may cause methemoglobinemia) 4. Use with caution in thrombocy-topenic/coagulopathic patients and in those who are hypertensive
What are the adverse effects of BAL?	1. HTN 2. Injection-related – sterile abscess, painful administration 3. Febrile reaction 4. Cholinergic symptoms – nausea, vomiting, salivation, lacrimation, rhinorrhea 5. Hemolysis in G6PD-deficient patients 6. Chelation of essential metals, resulting in deficiency
What are the typical dosing regimens for BAL?	1. Lead encephalopathy – 75 mg/m^2 IM q4 hrs for 5 days (must be followed by $CaNa_2EDTA$ 4 hrs after injection) 2. Inorganic arsenic/inorganic mercury poisoning – 3 mg/kg IM q4 hrs for 48 hrs, then q12 hrs for 7 to 10 days

DIMETHYL-P-AMINOPHENOL (DMAP)

What are some alternative names for this chemical?	4-DMAP, 4-dimethylaminophenolate

DMAP is used as an antidote for toxicity from which substance?

Cyanide

What is the clinical effect of DMAP?

Induces methemoglobinemia, which is often the first step in treating cyanide poisoning. In Germany, it is used instead of sodium nitrite for treating cyanide poisoning.

How does DMAP induce methemoglobinemia?

Catalyzes the transfer of electrons from Fe^{2+} (ferrous) iron to O_2. In the process, oxidized Fe^{3}_+ (ferric) iron is produced.

How does methemoglobinemia aid in the treatment of cyanide poisoning?

Cyanide has higher affinity for ferric iron than it does for cytochrome oxidase a_3 in the respiratory chain of mitochondria. This will free cytochrome a_3 and allow normal cellular respiration.

What is the dose of DMAP used for cyanide poisoning?

3.25 mg/kg is the recommended dose; therefore, 250 mg or 5 mL of 5% solution IV is a reasonable dose for an adult of unknown weight. It can be given IM, if necessary. It should only be administered to comatose patients in whom cyanide poisoning is a reasonable certainty.

What medication must be administered along with DMAP?

Sodium thiosulfate. It acts as a sulfhydryl donor to the rhodanese enzyme, which converts cyanide into thiocyanate (eliminated in the urine).

What advantage does DMAP have over the nitrites?

It works faster and can induce a greater degree of methemoglobinemia than sodium nitrite.

What are the adverse effects of DMAP?

Excessive methemoglobinemia and hemolysis

What are the possible clinical effects of methemoglobinemia?

Cyanosis, nausea, headache, dizziness, dyspnea, confusion, seizures

How is DMAP reversed, if necessary?

Methylene blue; however, this could theoretically release cyanide bound to methemoglobin, causing reexposure.

When should DMAP be avoided?

When there is a question of combined cyanide and CO exposure (as in smoke inhalation from a structure fire). DMAP-induced methemoglobinemia, in combination with significant carboxyhemoglobin, could markedly impair O_2 transport.

DIPHENHYDRAMINE

What are the clinical uses for diphenhydramine in the realm of toxicology?

1. Treatment of symptoms of histamine excess (e.g., urticaria)
2. Prophylaxis against hypersensitivity to antivenoms or antitoxins
3. Treatment of EPS due to neuroleptic drugs (e.g., dystonia)
4. Antipruritic agent (due to insect bites or plant exposures)

How is diphenhydramine administered?

PO, IV, IM, topically

What is the mechanism of action of diphenhydramine?

1. Histamine (H_1) receptor blockade
2. Anticholinergic activity
3. Sodium channel blockade

What are the contraindications for diphenhydramine administration?

1. Angle-closure glaucoma
2. Obstructive uropathy (e.g., from prostatic hypertrophy)
3. Preexisting anticholinergic symptoms

What is the typical dosing of diphenhydramine?

Depending on symptom severity, 25–50 mg in adults (1.25 mg/kg in children) IV/IM/PO q6 hrs

What are the acute side effects of diphenhydramine use?

CNS depression (may cause paradoxical agitation in children), AMS, hyperthermia, urinary retention, skin flushing, tachycardia, blurred vision

ETHANOL

For what toxins is ethanol used as an antidote?	Methanol and ethylene glycol
By what mechanism does ethanol work as an antidote?	Competitive inhibition of alcohol dehydrogenase blocks the conversion of toxic alcohols (i.e., methanol and ethylene glycol) to toxic metabolites.
What difficulties should be considered regarding the use of ethanol as an antidote?	1. IV solution is not FDA approved 2. IV solution is hyperosmolar 3. Frequent serum ethanol determinations are required to maintain therapeutic levels 4. Hypoglycemia may develop in children
If used as an antidote, what is the target serum ethanol level?	100 mg/dL. At this level, the metabolism of both methanol and ethylene glycol by alcohol dehydrogenase is completely blocked.
Following toxic alcohol ingestion, does ethanol remove the acidic metabolites?	No. Ethanol, at appropriate doses, will block the formation of toxic metabolites; however, once these metabolites are formed, only further metabolism or hemodialysis will remove them.
Describe the dosing of an ethanol infusion.	Generally, 10 mL/kg loading dose of 10% ethanol solution, then 1 to 2 mL/kg/hr maintenance dose, will keep serum ethanol concentrations at 100 mg/dL; however, rates of metabolism vary greatly.
Is ethanol dialyzable?	Yes; therefore, the infusion rate must be doubled for patients receiving hemodialysis.
The maintenance infusion rate must be adjusted for which patient populations?	1. Chronic alcoholics 2. Other patients with induced cytochrome enzymes 3. Patients receiving hemodialysis
What are some common complications of ethanol infusion?	Hypoglycemia (especially in children), phlebitis, inebriation

Are any laboratory tests important during ethanol infusion?	Serum ethanol level and blood glucose checks should be done every hour.
For what other poisoning may ethanol be an antidote?	SMFA. While data on human efficacy is limited, ethanol may supply the necessary acetate to overcome SMFA's inhibition of the TCA cycle.

FLUMAZENIL

What type of medication is flumazenil?	Benzodiazepine antagonist (1,4-imidazobenzodiazepine)
What is the mechanism of action of flumazenil?	Competitive inhibition of the benzodiazepine receptor with subsequent prevention of GABA potentiation in the CNS
Is flumazenil routinely indicated for benzodiazepine overdose?	No. It should not be administered as a nonspecific coma-reversal drug and should be used with extreme caution after intentional overdose.
Why should one avoid flumazenil in these circumstances?	It has the potential to precipitate withdrawal in benzodiazepine-dependent individuals and/or induce seizures in those at risk. Also, overdoses of benzodiazepines alone are rarely fatal. Fatalities can occur in mixed overdoses with other CNS depressants (e.g., ethanol, opioids, other sedatives) due to synergistic activity.
How is flumazenil most commonly used?	To treat iatrogenic benzodiazepine over-medication during procedural sedation or monitored anesthesia care
What is the adult dose of flumazenil?	0.5 to 5 mg (adults). Typically, begin with 0.2 mg IV over 30 sec, then titrate in 0.5 mg doses at 1 min intervals.
What is the time of onset of flumazenil?	1 to 2 min, peak effect in 6 to 10 min

What is the duration of action of flumazenil?	45 to 90 min. Patients will always need to be monitored for re-sedation, and additional doses may be necessary.
What are the risks associated with administering flumazenil?	Primarily seizures and benzodiazepine withdrawal, although cardiac dysrhythmias are possible
What groups of patients are more likely to develop seizures?	1. Chronic benzodiazepine use (habituated user) 2. Co-ingestant that lowers the seizure threshold (e.g., CAs, cocaine, methylxanthines, diphenhydramine) 3. Preexisting seizure disorder
What medication should be used to treat seizures induced by flumazenil?	Barbiturates are the first-line agents.
What is the preferred treatment of benzodiazepine overdose?	Airway management and supportive care with observation until symptoms resolve
In what type of overdose patient could flumazenil be considered?	Young children with no history of seizure disorder and who are on no chronic benzodiazepine therapy who present with respiratory depression after isolated benzodiazepine ingestion

FOLIC ACID

What is folic acid?	An essential B-complex vitamin (vitamin B_9)
Are folic acid and folinic acid the same compound?	No. Folinic acid is the activated form of folic acid and does not need to be activated by dihydrofolate reductase (DHFR) in order to be used in cellular processes. Folic acid requires further activation (by DHFR) before use.
How is folic acid used as a therapy for toxic ingestions?	As adjunctive therapy for the treatment of methanol ingestions

What is the mechanism of action of folate?	Enhances conversion of formic acid (toxic metabolite of methanol) to CO_2 and water
How should folate be administered to treat methanol ingestion?	IV
What dose of folate should be used to treat methanol ingestions?	Though no specific dose is widely accepted, the following are suggested: Adults – 50 mg IV q4 hrs × 6 doses Children – 1 mg/kg IV q4 hrs × 6 doses
Are there any contraindications to folate administration?	Known hypersensitivity

FOMEPIZOLE (4-METHYLPYRAZOLE, 4-MP)

What are other commonly encountered names for this antidote?	1. Antizol is the U.S. trade name. 2. 4-methylpyrazole (4-MP) is the chemical name.
What is the mechanism of action of 4-MP?	Competitive inhibition of alcohol dehydrogenase, which prevents certain alcohols from being converted to their more toxic metabolites
4-MP is indicated in preventing the toxic effects of which toxic alcohols?	Methanol and ethylene glycol
What are the indications for treatment with 4-MP?	1. Ethylene glycol or methanol level >20 mg/dL 2. Known ingestion of ethylene glycol or methanol (if a serum level cannot be obtained quickly) 3. Clinical suspicion of ethylene glycol or methanol ingestion and 2 of the following: pH <7.3, serum bicarbonate <20 mg/dL, or osmol gap >10 4. 4-MP can also be considered for patients with an unexplained acidosis (especially if there is an osmol gap) and for those who are clinically intoxicated with a negative serum ethanol.

What other antidote should be considered if 4-MP is not readily available for methanol or ethylene glycol poisonings?	Ethanol
How could 4-MP decrease the severity of disulfiram or disulfiram-like reactions to ethanol?	By blocking the formation of acetaldehyde by alcohol dehydrogenase. Acetaldehyde is responsible for many of the toxic effects of the disulfiram-ethanol reaction (i.e., flushing, diaphoresis, nausea, vomiting, tachycardia, hypotension).
Should 4-MP be used for isopropyl alcohol ingestions?	No. This would prolong the metabolism of isopropanol to its less toxic metabolite, acetone.
How is 4-MP dosed?	Loading dose of 15 mg/kg IV, then 10 mg/kg IV q12 hrs × 4 doses. Subsequent doses are given at 15 mg/dL if therapy extends beyond 48 hrs.
Should 4-MP dosing be altered if the patient is undergoing hemodialysis?	Yes. Dosing should be increased to q4 hrs during hemodialysis. <u>At start of dialysis</u> – if most recent dose was >6 hrs ago, give another dose <u>At end of dialysis</u> – if most recent dose was ≥3 hrs earlier, give full dose; if most recent dose was 1 to 3 hrs earlier, give half dose

GLUCAGON

What is glucagon?	A polypeptide hormone that is naturally produced in the pancreas and is currently synthesized by pharmaceutical companies
Why must glucagon be given parenterally?	It is destroyed in the GI tract and would have no effect if given PO.
What is the mechanism of action of glucagon?	1. Binds to specific glucagon receptors → activates adenylyl cyclase → ↑ cAMP production → ↑ cardiac inotropy and chronotropy, ↑ hepatic glycogenolysis and gluconeogenesis, GI smooth muscle relaxation

2. A metabolite of glucagon (miniglucagon) increases arachidonic acid in cardiac cells, which improves myocardial contractility, partly by increasing Ca^{2+} stores in the sarcoplasmic reticulum.

What was the original indication for glucagon?

Treatment of hypoglycemia when a patient cannot tolerate PO glucose and/or when IV glucose is unavailable

For what other indications is glucagon utilized?

1. Principally to ↑ BP as a primary treatment for beta-blocker poisoning and as adjunctive therapy for CCB poisoning
2. To correct myocardial depression after overdose with TCAs, quinidine, or procainamide
3. To facilitate passage of an esophageal foreign body

How does glucagon improve cardiac function in patients with beta-blocker or CCB poisoning?

<u>Beta-blocker</u> – bypasses blocked cardiac beta-adrenergic receptors to ↑ intracellular cAMP → activates protein kinase A → ↑ Ca^{2+} influx through voltage-sensitive calcium channels → ↑ sarcoplasmic reticulum Ca^{2+} stores
<u>CCB</u> – facilitates Ca^{2+} entry → may ↑ inotropy. It may also be used in conjunction with IV calcium and high-dose insulin therapy.

How soon are the effects of glucagon seen after administration?

1 to 2 min

How long do glucagon's cardiac effects persist?

10 to 15 min

How should glucagon be administered?

1. For hypoglycemia or facilitating passage of an esophageal foreign body, 1 mg IV is recommended.
2. For hypotension following an overdose, 50 to 150 μg/kg (5–10 mg) IV is recommended. If there is a positive

response, an infusion should be started due to glucagon's short duration of action. The infusion rate should be the amount of the effective bolus per hour (usually 5–10 mg/hr in adults), which can then be titrated to effect.

What must be remembered when reconstituting glucagon for injection?

Use saline or D5W to dissolve the glucagon. Previous packages in the U.S. contained phenol as a diluent. With the large doses used in treating an overdose, a toxic dose of phenol could be administered.

What are the adverse effects of glucagon use?

Nausea and vomiting are common, especially with larger doses; therefore, it should only be administered to patients with a protected airway. Glucagon may also cause hyperglycemia and hypokalemia.

GLUCOSE

What is glucose?

A 6-carbon carbohydrate used for energy by the body. The biologically active isomer (d-glucose) is also known as dextrose.

How is glucose administered?

PO, IV

When is glucose administration indicated?

Hypoglycemia, hyperkalemia, CCB toxicity, beta-blocker toxicity, undifferentiated AMS

Why is glucose used to treat hyperkalemia?

It is used as an adjunct to insulin therapy, which results in the shifting of potassium into cells.

Why is glucose administered in patients with undifferentiated AMS?

Hypoglycemia is a common cause of AMS.

How should glucose be used in a sulfonylurea overdose?

May be administered as intermittent boluses; however, continuous infusion of 5% to 10% dextrose may be more effective in maintaining euglycemia.

What is one potential problem when using glucose for a sulfonylurea overdose?

IV glucose infusion may induce further insulin release, resulting in paradoxical hypoglycemia.

How is glucose used for CCB and beta-blocker overdose?

Glucose and insulin are used together in a treatment called hyperinsulinemia-euglycemia therapy.

What is the mechanism behind hyperinsulinemia-euglycemia therapy?

CCBs cause insulin resistance in over-dose. Glucose provides the carbohy-drates necessary for cardiac metabolism, while high doses of insulin help to over-come the insulin resistance and allow glucose to enter the myocardial cells → ↑ cardiac inotropy.

What is the typical dose of glucose used for treating hypoglycemia?

Adults – 1 to 2 mL/kg of D50 solution
Children – 2 to 4 mL/kg of D25 solution

When is oral glucose contraindicated?

1. No secure airway
2. Inability to swallow
3. Hyperglycemia

What are toxic effects of glucose administration?

1. Hyperglycemia
2. Irritation/phlebitis at administration site when given IV (especially with rapid push)
3. Tissue necrosis if IV catheter infiltrates
4. Wernicke-Korsakoff syndrome in thiamine-deficient patients

HALOPERIDOL AND DROPERIDOL

What type of medications are droperidol and haloperidol?

Butyrophenone class neuroleptics (antipsychotics). Droperidol is considered "medium potency," while haloperidol is considered "high potency."

How do these drugs help mediate psychotic symptoms (mechanism of action)?

Dopamine receptor blockade (D2 receptors in the mesolimbic system of the brain)

For what are these medications most typically used in the emergency department?	Rapid tranquilization and treatment of acute psychosis
How is this accomplished?	The sedative properties are mediated through alpha 2-adrenergic receptor agonism, droperidol more so than haloperidol.
What side effects might be expected with dopamine receptor blockade?	Akathisia, dystonia, parkinsonian symptoms, and tardive dyskinesia. These are likely due to blockade of dopamine receptors in the nigrostriatal pathway.
Above what dose are these side effects more likely?	With >10 mg haloperidol (cumulative), the risk of EPS increases.
What cardiac side effects have been described for this class of medications?	QT prolongation and torsade de pointes
Which one received a "black box" warning from the FDA in 2001 because of the concern over QT prolongation?	Droperidol
Are these agents used as first-line agents for the sedation of patients with toxin-induced agitation?	No. Benzodiazepines are effective in managing agitation and have an excellent safety profile; however, occasionally small doses of haloperidol or droperidol may be helpful in managing severe agitation refractory to benzodiazepines.
What are some conditions for which haloperidol or droperidol may be useful?	1. Overdose that causes excessive dopaminergic stimulation (e.g., methylphenidate, pemoline) 2. Conditions in which hallucinations are potentially contributing to the agitation (e.g., delirium tremens)
What are some disadvantages to using haloperidol or droperidol to treat toxin-induced agitation?	1. May exacerbate hyperthermia by inhibiting diaphoresis due to an anticholinergic effect

2. Could worsen the condition if agitation was secondary to NMS
3. Could further prolong the QT interval if given for an overdose of a QT-prolonging agent

What other medication can be given in conjunction with haloperidol or droperidol to augment the sedative effects and provide rapid control?

Benzodiazepines (e.g., midazolam, lorazepam)

HISTAMINE-2 RECEPTOR ANTAGONISTS (H₂ BLOCKERS)

What are the toxicologic uses of H₂ blockers?

1. Toxin-induced gastritis (e.g., isopropyl alcohol)
2. Adjunctive therapy for the treatment of scombroid toxicity
3. Adjunctive therapy and/or pretreatment for allergic/anaphylactoid reactions

Why are H₂ antagonists useful for allergic symptoms?

Large amounts of histamine released during an allergic response may cause nausea and GI distress through stimulation of acid production. There are also a small number of H₂ receptors in the skin, smooth muscle, and heart.

Name the 4 H₂ receptor antagonists available in the U.S.

1. Cimetidine
2. Ranitidine
3. Famotidine
4. Nizatidine

What are the dosages for common H₂ blockers?

<u>Cimetidine</u> – 300 mg IV/PO/IM q8 hrs
<u>Ranitidine</u> – 50 mg IV/IM q8 hrs or 150 mg PO q12 hrs

For what other treatment can cimetidine potentially be used?

Cimetidine is an inhibitor of the P450 system. Theoretically, it may be used to block the production of toxic metabolites following the ingestion of substances whose metabolism through the P450 system generates toxins (e.g., APAP, carbon tetrachloride, *Amanita* mushrooms); however, studies have not demonstrated clinical efficacy in humans.

HYDROXOCOBALAMIN

What is hydroxocobalamin?	Synthetic precursor of vitamin B_{12}

For what is hydroxocobalamin indicated?

Given its safety profile, hydroxocobalamin should be administered to any patient suspected of having cyanide toxicity. It can be given empirically to victims of smoke inhalation with profound metabolic (lactic) acidosis, hemodynamic instability, or other signs of cyanide poisoning.

What is the mechanism of action of hydroxocobalamin?

Acts as a chelating agent for cyanide. Hydroxocobalamin combines with cyanide in an equimolar ratio to form cyanocobalamin. Cyanocobalamin is also known as vitamin B_{12}; it is nontoxic and renally eliminated.

How is hydroxocobalamin administered when treating cyanide poisoning?

5 g IV for adults, 70 mg/kg for children. This should be given over 15 min. It is supplied in 250 mL vials, each containing 2.5 mg of hydroxocobalamin, which are to be diluted in 100 mL of normal saline.

Which medicine should also be administered when treating a patient with hydroxocobalamin?

Sodium thiosulfate. Together, these agents have synergistic effects, increasing their antidotal efficacy; however, they should not be administered at the same time or through the same line, as thiosulfate will bind to hydroxocobalamin and render it inactive.

What are the adverse effects of hydroxocobalamin administration?

Good safety profile, overall. Allergic reactions have been reported but only in patients receiving long-term treatment for pernicious anemia. Virtually every patient receiving a 5 g dose will develop orange-red discoloration of the skin, mucous membranes, and urine, which typically resolves in 24 to 48 hrs. The discoloration of the serum may interfere with several laboratory tests. Also, a pustular rash has developed in some individuals receiving hydroxocobalamin.

Its appearance was delayed until ≥ 1 wk following infusion, and it resolved in 6 to 38 days.

What are the advantages of hydroxocobalamin over the traditional cyanide antidote kit?

As it does not induce methemoglobinemia, hydroxocobalamin is safe to administer to victims of smoke inhalation who are at risk for significant carboxyhemoglobinemia. This is important because smoke inhalation is the most commonly reported cause of cyanide poisoning, and the nitrite portion of the cyanide antidote kit is not typically administered in these cases. Also, hydroxocobalamin administration can cause transient HTN, which may be advantageous in the hemodynamically unstable patient.

HYPERBARIC OXYGEN

What is hyperbaric oxygen (HBO)?

A treatment modality in which a patient is placed in a sealed pressure chamber and breathes oxygen at a pressure >760 mmHg, or 1 atmosphere.

What are the physiologic effects of HBO?

1. ↑ partial pressure of O_2 in the blood (Henry's law)
2. ↓ size of undissolved gas bubbles (Boyle's law)

Name some other postulated effects of HBO therapy.

1. Stimulates fibroblast proliferation and angiogenesis (promotes wound healing)
2. WBC cytotoxicity is enhanced, and WBC vessel wall adherence is decreased.
3. Directly bactericidal to anaerobic bacteria and bacteriostatic to aerobic bacteria

For which toxicologic exposures has HBO therapy been advocated?

1. CO – may reduce cognitive sequelae in severe poisoning, but patient selection criteria are not well-defined. Indications that have been advocated (but not proven) include AMS,

pregnancy, age >36 yrs, exposure >24 hrs, cerebellar dysfunction, and carboxy-Hgb level >25%.

2. Cyanide – no proven role, may help if concomitant CO exposure (smoke inhalation)

3. Concentrated hydrogen peroxide ingestion with arterial gas embolism (AGE) – gastric mucosal perforation may allow gas bubbles to enter venous circulation and embolize to the brain, resulting in stroke symptoms

4. *Loxosceles* spider envenomation (brown recluse) – for wound healing of necrotic ulcers

5. Methemoglobinemia – if refractory to methylene blue, can support tissue oxygen demands independent of Hgb

6. Methylene chloride – indications similar to CO poisoning due to the development of CO as methylene chloride is metabolized

Why is HBO only a consideration in the above exposures?

Very little data exists to support HBO use, except in decompression illness (DCI) and AGE.

What are adverse effects of HBO?

1. O_2 toxicity–reactive oxygen species produce oxidant damage to membranes and cellular components

2. Pulmonary toxicity–type II alveolar cells have ↓ surfactant production, acute reversible exudative process. Continued hyperbaric exposure can result in permanent damage via fibrosis, fibroblast proliferation, and hyperplasia.

3. Lowers seizure threshold

4. Visual toxicity–reversible myopia, scotomata

5. Barotrauma–direct mechanical damage to tissue

How are oxygen toxicity symptoms managed?

1. ↑ air breaks between breathing 100% O_2

2. ↓ pressure/depth – the only variable to change in a monoplace (single patient) chamber, as it is filled with 100% O_2

What is an absolute contraindication to HBO?

Untreated pneumothorax (PTX) – will expand on ascent, potentially causing a tension PTX

What are relative contraindications to HBO therapy?

1. Prior chest surgery, resulting in air trapping and barotrauma
2. Lung disease – same as above
3. Viral infections – prevent middle ear/sinus pressure equalization
4. Recent middle ear surgery – same as above
5. Optic neuritis – possible ↑ optic nerve pathology
6. Seizure disorders – ↑ risk of seizures
7. High fever – ↓ seizure threshold
8. Congenital spherocytosis
9. Claustrophobia
10. Unstable patients (if using a monoplace chamber) – they are inaccessible if rapid interventions are needed
11. Disulfiram use – inhibits superoxide dismutase
12. Premature infants – risk of retrolental fibroplasia, causing blindness
13. Concurrent use of antineoplastic agents (e.g., doxorubicin, cisplatin, bleomycin)

Are all recompression chambers the same?

No. Monoplace chambers accommodate one supine patient and are filled entirely with 100% O_2, which the patient breathes during the entire treatment. Multiplace chambers accommodate two or more patients sitting upright or supine, along with an attendant, and are filled with ambient air consisting of 21% O_2. Tight-fitting aviation masks are utilized to administer 100% O_2 intermittently during the treatment, reducing the risk of oxygen toxicity. Portable recompression chambers may be used in remote or austere environments.

INAMRINONE (PREVIOUSLY AMRINONE)

What are the primary actions of inamrinone?

Inotropy and vasodilation

What is the mechanism of action of inamrinone?

1. Inhibition of myocardial cell phospho-diesterase activity → ↑ intracellular cAMP → ↑ inotropy
2. Vascular smooth muscle relaxation → ↓ preload and afterload

What are the primary toxicologic indications for inamrinone?

Treatment of CCB, beta-blocker, or mixed beta- and alpha-blocker overdose refractory to conventional management techniques

By what route, and in what dosage, is inamrinone administered?

Loading dose – 0.75 mg/kg IV over 2 to 3 min (may be repeated once in 30 min)
Infusion – 5 to 10 μg/kg/min IV

What is the approximate onset of action?

2 to 5 min

How long is the duration of action?

0.5 to 2 hrs following IV administration

What is the approximate half-life of inamrinone?

5 to 8 hrs (can be prolonged in patients with CHF)

In which organ is inamrinone metabolized?

Liver

What are the potential adverse effects of inamrinone?

Thrombocytopenia, dysrhythmias, hypotension, nausea, vomiting, injection site irritation, exacerbation of outflow tract obstruction in patients with hypertrophic subaortic stenosis

What, if any, are the contraindications to inamrinone usage?

Known hypersensitivity to inamrinone or to sulfites (metabisulfite is used as a drug preservative)

INSULIN

Insulin can be used for treating which toxicologic emergencies?	1. CCB toxicity with hypotension (possibly with dextrose) 2. Beta-blocker toxicity with hypotension (possibly with dextrose) 3. Vacor toxicity
What are contraindications for insulin use?	1. Hypoglycemia 2. Known hypersensitivity to insulin components
What cells increase glucose uptake when stimulated by insulin?	Skeletal muscle cells, cardiac myocytes, adipose tissue
What are the adverse effects of insulin?	1. Hypoglycemia 2. Hypokalemia 3. Local pain/irritation at the site of injection 4. Lipodystrophy at injection site (uncommon)
What is the serum half-life of regular human insulin?	~4 to 5 min
What substances may antagonize the effects of insulin?	1. Epinephrine 2. Corticosteroids 3. Glucose (PO or IV) 4. Glucagon
What are the effects of CCBs on insulin secretion?	1. CCB overdose causes insulin resistance. 2. CCBs block voltage-dependent (L-type) calcium channels within beta islet cells of the pancreas → ↓ Ca^{2+} influx → ↓ exocytosis of insulin stored in secretory granules → insulin deficiency
What is the effect of CCB overdose on myocardial metabolism?	The combination of insulin resistance with decreased systemic insulin production impairs myocardial glucose uptake, further depressing contractility.

What name is given to insulin therapy for CCB toxicity?

Hyperinsulinemic-euglycemic therapy

Why is insulin useful in treating the hemodynamic effects of CCB toxicity?

The blockade of insulin's effect by CCBs is competitive. Administration of high-dose insulin $\rightarrow \uparrow$ glucose uptake by cardiac myocytes $\rightarrow \uparrow$ myocardial function.

What is the mechanism of action of insulin in a beta-blocker overdose?

While hyperinsulinemic-euglycemic therapy has been shown to be efficacious in beta-blocker poisoning, the exact mechanism has not been well-defined.

What dosing of insulin should be provided to treat hypotension due to CCB or beta-blocker toxicity?

There is no universal dose. Supra-physiological doses of insulin, much higher than those used for the treatment of DKA, are required to overcome CCB-induced insulin resistance.

How should insulin be administered?

Recommended regimens vary. An infusion of regular insulin may be started and rapidly titrated up to 1 to 2 U/kg/hr as needed to support blood pressure. Blood sugar should be measured frequently, with IV dextrose administered to maintain euglycemia. With significant CCB toxicity, supplemental glucose is often not necessary. Patients may remain hyperglycemic despite massive insulin infusions. K^+ should also be monitored.

How long may it take before a therapeutic benefit is observed?

Up to 30 min. Additional supportive care should be employed until effects are seen.

What is the dose of insulin used for treating adults with hyperkalemia?

0.1 U/kg regular insulin IV (with 25 g IV D50)

Is there a simpler dosing recommendation that does not require calculations?

Begin with 5 to 10 U regular insulin IV (with D50 as above), then infuse 1 L of D20 with 40 to 80 U regular insulin over 2 to 4 hrs.

How often should glucose levels be monitored while treating hyperkalemia with insulin?	q30 min
Is there a way to use insulin to treat hyperkalemia if you have no insulin readily available?	Yes. By giving an IV dextrose load (25 g D50), the non-diabetic patient will respond by releasing endogenous insulin; this method is not as effective as administering exogenous insulin.
What is the mechanism for insulin's role in hyperkalemia?	Insulin → ↑ activity of skeletal muscle Na-K-ATPase → ↑ K^+ influx (thereby ↓ serum K^+)
After providing exogenous insulin, how long does it take for the serum potassium to fall?	~15 min
How long does the drop in potassium last?	Several hours
Is insulin safe to use during pregnancy?	Yes (category B). It does not cross the placenta.

IODIDE

What is iodide?	The anion (I^-) of iodine, which exists as 7 different species in aqueous solution – iodide, triiodide, hypoiodite ion, iodate ion, iodine cation, hypoiodic acid, and elemental iodine
What is the toxicologic indication for iodides?	Potassium iodide (KI) is indicated for preventing the development of thyroid cancer in those exposed to radioactive iodine.
Where is radioiodine found?	Commonly used in medical applications and in nuclear reactors
What is the time frame for administration of iodides in the setting of radioiodine exposure?	Optimally, it is given 1 hr prior to the exposure (as prophylaxis), but it may still be beneficial up to 4 hrs post-exposure.

What is the recommended dose and duration of therapy after exposure?

The doses recommended by the FDA are:
<u>Adults</u> – 130 mg
<u>Children</u> (3 to 18 yrs) – 65 mg
<u>Infants and children</u> (1 month to 3 yrs) – 32 mg
<u>Newborns</u> (0 to 1 month) – 16 mg
Daily dosing should continue until the risk of exposure is eliminated.

How do iodides work in the setting of a radiological exposure?

They are readily absorbed by the thyroid gland, saturating the gland with iodide and preventing uptake of any radioactive iodide.

Who benefits the most from treatment with KI?

Children have a far greater risk of developing cancer secondary to radioactive iodine exposure; therefore, adults over 40 yrs are generally not advised to take KI unless there is a projected thyroid dose of >5 Gray (500 rads). Children and pregnant, or lactating, women should receive prophylaxis for projected exposure of >5 rads.

How are iodides administered?

PO in salt form, most commonly as potassium iodide (KI)

Can iodide be given in pregnancy?

Yes; however, it is recommended that pregnant and lactating women take only 1 dose, as iodide readily crosses the placenta and is found in breast milk.

How else is iodide used?

Iodide salts were the mainstay of treatment for hyperthyroidism prior to the advent of thioamides. Historically, they were also used as antimicrobials.

IPECAC SYRUP

What is ipecac syrup?

An alkaloid oral suspension that induces vomiting

Where is this found in nature?

In plants belonging to the family *Rubiacea*

Name the two key components.	Emetine and cephaeline
How is ipecac used?	Historically, ipecac was used as an emetic in the case of a potentially poisonous ingestion or intentional overdose. Ipecac is no longer recommended for GI decontamination.
What is the mechanism of action of ipecac?	Emetine produces irritation of the gastric mucosa, while cephaeline causes stimulation of the medullary CTZ.
What is the time to onset of action of ipecac?	15 to 30 min
What are symptoms of acute ingestion of ipecac?	Nausea, vomiting, diarrhea
What are the cellular effects of chronic use?	Emetine-mediated inhibition of protein synthesis in skeletal muscle

ISOPROTERENOL

What is isoproterenol?	Sympathomimetic drug that targets beta-adrenergic receptors
What is the mechanism of action of isoproterenol?	Stimulates beta 1- and beta 2-adrenergic receptors → ↑ chronotropy and inotropy, as well as bronchodilation, vasodilation, and hepatic glycogenolysis
What are toxicologic indications for isoproterenol use?	Refractory drug-induced torsade de pointes (TdP)
Where is isoproterenol metabolized?	Primarily by COMT in the liver
What is the half-life of IV isoproterenol?	2.5 to 5 min
What contraindications prevent administration of isoproterenol?	VF, VT (except TdP), and history of *congenital* long QT syndrome. History of ischemic heart disease is a relative

contraindication, as these patients may not tolerate an ↑ HR.

What is the recommended dose of isoproterenol used for treating TdP?

Adults – 2 μg/min initially, then titrate to patient response (2 to 10 μg/min) Children – 0.1 μg/kg/min initially (effective dose is typically 0.2 to 2 μg/kg/min)

What is the goal of isoproterenol therapy in TdP?

Suppression of TdP. This is generally achieved when the patient's HR is 90 to 140 beats/min.

What is the mechanism by which isoproterenol treats TdP?

Not fully understood. Isoproterenol appears to suppress TdP by ↑ HR, which helps to homogenize repolarization among myocardial cells.

LEUCOVORIN

What is the common name for folinic acid?

Leucovorin

What is leucovorin?

The metabolically active form of folic acid

How is folic acid activated?

Folic acid is converted, by dihydrofoliate acid reductase (DHFR), to tetrahydrofolic acid, which is a precursor of folinic acid.

What is the mechanism of action of folinic acid?

Acts as a cofactor for production of purine nucleotides and thymidylate in the formation of DNA

What are the uses of leucovorin?

1. Treatment of methanol poisoning
2. Rescue therapy for high-dose methotrexate therapy
3. Treatment of methotrexate overdose
4. Treatment of trimethoprim- and pyrimethamine-induced bone marrow suppression

How does leucovorin overcome methotrexate toxicity?

Methotrexate inhibits the formation of tetrahydrofolate, which halts DNA synthesis. Leucovorin overcomes this blockade by supplying the necessary folinic acid for purine synthesis.

What is the dosing of leucovorin after methotrexate overdose?

Initial dose of leucovorin should be $\geq$ the amount of methotrexate ingested. Generally, an initial dose of 100 mg/m^2 of leucovorin will be sufficient for all but the most severe poisonings. This dose should optimally be given within 1 hr of ingestion. Subsequent doses of leucovorin may be adjusted based on methotrexate levels.

At what point can leucovorin therapy be stopped after methotrexate overdose?

When methotrexate blood levels are <0.01 μmol/L and there are no signs of bone marrow suppression

What are some adverse effects of leucovorin?

1. Hypercalcemia may result from the calcium salt.
2. Intrathecal administration can result in neurotoxicity and death.
3. Seizures have been reported.

LIDOCAINE

What are the toxicologic indications for lidocaine?

Suppression of refractory ventricular dysrhythmias induced by cardiac toxins, particularly cardiac glycosides and possibly CAs (controversial)

What is the mechanism of action of lidocaine?

Inhibits fast sodium channels without prolonging the QRS (type Ib antidysrhythmic) → slows phase 0 of action potential

How does lidocaine abolish ventricular dysrhythmias?

By depressing conduction in aberrant tissue and, thus, stopping re-entrant circuits

What is the effect of lidocaine on the SA and AV nodes?

Minimally suppresses conduction

When is lidocaine contraindicated?

Adams-Stokes syndrome, Wolff-Parkinson-White syndrome, AV block, bradycardia, hypotension, hypersensitivity to lidocaine or amide anesthetics

What are some toxic CNS side effects of lidocaine?

Dizziness, confusion, agitation, seizures, coma

What are some toxic cardiac side effects of lidocaine?	Worsened dysrhythmias, AV block, bradycardia, cardiac arrest
Where is lidocaine metabolized?	Liver
What is the typical dose of lidocaine used for treating dysrhythmias?	1 mg/kg IV
What is the maximum safe dose of lidocaine for local anesthesia?	Without epinephrine – 3 to 5 mg/kg (~30 mL of 1% solution) With epinephrine – 7 mg/kg (~50 mL of 1% solution)
What is the maximum safe dose of systemic lidocaine for dysrhythmias?	3 mg/kg total
What increases risk factors for lidocaine toxicity?	1. Liver dysfunction (lidocaine is metabolized in the liver) 2. Low protein states (lidocaine is protein-bound) 3. Certain medications – cimetidine, ciprofloxacin, clonidine, phenytoin, beta-blockers

MAGNESIUM

For what toxin-induced conditions is magnesium indicated?	1. Torsade de pointes induced by agents that prolong the QT interval 2. Hypercalcemia 3. Treatment of soluble barium (i.e., barium carbonate) ingestions 4. Digoxin toxicity (functions at the Na-K-ATPase to indirectly antagonize the drug) 5. Hypomagnesemia caused by ingestion of fluorides (e.g., hydrofluoric acid, ammonium bifluoride)
What is the mechanism of action of magnesium?	Competitive antagonism of cellular Ca^{2+} influx, which may decrease the likelihood of delayed after-depolarizations and inhibit presynaptic ACh and catecholamine release. Too large a dose of magnesium

will, therefore, impair muscle contraction, leading to paralysis and ileus, and interfere with cardiac conduction.

Why is magnesium administration potentially helpful after a digoxin overdose?

Magnesium can theoretically ↑ Na-K ATPase activity, directly interfering with digoxin. Also, by ↓ Ca^{2+} influx, it may suppress delayed after-depolarizations and, therefore, lessen the risk of dysrhythmias. This is only a temporizing measure until digoxin immune Fab can be administered.

What dose of magnesium is given for barium ingestions, and how does it work?

Magnesium can be given PO to convert soluble barium to insoluble barium sulfate. Recommended doses include:
Adults – 30 g PO (or by NG tube)
Children – 250 mg/kg PO (or by NG tube)

Magnesium can be used to treat what aquatic envenomation?

IV magnesium has been used to treat Irukandji syndrome caused be envenomation by the jellyfish *Carukia barnesi*. It is theorized that magnesium will ↓ catecholamine release, reducing the HTN, agitation, and pain caused by this syndrome.

What initial dose of magnesium is typically administered?

2 g magnesium sulfate over 10 to 20 min (to avoid hypotension)

What are some of the side effects of magnesium administration?

1. GI irritation if given PO
2. Blunted deep tendon reflexes
3. Impairment of cardiac function, leading to bradycardia and hypotension
4. Diaphoresis and flushing

In which patient populations should magnesium be used with caution?

Patients with renal disease, hypotension, and/or AV block

METHYLENE BLUE

What is methylene blue?

An alkaline thiazine dye

What is the toxicologic indication for methylene blue?

Symptomatic methemoglobinemia, which typically occurs at levels >20%

How is methylene blue administered, and what are the potential adverse effects?

IV administration is irritating and painful. Local tissue damage is possible, even without extravasation.

How is it dosed?

<u>Adults/Children</u> – 1–2 mg/kg IV over 5 min, followed by a fluid bolus to minimize local irritation
<u>Neonates</u> – 0.3–1 mg/kg
Repeat dosing may be required in cases of continued absorption of the etiologic agent.

What is the time to onset of action?

Within 30 min

What is the mechanism of action of methylene blue?

Methylene blue is reduced to leukomethylene blue in the presence of NADPH and NADPH methemoglobin reductase. Leukomethylene blue then reduces methemoglobin to hemoglobin.

What enzyme must be present for methylene blue to work properly as an antidote?

G6PD. It is a component of the hexose monophosphate pathway that generates the NADPH necessary for reduction of methylene blue to leukomethylene blue.

Name an undesired potential effect of methylene blue.

Paradoxical production of methemoglobinemia by oxidation of Hgb (at high doses or with dysfunctional NADPH methemoglobin reductase)

Does methylene blue cause any urinary symptoms?

Yes, blue-green discoloration of the urine with possible dysuria

Is methylene blue effective in patients with G6PD deficiency?

It is impossible to know before a trial dose is given. Those with an African subtype generally have enough G6PD activity to respond to methylene blue, whereas those with a Mediterranean subtype are unlikely to respond. In the latter case, other options, such as exchange transfusion and HBO, should be considered.

NALOXONE, NALTREXONE, AND NALMEFENE

What do these medications have in common?	They are all opioid antagonists.
What are the differences among these medicines (generally)?	Route of administration and duration of action
Which medication is typically used in the setting of *acute* opioid toxicity?	Naloxone
In the patient with AMS, what two signs should raise your suspicion for opioid toxicity?	1. Miosis 2. Respiratory depression
Name five different routes of administration for naloxone.	IV, IM, SQ, ET, intranasal
What is the dose of naloxone?	0.4–2 mg titrated slowly as the initial starting dose
How is naloxone administered?	0.4 mg of naloxone is mixed with 10 mL of normal saline and given slowly (i.e., 1 mL/min) IV until clinical effects are seen.
What are the effects of administering a larger than necessary dose to a patient with acute opioid intoxication?	1. Acute opioid withdrawal 2. Unmasking effects of co-intoxicants (e.g., cocaine)
What is the clinical goal in the administration of naloxone?	Improved respiratory effort without signs or symptoms of withdrawal
How long should overdose patients be monitored after reversal of CNS depression with naloxone?	The half-life of naloxone is ~30–60 min. Patients should be monitored for ~5 half-lives (4 hrs) to make certain that re-sedation does not occur.

What condition can significantly prolong the half-life of naloxone and subsequently delay the clinical appearance of re-sedation?	Renal failure
How can symptoms of re-sedation be treated?	Continuous naloxone infusion. Generally, two-thirds of the initial reversal dose per hour will maintain adequate arousal.
What opiates may require larger than usual doses to reverse?	Methadone, fentanyl, diphenoxylate, propoxyphene, pentazocine
How is nalmefene administered?	Parenterally
How is nalmefene different from naloxone?	It is a long-acting antagonist, with a duration of action of ~4 hrs.
Why might this be an advantage?	1. Fewer changes in the patient's level of consciousness 2. Limited need to re-dose the medication
Why might this be a disadvantage?	Precipitation of prolonged withdrawal symptoms
What is different about naltrexone?	While it is also a long-acting antagonist, it is administered PO instead of parenterally.
What is its primary indication?	Long-term opioid detoxification (outpatient addiction management)

NEUROMUSCULAR BLOCKERS

How are neuromuscular blockers classified?	Broadly classified as depolarizing (DNMB) and non-depolarizing (NDNMB) based on their activity at the postsynaptic ACh receptor of the neuromuscular junction
What are some common neuromuscular blockers?	1. DNMB – succinylcholine 2. NDNMB (aminosteroids) – mivacurium, tubocurarine, pancuronium, vecuronium 3. NDNMB (benzylisoquinolinium diesters) – atracurium, cisatracurium

What are the toxicologic indications for neuromuscular blockers?

1. To facilitate paralysis and orotracheal intubation in patients with hypoxia or lack of airway protection and in those requiring other life-saving procedures
2. To ↓ muscular hyperactivity, along with associated hyperthermia and rhabdomyolysis, in refractory strychnine poisoning and tetanus
3. To ↓ muscular hyperactivity, along with associated hyperthermia and rhabdomyolysis, in refractory NMS, serotonin syndrome, and uncoupling syndromes

What is the mechanism of action of succinylcholine?

1. Binds postsynaptic ACh receptor → membrane depolarization → muscle fasciculations
2. As depolarization continues, the muscle is temporarily insensitive to ACh → phase I block.

What is the mechanism of action of NDNMBs?

Competitive inhibition of postsynaptic ACh receptors

What are some adverse effects from neuromuscular blockers?

1. Histamine release
2. Anaphylactic shock (most commonly with rocuronium)

Why should long-acting NMBs be avoided in the toxicologic patient?

They may hide the physical manifestations of seizures.

What testing modality should be available for chemically paralyzed patients with toxin-induced seizures?

EEG monitoring

How is succinylcholine metabolized?

Plasma cholinesterase (primary) and alkaline hydrolysis (minimal)

What are some contraindications for the use of succinylcholine?

1. Hyperkalemia
2. Known plasma cholinesterase deficiency

3. ↑ ICP or IOP
4. History of malignant hyperthermia
5. History of recent severe burn or crush injury
6. History of progressive neuromuscular disease
7. OP or carbamate poisoning

What is the dosing of common NMBs?

Succinylcholine – 1 to 1.5 mg/kg IV
Vecuronium – 0.1 mg/kg IV
Rocuronium – 0.6 mg/kg IV

How are NDNMBs metabolized?

<u>Aminosteroids</u> (e.g., pancuronium, vecuronium, pipecuronium) – hepatic metabolism
<u>Synthetic benzylisoquinolinium drugs</u> (e.g., tubocurarine, metocurine) – eliminated renally or metabolized by plasma cholinesterase

How can neuromuscular blockade by NDNMBs be reversed?

AChE inhibitors can be given to ↑ junctional ACh levels.

What drugs can be used to reverse NDNMBs?

1. Neostigmine, pyridostigmine, and edrophonium ↑ ACh levels.
2. Atropine can be given to limit bradycardia.

Why are AChE inhibitors contraindicated for succinylcholine reversal?

They inhibit plasma cholinesterase, prolonging the effects of succinylcholine.

What are some adverse effects of neuromuscular blockers?

1. Prolonged weakness due to accumulated metabolites or lengthened drug activity
2. Post-op respiratory problems due to paralysis/weakness of diaphragm
3. Malignant hyperthermia

OCTREOTIDE

What is octreotide?

Somatostatin peptide analog that inhibits endogenous insulin secretion

What are the toxicologic indications for its use?

Treatment of hypoglycemia caused by sulfonylurea or quinine toxicity

What is the mechanism of action of octreotide?

1. $\downarrow$ cellular Ca^{2+} influx by a G-protein-mediated process $\rightarrow$ inhibits insulin release
2. Stimulates G_i-coupled receptor $\rightarrow$ $\downarrow$ adenylate cyclase activity $\rightarrow$ $\downarrow$ cAMP production $\rightarrow$ inhibits insulin release

When should octreotide be used to treat drug-induced hypoglycemia?

When hypoglycemia is refractory to IV dextrose

What is the dosage of octreotide used for treating drug-induced hypoglycemia?

<u>Adults</u> – 50 μg SQ/IV q6 hrs
<u>Children</u> – 4 to 5 μg/kg/day SQ/IV divided q6 hrs (max 50 μg per dose)

How is octreotide packaged, and which formulation should be used?

As an injectable liquid and as a depot formulation. Do not use the depot formulation for toxicologic indications.

What adverse effects can octreotide cause?

1. Potential for hypoglycemia (octreotide also inhibits glucagon secretion, which may outlast the inhibition of insulin secretion)
2. Local irritation at injection site
3. GI distress
4. Anaphylactoid reactions (rare)

PENICILLAMINE

What is D-penicillamine?

A penicillin metabolite initially identified in the urine of patients taking penicillin. It was later found to be an effective chelating agent.

What are the primary indications for D-penicillamine therapy?

Chronic exogenous copper toxicity and Wilson's disease. D-penicillamine may be beneficial in acute copper poisoning, but its efficacy has not been validated.

Are there other indications for D-penicillamine therapy?

Treatment of lead, arsenic, and mercury toxicity, although it is considered a second-line therapy. Due to adverse effects seen with its use for lead chelation, it has been supplanted by succimer. It should be used only when succimer or BAL + CaNa$_2$EDTA cannot be tolerated.

How is D-penicillamine dosed?

1 to 1.5 g/day PO divided q6 hrs

How is D-penicillamine excreted?

Renally

What are some potential adverse effects of D-penicillamine?

1. Aplastic anemia or agranulocytosis
2. Renal disease
3. Pulmonary disease
4. Hepatitis and pancreatitis
5. Chelation of other essential metals
6. Hypersensitivity reaction, especially in those with penicillin allergy (25% in this population)
7. Chronic use – cutaneous lesions, immune dysfunction

How does D-penicillamine alter the sensation of taste?

Through chelation of zinc

What other uses exist for D-penicillamine?

1. Treatment of Wilson's disease – chelates copper for renal excretion
2. Rheumatological disorders – immunosuppressant action
3. Cystinuria – binds cystine, increasing its solubility

PHENTOLAMINE

What is phentolamine?

An IV vasodilator

How does phentolamine work?

Competitive antagonism at peripheral alpha 1-adrenergic receptors

What are the general toxicologic indications for phentolamine?

Hypertensive crisis that results from alpha-adrenergic receptor stimulation

For what specific toxins is phentolamine typically used?

1. Sympathomimetic toxicity (e.g., cocaine, amphetamines, ergot alkaloids)
2. MAOI drug interactions/tyramine crisis

3. Limb-threatening ischemia secondary to vasoconstrictor extravasation
4. Alpha-2 agonist withdrawal syndrome

Why is phentolamine useful for cocaine-induced chest pain?

Has been shown to ↓ cocaine-induced coronary artery vasoconstriction

How is it dosed and administered?

1 to 5 mg IV bolus repeated until resolution of symptoms or induction of hypotension. Exact dosing is toxin-dependent. It may also be administered as an IV infusion. In areas of ischemia induced by infiltrated vasopressors, infiltration of 0.5 mg of phentolamine can speed recovery.

What is the typical onset of action?

Within 2 min when given IV

What are the adverse effects of phentolamine therapy?

Hypotension and reflex tachycardia

PHENYTOIN AND FOSPHENYTOIN

What is phenytoin?

An anticonvulsant of the hydantoin structural class (related to the barbiturates)

What is fosphenytoin?

Phenytoin with a phosphate group attached to the hydantoin anhydride nitrogen (promotes water solubility)

What is the mechanism of action underlying phenytoin's therapeutic effect?

Voltage-gated sodium channel blockade

In what cardiac drug toxicity has phenytoin use been reported to be of benefit?

Cardiac glycoside-induced dysrhythmias

How does phenytoin exert its antidysrhythmic effect?

Phenytoin is a type 1b antidysrhythmic (sodium channel blocker that does not prolong QRS duration). It suppresses ventricular irritability without slowing AV nodal conduction.

In what types of drug toxicities has phenytoin use been found to increase toxicity?	Cocaine, lidocaine, theophylline
What is the typical IV dose of phenytoin?	15 to 20 mg/kg
What is the maximum rate of phenytoin infusion?	50 mg/min. Rates greater than this are associated with hypotension and CV collapse. This is likely related to the propylene glycol diluent.
What side effects are associated with phenytoin use?	Stevens-Johnson syndrome, anticonvulsant hypersensitivity syndrome, systemic lupus erythematosus-like syndrome, blood dyscrasias, hepatitis drug-drug interactions, gingival hyperplasia, "purple glove syndrome" (not associated with fosphenytoin)
What is "purple glove syndrome"?	Limb (usually hand) ischemia, swelling, and discoloration related to the IV infusion of phenytoin. Compartment syndrome and necrosis are possible sequelae.

PHYSOSTIGMINE AND NEOSTIGMINE

What enzymes are antagonized by physostigmine and neostigmine?	AChE and butylcholinesterase
What physiological effect does this have?	1. Reverses anticholinergic effects 2. Can lead to cholinergic toxidrome
How do physostigmine and neostigmine differ?	Physostigmine is a tertiary amine, while neostigmine is a quaternary amine.
What does this mean physiologically?	Physostigmine crosses the blood-brain barrier, and neostigmine does not.

What does this mean clinically?	Physostigmine affects the CNS, while neostigmine has strictly peripheral effects.
What are the toxicologic uses of physostigmine?	1. Treatment of anticholinergic toxidrome 2. Differentiation of anticholinergic delirium from other disease entities (e.g., meningitis, encephalitis, psychosis) 3. Reversal of anticholinergic effects during surgery
How can neostigmine be used therapeutically?	To reverse effects of NDNMBs
What dose of physostigmine is recommended in the treatment of an anticholinergic toxidrome?	0.5 to 2.0 mg slow IV push (2 mg in 10 mL normal saline given at 1 mL/min)
What are the possible adverse effects of treating anticholinergic patients with physostigmine?	Seizures, bradycardia, asystole (particularly in CA overdose), cholinergic excess
What would you expect to happen if you gave succinylcholine to a patient who had received physostigmine?	The effect of succinylcholine would last much longer than normal
What would be the antidote for a physostigmine or neostigmine overdose?	Atropine

PRALIDOXIME (2-PAM) AND OTHER OXIMES

What is pralidoxime (2-PAM)?	Pralidoxime chloride, or Protopam (2-PAM), is a member of the oxime group used to reactivate AChE after inhibition by OPs. 2-PAM is the only oxime approved in the U.S.
To whom is 2-PAM administered?	To patients who have suspected OP/nerve agent (NA) poisoning and are

demonstrating moderate (i.e., fascicula-tions, vomiting, respiratory difficulty) to severe toxicity. Atropine is also adminis-tered for its antimuscarinic properties ($\downarrow$ bronchorrhea and wheezing), while 2-PAM can treat both nicotinic and mus-carinic effects.

How should 2-PAM be administered?

IV/IM. The preferred route is IV, although IM administration with a Mark I auto-injector is acceptable in the field prior to establishing an IV line. The initial dose should be given as quickly as possible to prevent aging (permanent inactivation of the AChE molecule).

What is the dose for 2-PAM?

Initially, 1 to 2 g (20 to 50 mg/kg in children, max 2 g) diluted in 100 mL NS given over 15 to 30 min. It is important to note that 2-PAM is rapidly excreted by the kidney with a half-life of 90 min; therefore, a continuous infusion is often recommended after the loading dose to maintain therapeutic levels. The current WHO recommendation is a >30 mg/kg bolus followed by an >8 mg/kg/hr infusion. A reasonable treatment regimen for severely poisoned adult patients would be 2 g IM or slow IV infusion over 15 to 30 min, followed by a 500 mg/hr infusion.

How is 2-PAM delivered when using Mark I kits?

Each Mark I auto-injector delivers 600 mg 2-PAM + 2 mg atropine. Three Mark I auto-injectors are recommended to treat severely poisoned patients. This delivers 1.8 g of 2-PAM, which is nearly the max recommended initial dose of 2 g; there-fore, if after administration of 3 Mark I kits a patient is still exhibiting respira-tory distress, further treatment should include only the atropine portion of subsequent Mark I kits to avoid exces-sive 2-PAM administration.

Is there a therapeutic window of administration time for 2-PAM?

Early administration is advocated to prevent the OP-AChE complex from undergoing hydrolysis, losing one of the OP alkyl groups and forming an irreversible covalent bond between toxin and enzyme. This "aging" process is variable, depending on the specific agent. For example, NA aging ranges from 2 to 6 min for soman (GD) to 48 hrs for VX. For the insecticide malathion, it is ~3.5 hrs, and for parathion, it is 33 hrs.

What is the mechanism of 2-PAM?

OPs form a covalent bond with the active site of AChE, preventing it from inactivating ACh. 2-PAM is attracted to the active site of AChE, and its nucleophilic oxime moiety will attack the phosphate atom of the OP, displacing it from the active site and reactivating the enzyme.

Are there side effects of 2-PAM?

1. Rapid administration may cause HTN, tachycardia, laryngospasm, muscle rigidity, and transient neuromuscular blockade.
2. Use in myasthenic patients may precipitate a crisis.

Is 2-PAM indicated for carbamate poisoning?

No. AChE poisoned by carbamates does not undergo aging; however, it is reasonable to consider administration of pralidoxime to a patient presenting with cholinergic crisis of unknown etiology.

PROPOFOL

What is propofol?

A sedative-hypnotic agent

What are the effects of propofol?

Amnesia and sedation, but not analgesia

How is it administered?

As an emulsion, due to the fact that it is an oil at room temperature

Where does propofol act?

Activates the chloride channel at the $GABA_A$ receptor and antagonizes the NMDA receptor

Where is propofol metabolized?

In the liver by cytochrome P450

How is propofol used in the toxicologic patient?

As a sedative agent to induce/maintain anesthesia, as an anticonvulsant, and secondary to its activity at the GABA receptor, it may be beneficial in ethanol withdrawal

In what patient populations is propofol use contraindicated?

1. Patients <3 yrs old
2. Hyperlipidemic states
3. Patients with hypersensitivity to soybeans or eggs

What is the main risk of propofol excess?

Over-sedation

What signals over-sedation with propofol in the conscious sedation patient?

Hypoventilation, hypoxia, hypotension

When should a lower dose of propofol be used to prevent over-sedation?

With concomitant use of benzodiazepines, opiates, or other CNS depressants

How long does it take for propofol to wear off?

<2 min

What is propofol infusion syndrome?

Mostly seen in children after long-term propofol infusion (>48 hrs at ≥5 mg/kg/h), it consists of heart failure, rhabdomyolysis, severe metabolic acidosis, and renal failure.

What do you want to avoid when giving propofol to the elderly?

Rapid bolus doses (higher risk of adverse reactions)

What are other adverse effects of propofol use?

Pancreatitis, discolored (green) urine, metabolic acidosis, hyperlipidemia, seizures, burning at IV site, cardiac conduction disturbances, bronchospasm, acute renal failure

PROPRANOLOL

What is the mechanism of action of propranolol?	Competitive blockade of beta 1- and beta 2-adrenergic receptors (i.e., non-selective beta-blocker)
How is propranolol typically used in toxicology?	To control the effects of excessive beta-adrenergic stimulation
What are some specific indications for propranolol in toxicology?	1. Methylxanthine-induced dysrhythmias (theoretical) 2. Thyroid hormone-induced tachycardia and dysrhythmias – ↓ HR and prevents dysrhythmias, also blocks peripheral conversion of T4 → T3 3. Halogenated hydrocarbon-induced myocardial sensitization and subsequent dysrhythmias
How does propranolol treat methylxanthine-induced hypotension?	Methylxanthines activate beta 1- and beta 2-adrenergic receptors, resulting in tachycardia and peripheral vasodilation. Beta 1-adrenergic blockade ↓ HR → improved ventricular filling during diastole. Beta 2-adrenergic blockade prevents peripheral vasodilation. This is theoretical, as definitive evidence is lacking.
In what situations should propranolol be used with extreme caution?	1. Comorbid asthma/other respiratory diseases – beta 2-adrenergic blockade can cause bronchoconstriction 2. CHF – cardiodepressant effects can worsen heart failure 3. Ethanol intoxication – can disguise tremors and tachycardia resulting from alcoholic hypoglycemia
What are the adverse effects of propranolol therapy?	1. Bradycardia, hypotension, CHF 2. Precipitation of bronchospasm in susceptible individuals 3. Induction of unopposed alpha-adrenergic stimulation with subsequent HTN in patients poisoned with sympathomimetics

Should propranolol be given to patients with sympathomimetic-induced hypertension?	No. Propranolol blocks only beta-adrenergic receptors. Unopposed alpha-adrenergic effects may result in worsening HTN.
What is the typical IV dose of propranolol?	Adults – 0.5 to 3 mg Children – 0.01 to 0.1 mg/kg (max 1 mg)

PROTAMINE

What is the primary indication for protamine?	Heparin reversal
From what is protamine derived?	Salmon sperm/testes
How is protamine administered?	IV
What is the mechanism of action of protamine?	Once hydrolyzed, basic (cationic) amino acids of the protamine peptide form ionic bonds with heparin, thereby neutralizing it and causing dissociation of heparin and antithrombin III.
Does protamine work on LMWHs?	Partially, reduces ~60% of the anti-factor Xa effect
What is the "rebound effect"?	Heparin anticoagulation within 8 hrs after receiving an apparently adequate dose of protamine
What are the three types of adverse reactions possible after protamine administration?	1. Systemic hypotension 2. Anaphylactoid reactions 3. Rare, but potentially fatal, pulmonary HTN
Why is protamine administered slowly?	To prevent rate-related hypotension and hypersensitivity reactions. Whenever administering protamine, have all equipment and medications to treat an acute allergic reaction readily available.
Pretreatment with what drug can limit the adverse hemodynamic affects?	Indomethacin

What are the risk factors for an adverse reaction to protamine?

1. Prior exposure to protamine
2. Vasectomy/infertile male
3. Allergy to fish
4. Use of NPH insulin
5. Any prior medication allergy
6. Rapid infusion rate

Upon what parameter is the dose of protamine based?

Amount of heparin remaining in the body, based on dose received and time since administration. One mg of protamine will bind 100 U of unfractionated heparin. For overdoses involving an unknown amount of heparin, 25 to 50 mg may be given slowly over 15 min. PTT should be monitored for up to 8 hrs to determine the need for additional dosing.

What doses should be given 0 to 30 min after heparin administration? 30 to 60 min after? 2 hrs after?

1. 0 to 30 min – 1 to 1.5 mg/100 U heparin
2. 30 to 60 min – 0.5 to 0.75 mg/100 U heparin
3. ≥2 hrs – 0.25 to 0.375 mg/100 U heparin

PRUSSIAN BLUE

How is Prussian blue administered?

PO

What is Prussian blue?

A crystal lattice of iron and cyanide, initially synthesized as a pigment in 1704

What are its indications?

1. Thallium toxicity
2. Radiocesium exposure (i.e., "dirty bombs")

What is the mechanism of action of Prussian blue?

Potassium ions are typically bound in the lattice upon administration. Large univalent cations (e.g., thallium, cesium) are preferentially bound, becoming trapped within the crystal lattice. This interrupts enterohepatic and entero-enteric recirculation of these toxins and enhances their elimination.

What physiologic state may hinder Prussian blue's effectiveness?	Ileus. Consider promotility agents.
What are the common side effects of Prussian blue administration?	Hypokalemia and constipation. It is recommended that Prussian blue be dissolved in 50 mL of 15% mannitol to act as a cathartic.
How is Prussian blue dosed?	1. Adult – 3 g q8 hrs 2. Children (ages 2 to 12) – 1 g q8 hrs
What will turn blue following administration?	Feces, sweat, tears
Is cyanide poisoning a concern after Prussian blue administration?	No. Cyanide release is minimal.

PYRIDOXINE (VITAMIN B₆)

What is pyridoxine?	1 of 8 water-soluble B vitamins
What are the toxicologic indications for pyridoxine?	1. Seizures induced by hydrazine toxicity (i.e., hydrazine, monomethylhydrazine, gyromitrin, INH), cycloserine toxicity and theophylline toxicity 2. Ethylene glycol toxicity – drives glyoxylic acid (toxic) → glycine (nontoxic) 3. May help dyskinesias caused by dopamine agonists (e.g., L-dopa)
How does pyridoxine help to treat hydrazine-induced seizures?	Administration of pyridoxine overcomes the competitive inhibition of pyridoxine phosphokinase by hydrazine, allowing for the production of GABA.
What are the doses of pyridoxine for the above clinical indications?	1. INH toxicity – 1 g IV per g INH (give 5 g initially if INH amount unknown), rate 1 g/min 2. Monomethylhydrazine toxicity – 25 mg/kg IV 3. Ethylene glycol toxicity – 50 mg IV/IM q6 hrs until resolution 4. Cycloserine poisoning – 300 mg/day

Which type of mushroom contains the toxin monomethylhydrazine?	*Gyromitra esculenta* mushrooms contain the toxin gyromitrin (monomethylhydrazine).
What is the one possible side effect of chronic pyridoxine supplementation?	Peripheral neuropathy (inhibits myelin production at the dorsal root ganglion). This has been reported in patients taking as little as 200 mg daily × 1 month.
How does this neuropathy present?	Poor coordination and ↓ light touch/temperature/vibratory sensation

SILIBININ OR MILK THISTLE (*SILYBUM MARIANUM*)

What is milk thistle?	A plant with active flavonoids
What is the functional extract of milk thistle?	Silymarin
What is the active component of silymarin?	Silibinin
For what natural toxic ingestion is milk thistle advocated as a treatment?	Mushroom poisoning with *Amanita phalloides*. Although no studies definitively document its efficacy following *Amanita* mushroom poisoning, silymarin has few side effects and is considered a beneficial therapy.
Why is milk thistle sold in herbal stores?	Considered to provide liver protection
What is the mechanism of silibinin?	Appears to block uptake of amatoxin into the hepatocyte. It also may increase ribosomal protein synthesis and works as an antioxidant.
How is silymarin typically dosed?	20 to 50 mg/kg day IV, optimally started within 48 hrs of mushroom exposure
Are there any adverse effects of silymarin?	Nausea/GI upset. Allergic reactions may occur in ragweed-sensitive patients.
Has milk thistle been FDA-approved for these treatments?	No

SUCCIMER (DMSA)

What is DMSA?	Dimercaptosuccinic acid, a water-soluble analog of BAL
How is DMSA administered?	PO
What is the dosing schedule?	350 mg/m^2 or 10 mg/kg PO q8 hrs × 5 days, then q12 hrs × 2 wks
What are the advantages of succimer over CaNa$_2$EDTA or BAL?	1. PO route available 2. Better tolerated, particularly by children 3. Fewer contraindications
For what indications is DMSA currently used?	1. Primary use is for lead poisoning without encephalopathy 2. Investigational for arsenic/mercury toxicity
At what serum lead levels should chelation be initiated in children?	>45 µg/dL. Below this level there is no evidence of efficacy, and it may be harmful.
What is the mechanism of action of DMSA?	As an analogue of BAL, it chelates heavy metal ions to form an excretable complex.
What are the adverse effects of DMSA?	Rare reports of nausea, vomiting, diarrhea, transient transaminitis, and dermatitis. Also, there is minimal chelation of essential metals, such as zinc and copper.
How is DMSA eliminated?	1. Primarily excreted in urine as an unchanged drug or as disulfides 2. Bile
Should DMSA be used in severe lead intoxication?	No. DMSA is only indicated for PO use. BAL is the preferred chelator in the encephalopathic patient.

THIAMINE (VITAMIN B$_1$)

What is thiamine?	1 of 8 water-soluble B vitamins that serves as an essential cofactor for carbohydrate metabolism, often as thiamine

pyrophosphate (TPP) during oxidative decarboxylation reactions

What are the complications of thiamine deficiency?

1. Beriberi (dry or wet)
2. Infantile beriberi (if breastfeeding mother is thiamine-deficient)
3. Wernicke-Korsakoff syndrome

What are some risk factors for thiamine deficiency?

Alcoholism, anorexia nervosa, hyperemesis gravidarum, loop diuretics, gastric bypass

For what indications is thiamine used?

1. Beriberi (dry and wet)
2. Treatment and prevention of Wernicke's encephalopathy
3. Ethylene glycol poisoning

When is thiamine used empirically?

When administering glucose in any alcoholic patient with AMS. This ostensibly prevents worsening of Wernicke-Korsakoff syndrome by bolstering thiamine levels before glucose metabolism depletes them. Thiamine administration should also be considered in any patient presenting with AMS or with coma, especially if at risk for malnutrition.

When treating a patient with AMS, should dextrose be withheld until thiamine is administered?

No. Do not withhold dextrose while awaiting delivery of thiamine. Thiamine should be administered with glucose or soon after glucose administration if thiamine deficiency is suspected.

What is the classic clinical triad for Wernicke's encephalopathy?

1. AMS
2. Ophthalmoplegia
3. Ataxia

How often is this triad seen?

10% to 15% of cases

What diagnostic criteria should be used?

Consider the diagnosis in a patient with two of the following four conditions:
1. Nutritional deficiency
2. Ocular findings (often nystagmus)
3. Ataxia
4. AMS

What is the dose of thiamine?	100 mg IV
How soon after administration of thiamine do symptoms begin to improve?	Symptoms may begin to improve within hours to days; however, many patients have persistent deficits.
What is Korsakoff's syndrome?	A syndrome characterized by anterograde amnesia and confabulation, it usually becomes evident after treatment of Wernicke's encepholapathy. It can be prevented by early treatment of Wernicke's, but once it develops, thiamine administration may have little to no effect.
What is the main complication of giving thiamine to a patient with wet beriberi?	Acute pulmonary edema due to rapid increase in afterload
By what mechanism does thiamine reduce toxicity after an ethylene glycol ingestion?	Thiamine functions as a cofactor in the conversion of glyoxylic acid to alpha-hydroxy-beta-ketoadipate (a nontoxic metabolite).

VASOPRESSORS

What is the mechanism of action of phenylephrine?	Direct stimulation of alpha 1-adrenergic receptors → vasoconstriction, ↑ PVR and ↑ BP
What are the toxicologic indications for phenylephrine?	Hypotension secondary to an overdose of vasodilatory agents (e.g., alpha-1 antagonists, dihydropyridine CCBs)
What is the typical dose of phenylephrine?	0.5 μg/kg/min IV infusion, titrate up to 5 to 8 μg/kg/min IV, as needed to improve BP
What are the positive hemodynamic effects of phenylephrine?	Stimulation of peripheral alpha-adrenergic receptors → vasoconstriction and corresponding ↑ SBP and DBP

What are the negative hemodynamic effects of phenylephrine?

As there is no effect on beta-1 receptors, phenylephrine does not ↑ chronotropy or inotropy; therefore, the vasoconstriction may ↓ cardiac output and/or cause reflex bradycardia.

Why would administration of phenylephrine be favored for increasing BP in a CA-toxic patient who is hypotensive despite adequate fluid resuscitation and sodium bicarbonate?

CAs are alpha-1 antagonists, adding to their ability to induce hypotension. In addition, CAs are anticholinergic agents, causing tachycardia. Phenylephrine will counteract the alpha-1 blockade without worsening the tachycardia.

What is the mechanism of action of norepinephrine?

Direct alpha- and beta 1-adrenergic receptor agonism, with a relatively stronger effect on the alpha receptor

How is norepinephrine administered?

IV (large bore)

Why should norepinephrine be infused into large veins?

Extravasation may lead to tissue necrosis

What is the effect of norepinephrine on the heart and vasculature?

Peripheral vasoconstriction and ↑ venous return (preload). Weak beta-1 receptor effects → ↑ chronotropy and inotropy with coronary artery dilation.

What are the indications for norepinephrine?

Hypotension refractory to other conventional modalities (i.e., glucagon, calcium, hyperinsulinemia-euglycemia therapy) secondary to toxicity from cardio-depressant or vasodilatory drugs (e.g., alpha-blockers, beta-blockers, CCBs)

How much norepinephrine should be administered when treating a patient experiencing severe hypotension secondary to drug intoxication?

Begin with 1 μg/min, then titrate to effect. Typical dose is 8 to 20 μg/min.

What is the pediatric dosing for hypotension and shock?

Begin with 0.05 to 0.1 μg/kg/min, then titrate to hemodynamic improvement (max 1 to 2 μg/kg/min).

What are some reported side effects of norepinephrine?

1. HTN
2. Tachydysrhythmias
3. Nausea and vomiting
4. Headache, anxiety, tremor
5. End-organ ischemia
6. Extravasational ischemia/necrosis
7. Possible allergic/anaphylactic reactions in patients sensitive to sulfite preservatives

How is epinephrine administered?

IV, IM, SQ, ET, inhaled

What are the toxicologic indications for epinephrine?

1. Hypotension refractory to other conventional modalities (i.e., glucagon, calcium, hyperinsulinemia-euglycemia therapy) secondary to toxicity from cardio-depressant drugs (e.g., CCBs, beta-blockers)
2. Treatment of anaphylactic/severe anaphylactoid reactions
3. Cardiac arrest

How is epinephrine metabolized?

Largely by COMT and MAO in the liver, then excreted renally

What is the half-life of epinephrine?

~2 min

What is the mechanism of action of epinephrine?

1. Direct stimulation of alpha 1-, beta 1- and beta 2-adrenergic receptors → ↑ cAMP
2. Stabilizes mast cells and prevents histamine release

What is the typical dose of epinephrine?

1. Allergic reaction/anaphylaxis – typical adult dose is 0.3 to 0.5 mg IM/SQ (0.01 mg/kg in children, max 0.5 mg)
2. Hypotension – initially 1 μg/min (0.01 μg/kg/min in children), then titrate to effect

What are the positive hemodynamic effects of epinephrine?	1. Beta 1-adrenergic agonism → ↑ myocardial inotropy and chronotropy → ↑ cardiac output. 2. Peripheral alpha-adrenergic receptor agonism → vasoconstriction with corresponding ↑ SBP and DBP.
What are the negative hemodynamic effects of epinephrine?	1. Induces irritability of the autonomic conduction system and increases the incidence of dysrhythmias 2. HTN with subsequent ICH, acute pulmonary edema, and ACS
What laboratory abnormalities are expected during treatment with epinephrine?	Hyperglycemia, hypokalemia, hypophosphatemia, and leukocytosis
How does a patient's pH affect the hemodynamic impact of epinephrine?	Acidemia ↓ CV effects
What adverse reactions can occur with epinephrine administration?	Anxiety, headache, tachycardia, palpitations, tremor
What is dopamine?	An endogenous catecholamine that functions as an adrenergic receptor agonist and neurotransmitter. It is produced synthetically and may be given IV for its vasoconstrictive and inotropic properties.
How can dopamine be used in the toxicologic patient?	1. Hypotension that is refractory to fluid resuscitation and is due to ↓ cardiac output or peripheral vasodilation 2. Bradycardia refractory to atropine/pacing
Where is dopamine metabolized?	Liver, kidneys, and plasma by MAO and COMT
What is the half-life of dopamine?	~2 min
What is the mechanism of action of dopamine?	Dose-dependent. It specifically stimulates alpha-adrenergic, beta 1-adrenergic,

and dopaminergic receptors. Beta 1-adrenergic receptors are favored at low doses, while alpha-adrenergic effects predominate at higher doses.

What is one drawback to the use of dopamine?

Dopamine exerts much of its vasoconstrictive effects indirectly (by inducing norepinephrine release); therefore, outcome may be variable in the toxicologic patient. Direct-acting agents (i.e., norepinephrine, phenylephrine, epinephrine) are generally preferred.

What dose can achieve therapeutic effects?

Low (0.5 to 2 μg/kg/min) – dopaminergic effects (i.e., renal and mesenteric vasodilation)
Moderate (2 to 10 μg/kg/min) – beta effects (i.e., ↑ inotropy and chronotropy)
High (10 to 20 μg/kg/min) – alpha effects (i.e., vasoconstriction)

When does dopamine reach therapeutic effect?

Onset in 5 min, duration up to 10 min

How is dopamine administered?

IV infusion

VITAMIN K₁ (PHYTONADIONE)

What is vitamin K?

A fat-soluble vitamin found in certain types of plants and produced in the intestine by bacteria. Vitamin K is essential to life.

How many forms of vitamin K are there?

3 (2 natural, 1 synthetic)

What are the forms?

1. K_1 (phylloquinone) – plants, cow's milk, soy oil
2. K_2 (menaquinone) – synthesized by intestinal bacteria
3. K_3 (menadione) – synthetic

In what food sources is vitamin K most abundant?

Leafy vegetables (e.g., spinach, celery), cheese, cow's milk, liver

For synthesis of what specific coagulation factors does the liver require vitamin K?	II, VII, IX, X
Can vitamin K be used as an antidote for any toxic ingestion?	1. Warfarin toxicity 2. Ingestion of anticoagulant (superwarfarin) rodenticides (i.e., hydroxycoumarins and indandiones)
Why is vitamin K effective as an antidote?	Both warfarin and the superfarwarins cause coagulopathy by inhibiting the enzyme vitamin K_1 reductase, which reduces vitamin K_1 2,3-epoxide to vitamin K_1 hydroxyquinone. The latter is used in coagulation factors (II, VII, IX, X). Vitamin K supplementation supplies the active cofactor for the generation of coagulation factor synthesis.
Which form of vitamin K will not work as an antidote?	Vitamin K_3
Should vitamin K be administered to suspected warfarin or superwarfarin rodenticide overdoses?	No. Following an acute overdose, do not give vitamin K prophylactically, as this may mask a clinically significant ingestion. Follow PT/INR in 48 hrs to evaluate for developing toxicity. Initiate treatment only when PT is prolonged or the patient is actively bleeding.
By what routes can vitamin K be administered?	PO, IV, IM (not recommended due to potential for hematoma)
What is the potential complication of IV vitamin K therapy?	IV vitamin K may cause anaphylactoid reactions
What is the goal of vitamin K therapy?	Restore the PT to normal in the case of rodenticides and to therapeutic range in the case of patients receiving anticoagulant therapy
How long will it take for vitamin K to exert its full effect?	8 to 24 hrs. For control of acute hemorrhage, FFP 10 to 15 mL/kg may be given to restore coagulation factors.

OTHER

What is metoclopramide?	A promotility and antiemetic agent used to treat toxin-induced nausea and prevent ileus
What is the mechanism of action of metoclopramide?	1. Antagonism at dopamine (D2) receptors in the CTZ (responsible for nausea/vomiting) 2. ↑ GI motility (including contractions of the small intestine) by stimulating $5HT_4$ receptors
What are the typical side effects of metoclopramide?	Sedation and EPS
How is metoclopramide typically dosed?	<u>Adults</u> – 10 to 20 mg IM/IV <u>Children</u> – 0.01 mg/kg/dose in children (max 20 mg)
What is mannitol?	An osmotic diuretic that has been used to prevent renal dysfunction in patients with rhabdomyolysis
What are the potential toxicologic uses of mannitol?	1. Treatment of neurologic dysfunction in ciguatera poisoning 2. Diluent for the delivery of Prussian blue (to act as a cathartic) 3. Prevention of renal dysfunction in patients with toxin-induced rhabdomyolysis 4. Treatment of ↑ ICP in patients with drug-induced or idiopathic intracranial HTN (pseudotumor cerebri)
What are the adverse effects of mannitol?	1. Fluid overload (due to rapid expansion of intravascular volume) 2. Electrolyte abnormalities (e.g., hyponatremia) due to movement of water into the extracellular space, as well as the creation of a hyperosmolar state 3. Renal failure with high doses (thought to be caused by renal vasoconstriction and ↓ renal perfusion)

What is apomorphine?

A morphine derivative that was previously used as an emetic agent but is no longer used for this purpose in humans

Why was apomorphine use abandoned by toxicologists?

The CNS depression caused by this agent significantly increased the risk of aspiration following its desired effect of inducing emesis.

In what toxicologic situations was apomorphine previously indicated?

GI decontamination following toxic ingestions. It was preferred over syrup of ipecac in agitated patients, as apomorphine can be given SQ.

What are contraindications to apomorphine administration?

1. Concurrent use of serotonin ($5HT_3$) receptor antagonists (e.g., ondansetron)
2. Known hypersensitivity reaction to apomorphine or the metabisulfite preservative

What is the mechanism of action of apomorphine?

Dopamine (D2) receptor agonism in the CTZ

What are the adverse effects seen with apomorphine administration?

CNS depression, injection site irritation, headache, priapism, orthostatic hypotension, QT prolongation, nausea, and vomiting

What is methocarbamol?

Carbamate derivative of guaifenesin

What formulations are available for methocarbamol?

IM, IV, PO

What is the action of methocarbamol?

Skeletal muscle relaxation through CNS depression

What are the toxicologic uses of methocarbamol?

Adjunctive therapy for muscle spasms induced by black widow spider envenomation, tetanus, and strychnine poisoning

What is the half-life of methocarbamol?

1 to 2 hrs

Where is methocarbamol metabolized?

Liver

What is the IV dosage for adults?

Typical adult dosing is 1 to 2 g (15 mg/kg in children) IV over 5 min, followed by continuous infusion of 0.5 g (10 mg/kg in children) over 4 hrs. This infusion may be repeated q6 hrs. Recommended daily doses should not exceed 3 g.

In what patient population should methocarbamol be used with caution?

Those with hepatic or renal impairment, seizure disorder, or history of myasthenia gravis

What are the side effects of methocarbamol administration?

Sedation, hypotension, nausea, vomiting, possibly allergic reaction

What is sodium polystyrene sulfonate (SPS)?

A cation-exchange resin typically used in the treatment of hyperkalemia

How can SPS be used as an antidote?

SPS has been shown to bind lithium and enhance its elimination in animal studies. It may be useful in lithium poisoning, especially if given PO soon after exposure.

What electrolyte must be monitored after SPS administration?

Potassium, as SPS may induce hypokalemia

What are IV fat emulsions (IFE)?

Also known as intralipid, it is a mixture of triglycerides, phospholipids, and choline that has been studied as an antidote for certain drug intoxications.

How is IFE used in toxicology?

While still under investigation, studies have shown efficacy for treating bupiva-caine, verapamil, and clomipramine toxicity in animal models.

What is the proposed mechanism of action of IFE?

Proposed mechanisms include acting as a lipid sink for fat-soluble drugs, providing a substrate for myocardial energy, and modulating ion channels.

What are the potential limitations of IFE therapy?

Fat emboli syndrome, increased absorption of the toxin from the GI tract, interaction with other antidotes, egg/soy allergies, liver disease, disorders of lipid metabolism

What is diazoxide?

A thiazide which has no diuretic activity but acts as a vasodilator

Diazoxide has been used as an antidote for poisoning with which type of medication?

Sulfonylureas

What is the mechanism of action of diazoxide?

Opens ATP-sensitive potassium channels on pancreatic beta cells → hyperpolarization → ↓ insulin release. This directly interferes with the sulfonylurea mechanism of action, which is to close these potassium channels.

What are the adverse reactions to diazoxide administration?

Hypotension, tachycardia, and sodium and water retention. For this reason, diazoxide is only used if the patient's hypoglycemia is refractory to IV glucose and if octreotide is unavailable.

For what poisoning is nicotinamide indicated?

Nicotinamide (vitamin B_3) has been used to prevent toxicity due to Vacor (PNU) ingestion; however, a parenteral form of nicotinamide is no longer available in the U.S. and now must be substituted with niacin. Niacin is less effective and may cause vasodilation and impaired glucose tolerance. As both of these can exacerbate the effects of Vacor poisoning, substitution with niacin is controversial.

Chapter 10

Visual Diagnosis in Medical Toxicology

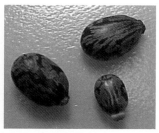

A 4-year-old boy is found chewing on the seed pictured. What toxin is he at risk of absorbing?

Ricin

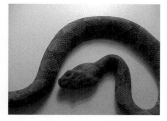

The snake pictured bit a 15-year-old girl on the foot. What complication of snake envenomation is the patient most at risk for contracting?

Copperhead (*Agkistrodon contortrix*) induced tissue necrosis

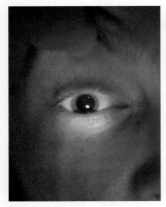

A 22-year-old man is on a cruise and touches his eye after placing a patch on his skin for motion sickness. What agent was contained within the patch?

Scopolamine

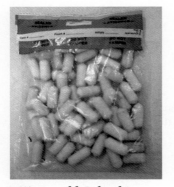

A 35-year-old Columbian female is caught in the airline restroom with this bag in her possession. How would drug traffickers refer to her?

As a "body packer." These packets are double-wrapped condoms filled with co-caine that are then swallowed by the "body packer."

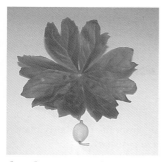

The plant pictured contains what toxin?

Podophylline, found within the mayapple plant (*Podophyllum peltatum*)

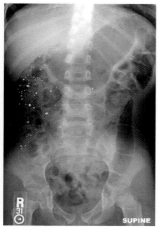

A young boy is found chewing on paint chips in his 100-year-old home. What toxin, evident on this x-ray, is he at risk of absorbing?

Lead

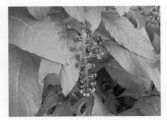

After eating the berries from the plant pictured, what abnormality may be seen on a CBC?

Leukocytosis, from the pokeberry plant (*Phytolacca americana*)

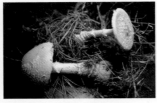

Following ingestion of this mushroom, what organ dysfunction may occur?

Liver dysfunction from *Amanita phalloides*

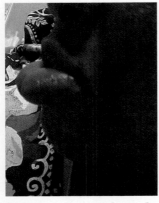

The woman pictured noted that her lower lip was swollen. What group of antihypertensive agents is responsible?

Angiotensin-converting enzyme inhibitors (ACE inhibitors), causing angioedema

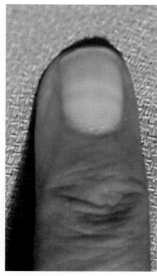

What is the name for this nail finding induced by arsenic poisoning?

Mees' lines

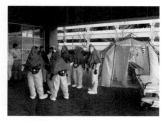

For what purpose is the tent visualized in the picture utilized?

Decontamination

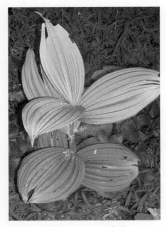

What is the name of this poisonous plant?

False hellebore (*Veratrum viride*)

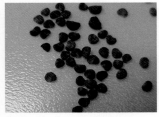

A teenager was found chewing and ingesting the seeds pictured. What substance was he attempting to derive from these seeds?

Lysergic acid amide (a relative of LSD), from Hawaiian baby woodrose seeds (*Argyreia nervosa*)

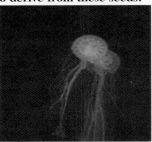

This creature uses what envenomation apparatus to deliver its marine toxin?

Nematocyst from jellyfish (class Scypho-zoa of the phylum Cnidaria)

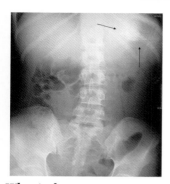

What is the name given to the radiopacity visualized in the stomach?

Bezoar

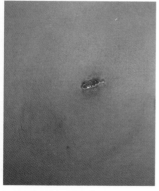

A mechanic's high-pressure grease gun discharges and strikes his skin in the area noted. What is the correct management of this injury?

Emergent surgical debridement due to the deep penetration of grease through his tissues

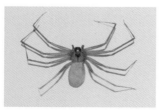

What is the name of the spider pictured?

Brown recluse (*Loxosceles reclusa*)

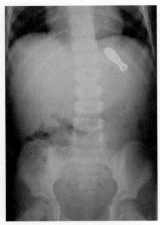

After ingestion of the lead foreign body pictured here, what is the next appropriate step in management?

Endoscopic removal

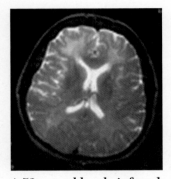

A 53-year-old male is found comatose in an unventilated home with a running gasoline-powered generator. A head CT is performed, and the results are pictured. What toxin is most likely responsible?

Carbon monoxide with bilateral lesions of the globus pallidus

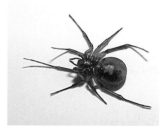

**The spider in the picture
bites a college student. What
muscle complaint may he
develop?**

Muscle spasms due to envenomation
by this black widow spider
(*Latrodectus spp.*)

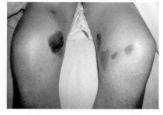

**A 23-year-old male overdoses
on phenobarbital. He is
found comatose with the
findings pictured. What
complication is he at risk for
developing?**

Rhabdomyolysis, with this case manifesting pressure necrosis of the skin

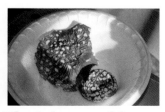

**What is the name of the
mushroom pictured?**

Fly agaric mushroom (*Amanita muscaria*)

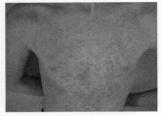

A young child who has been taking amoxicillin for the past 5 days is noted to develop the findings pictured. What is this reaction?

Acute allergic reaction

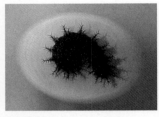

A child begins to scream after picking up the insect noted. He develops pustules at the sites of contact with his skin. What is the name of this caterpillar?

Buck moth caterpillar (*Hemileuca maia*)

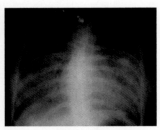

A young child swallows lamp oil and presents with dyspnea and cough. What is the etiology of his findings?

Aspiration pneumonia

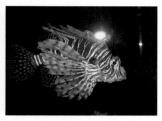

A pet store owner is stung by his pet lionfish. He has excruciating pain in his hand. What initial therapy should be performed?

Warm water immersion

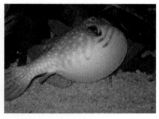

The fish pictured is eaten by a local fisherman. He develops rapid-onset ascending paralysis. What toxin is responsible?

Tetrodotoxin, from the pufferfish (family Tetradontidae)

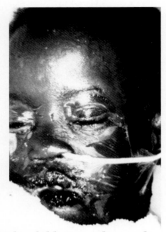

The child pictured recently had their phenytoin dose increased and subsequently developed a progressive rash. What is the name of the condition pictured?

Stevens-Johnson syndrome

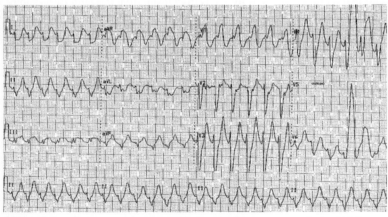

What class of antidepressants may be responsible for the ECG findings noted in the picture?

Cyclic antidepressants with the ECG manifesting tachycardia secondary to anticholinergic effects and QRS prolongation secondary to cardiac sodium channel blockade

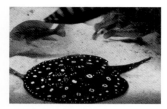

The marine animal pictured has an envenomation apparatus located where?

In the tail of the stingray (family Dasyatidae)

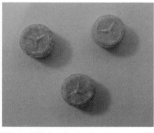

What illicit drug is pictured?

Ecstasy (methylenedioxymethamphetamine)

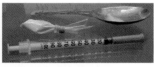

A 34-year-old is found with this paraphernalia in his pocket and presents with altered mental status, a new murmur, and fever. What condition must be ruled out in this patient?

Endocarditis

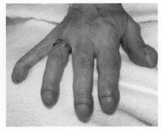

Chronic use of what laxative causes the condition pictured?

Senna, causing finger clubbing

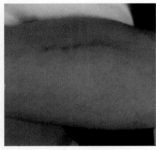

What are the findings noted in the picture?

"Track marks" from IV drug use

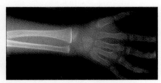

The markedly radiopaque metaphyseal lines seen in this radiograph are caused by exposure to which heavy metal?

Lead

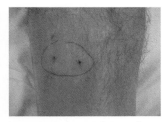

A patient's arm is bitten by a poisonous snake. Besides the two puncture wounds noted, no pain or edema develops at the site. This is known as what type of bite?

Dry bite (occurs in 10% to 20% of snake bites), meaning that no venom is introduced

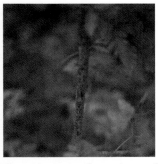

The poisonous plant pictured smells like a carrot. What is the name of this plant?

Poison hemlock (*Conium maculatum*)

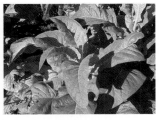

A young female presents with nausea, vomiting, tachycardia, and hypertension after picking this plant without gloves. What toxicity is she manifesting?

Nicotine toxicity due to "green tobacco sickness"

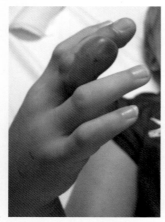

A poisonous snake bites a child's finger. What first aid procedures should be *avoided*?

Ice, tourniquet, suction, excision, incision

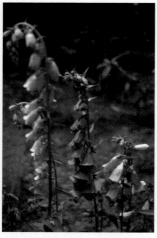

An herbalist ingests the plant pictured and presents with hypotension, bradycardia, and hyperkalemia. What is the appropriate antidote?

Digoxin immune Fab, for toxic ingestion of foxglove (*Digitalis purpurea*)

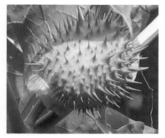

What syndrome would develop from ingestion of the seeds of the plant pictured?

Anticholinergic toxidrome, from jimson-weed (*Datura stramonium*) toxicity

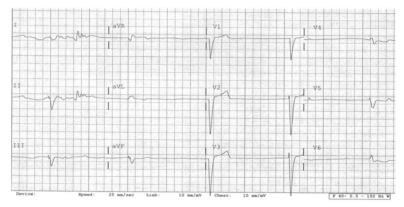

Would hypoglycemia or hyperglycemia be expected in a calcium channel blocker (CCB) poisoned patient presenting with the ECG pictured?

Hyperglycemia, due to CCB's ability to block peripheral insulin receptors

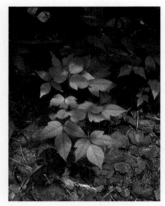

The plant pictured causes what type of allergic reaction?

Type 4 allergic reaction, by poison ivy (*Toxicodendron radicans*)

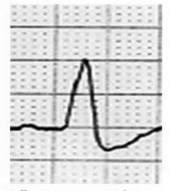

Following a propoxyphene overdose, this QRS complex is noted on the ECG. What is the treatment of choice for this finding?

Sodium bicarbonate

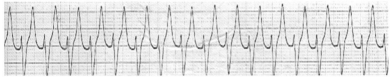

A cocaine overdose victim presents to the ED. His initial rhythm strip is shown. What electrolyte abnormality may be accounting for the finding(s) noted?

Hyperkalemia with characteristic changes consisting of peaked T waves, QRS prolongation, and loss of P waves

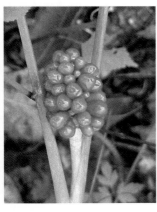

A child bites the seeds of the plant pictured and develops immediate pain and swelling of his lips. What is the cause of these clinical findings?

Calcium oxalate crystals, from the Jack-in-the-pulpit plant (*Arisaema triphyllum*)

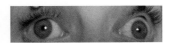

A 22-year-old female presents with the findings pictured, along with CNS and respiratory depression, after injecting illicit drugs. What is the most likely etiology?

Opioid toxicity, causing miosis and dysconjugate gaze (note the asymmetric pupillary light reflex)

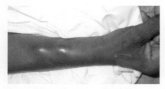

What is the name of the findings noted in this picture of a drug abuser?

"Skin popping," the subcutaneous injection of a drug, causing abscesses

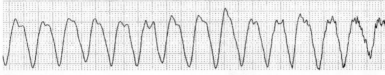

What is the most likely electrolyte channel inhibited in an overdose patient presenting with the rhythm strip pictured?

Cardiac sodium channel, which leads to QRS prolongation

Abbreviations

5-HT	5-Hydroxytryptamine (serotonin)
ABG	Arterial blood gas
ACh	Acetylcholine
AChE	Acetylcholinesterase
ACS	Acute coronary syndrome
ALT	Alanine aminotransferase
AMI	Acute myocardial infarction
AMS	Altered mental status
APAP	*N*-acetyl-*p*-aminophenol (acetaminophen)
aPTT	Activated partial thromboplastin time
ARDS	Acute (adult) respiratory distress syndrome
ASA	Acetylsalicylic acid (aspirin)
AST	Aspartate aminotransferase
ATP	Adenosine triphosphate
AV	Atrioventricular
BAL	British anti-Lewisite
BP	Blood pressure
BUN	Blood urea nitrogen
CA	Cyclic antidepressant
cAMP	Cyclic adenosine monophosphate
CBC	Complete blood count
CDC	Centers for Disease Control and Prevention
cGMP	Cyclic guanosine monophosphate
CHF	Congestive heart failure
CNS	Central nervous system
CO	Carbon monoxide
COMT	Catechol-*O*-methyltransferase
COPD	Chronic obstructive pulmonary disease
CPK	Creatine phosphokinase
CSF	Cerebrospinal fluid
CTZ	Chemoreceptor trigger zone
CV	Cardiovascular
CVA	Cerebrovascular accident
CXR	Chest x-ray
DBP	Diastolic blood pressure
DIC	Disseminated intravascular coagulation
DKA	Diabetic ketoacidosis
DM	Diabetes mellitus
ECG	Electrocardiogram

EEG	Electroencephalogram
EPS	Extrapyramidal symptoms
ET	Endotracheal
FDA	Food and Drug Administration
FFP	Fresh frozen plasma
G6PD	Glucose-6-phosphate dehydrogenase
GABA	Gamma-aminobutyric acid
GI	Gastrointestinal
GU	Genitourinary
HDL	High-density lipoprotein
Hgb	Hemoglobin
HIV	Human immunodeficiency virus
HMG-CoA	3-Hydroxy-3-methylglutaryl-coenzyme A
HTN	Hypertension
IARC	International Agency for Research on Cancer
ICH	Intracranial hemorrhage
ICP	Intracranial pressure
IM	Intramuscular
INR	International normalized ratio
IOP	Intraocular pressure
IV	Intravenous
LD_{50}	Dose of a particular toxin which is lethal in 50% of the tested population exposed
LFT	Liver function test
LMWH	Low-molecular-weight heparin
LSD	Lysergic acid diethylamide
MAO	Monoamine oxidase
MAOI	Monoamine oxidase inhibitor
MRI	Magnetic resonance imaging
NADH	Nicotinamide adenine dinucleotide (reduced)
NADPH	Nicotinamide adenine dinucleotide phosphate (reduced)
NAPQI	N-acetyl-p-benzoquinoneimine
NATO	North Atlantic Treaty Organization
NG	Nasogastric
NMDA	N-methyl-D-aspartate
NMS	Neuroleptic malignant syndrome
NSAID	Nonsteroidal anti-inflammatory drug
OP	Organophosphate
OTC	Over-the-counter
PCP	Phencyclidine
PNS	Peripheral nervous system
PO	Oral (Latin *per os*)
PPE	Personal protective equipment

PPV	Positive pressure ventilation
PR	Rectally (Latin *per rectum*)
PT	Prothrombin time
PTT	Partial thromboplastin time
PVC	Polyvinyl chloride, premature ventricular contraction
RAD	Right axis deviation
RBC	Red blood cell
RFT	Renal function test
RSI	Rapid sequence induction
SA	Sinoatrial
SBP	Systolic blood pressure
SMFA	Sodium monofluoroacetate
SQ	Subcutaneous
SSRI	Selective serotonin reuptake inhibitor
SVT	Supraventricular tachycardia
TCA	Tricarboxylic acid cycle (Krebs cycle, citric acid cycle)
UA	Urine analysis
US	United States
UV	Ultraviolet
VF	Ventricular fibrillation
VT	Ventricular tachycardia
WBC	White blood cell
WHO	World Health Organization
WWI	World War I
WWII	World War II

Index

A. *phalloides,* 404
Abdominal pain, 51, 148, 286
Absolute lymphocyte count, 246
Acarbose, 87
Acetaldehyde, 140
Acetaminophen, 15*t*, 17–19
  acidosis and, 19
  definition of, 17–19
  four hour treatment level, 19
  half-life of, 17
  labeling of, 17
  liver and, 18
  metabolite, 17
  plasma, 18
  poisoning, 18
  toxicity, 17
    high risk for, 18
Acetate, 140
Acetone, 214
Acetylcysteine, 444–446
Acidic agents, 176
Acidosis
  acetaminophen and, 19
  elevated anion gap metabolic, 184
  high anion gap metabolic, 193, 232
  lactic, 55, 84, 210
  metabolic, 112, 202, 207, 283
  non-anion gap, 253
Acids, 154–156. *See also* Hydrofluoric acid
  boric, 165–166
  calcium disodium ethylenediaminete-
      traacetic, 460–461
  commons uses of, 154
  dichlorophenoxyacetic, 313
  dimercaptosuccinic, 519
  DMPS, 470–471
  domoic, 396
  environmental/industrial toxins,
      154–156
  exposure, 176
  folic, 479–480
  folinic, 218
  glycolic, 193
  glyoxylic, 193

  ibotenic, 408–409
  ingestion, 155
  injuries from, 154
  lysergic, 345, 536
  ocular, 155
  selenious, 301
  soluble oxalic, 229
  tissue damage caused by, 154
  valproic, 124–125
Acneiform eruptions, 168
Acrodynia, 294
Actinomycin-D, 66
Activated charcoal, 13, 305, 463
Acute allergic reaction, 541
Acute amphetamine intoxication, 133
Acute arsenic intoxication, 263–264
Acute arsenic poisoning, 264
Acute benzene poisoning, 164
Acute botulism, 382
Acute inhalation, 253
Acute lung injury, 249
Acute nerve poisoning, 353
Acute oral ricin poisoning, 357
Acute pyrethrin, 329
Acute Radiation Syndrome (ARS), 245
Acute renal failure, 179
Acute toxicity, 159
Acute vesicant exposure, 362
Adams-Stokes syndrome, 498
Adenosine blockade, 115
ADHD. *See* Attention deficit
      hyperactivity disorder
Adipose tissue, 188
Adrenergic neuron terminals, 109
Aeromonas hydrophila, 468
Aerosol propellants, 181
Aerosolized benzodiazepines, 345
Aerosolized carbonaceous particulate
      matter, 248
Aflatoxins, 364, 414
Africanized honeybee (AHB), 378
Agent 15, 356
Agent orange, 189, 314
Aging, 326, 351

AHB. *See* Africanized honeybee
Airway management, 26
AKA. *See* Alcoholic ketoacidosis
Akathisia, 53, 485
Albuterol, 58
Alcohol. *See also* Drugs
  dehydrogenase, 139, 140, 195, 217
  intoxication, 4, 140
  rubbing, 214
  toxic, 5
Alcoholic ketoacidosis (AKA), 140
Aldehyde dehydrogenase, 402
Alkali acid injuries, 154
Alkaline, 156
  sodium, 190
  thiazine dye, 500
Alkaloids, 379
  anticholinergic, 415
  pyrrolizidine, 430
  rauwolfia, 109–110
  vinea, poisoning, 431
Allergic reaction
  acute, 541
  type 4, 549
Alpha 1-adrenergic blockade, 54
Alpha-adrenergic receptors, 72
Alpha-glucosidase, 3, 87
Alpha-latrotoxin, 368
Alpha-naphthylthiourea (ANTU), 331
Aluminum
  emanation of, 256
  exposure, 256
  hydroxide, 186
  phosphide, 258
  toxicity, 256
Amanita
  mushroom, 445
  phalloides, 534
Amantadine, 20–21
Amatoxin, 405
Amblyomma americanum, 376
Amblyopia, 50
American Academy of Clinical
    Toxicology, 462
American Revolutionary War, 416
Aminoglycosides, 28, 383
Aminophylline, 115
Aminosteroids, 505
Amitriptyline, 33

Ammonia, 156–158, 176
  aqueous, 157
  inhalation of, 157
Ammonium bifluoride, 197
Amotivational syndrome, 147
Amoxapine, 33, 36
Amoxicillin, 29, 374
Amphetamines, 132–133
Amphibians, 366–367
Amphibole, 161
Ampicillin, 29
Amygdalin, 418
Amyl nitrate pearls, 184, 465
Anaerobic metabolism, 210
Anaphylaxis, 436
Anemia, 256
  aplastic, 507
  functional, 225
  hemolytic, 128
  hypochromic, 256
  megaloblastic, 103
Anesthetics, 21–23
  effect, 8
  local, 23–25
Angina pectoris, 100
Angioedema, 25, 26
Angiotensin receptor blockers, 26–27
Angiotensin-coverting enzyme inhibitors,
    25–26, 534
  related angioedema, 26
Anhydrosis, 48
Anion gap, 3–4
  metabolic acidosis, 105, 163, 184, 202
    elevated, 184
    high, 193, 232
  negative, 158
  poisoning testing, 3–4
Annual radiation dose limits, 247
Antacids, 97
Anthracyclines, 66
Anthrax spores, 364
Antibacterial agents, 27–30
  symptoms from, 27
Antibiotics, 209, 374
Anticholinergics, 30–32
  alkaloids, 415
  delirium, 510
  plants, 415–416
  toxidrome, 31, 139, 548

Anticoagulants, 331–333
  effects, 51
  poisoning, 332
Anticonvulsants, 32–33
Antidepressants, 33–43
  atypical, 41
  cyclic, 543
  tricyclic, 64
Antidiarrheal agents, 43–44
Antidotes, 14–15
Antidysrhythmic agents
  type I, 118–121
  type II, 121–122
  type III, 122–123
  type IV, 123–124
Antiemetics, 53
  therapy, 166
Antifungal agents, 45–47
Antihistamines, 30, 47–49
Antihyperintensives, 77
Antihyperlipidemia agents, 49–51
Antimalarial agents, 51–52
Antimony, 258–261
  fumes, 259
  ingestion, 259
  poisoning, 259
  spots, 260
Antimotility agents, 43
Antiperspirants, 256
Antipsychotic agents, 52–54
Antiretroviral agents, 54–55
Antisecretory agents, 43
Antiseptics, 158–161
Antispasmodics, 30
Antitoxins, 457
  administration, 457
  botulinum, 383, 456–457
Antivenom
  administration, 446, 449
  crotalidae polyvalent, 449
  for scorpions, 447
  therapy, 369
Antiviral agents, 54–55
Ants, 378
ANTU. *See* Alpha-naphthylthiourea
Aplastic anemia, 507
Apomorphine, 528
Aquatic envenomation, 500
Aqueous ammonia, 157

Argyria, 303
Aromatic odor, 234
Arrhythmias, 8
ARS. *See* Acute Radiation Syndrome
Arsenic, 262–265
Arsine, 262–265
Arthropods, 367–371. *See also* Spiders
Aryl hydrocarbon receptor, 189
Asbestos, 161–162
Asphyxia, 227
Aspiration pneumonia, 541
Aspirin tablets, 111
Ataxia, 32, 57, 77, 129
Atrazine, 318
Atropa belladonna, 415
Atropine, 30, 149, 353, 450–451
Attention deficit hyperactivity disorder
  (ADHD), 33
Atypical antidepressants, 41
Australian funnel-web spiders, 380
Autonomic instability, 38
Autumn crocus, 69
Avermectins, 330
Ayurvedic medicines, 392
Azide, 162–163
Azole antifungals, 47
Azoxystrobin, 313

Babesiosis, 375
Baby woodrose seeds, 536
Bacillus cereus, 387
Baclofen, 114
Bacterial food poisoning, 407
Bad trip, 143
Bagging, 144
BAL. *See* Dimercaprol
Barbiturates, 55–56, 113, 451–452, 479
  administration, 452
  burns, 56
  in drug tests, 56
  mechanism of action of, 56
Baritosis, 267
Barium, 265–267
  containing radiologic contrast, 266
  ingestion, 266, 500
Bark scorpion, 447
Batrachotoxins, 367
Bazett's formula, 7

Bees, 378
Benzene, 163–165
  chronic exposure, 164
Benzocaine, 23
Benzodiazepines, 2, 15*t*, 49, 56–58, 113, 135, 169
  aerosolized, 345
  chronic, 479
  iatrogenic, 478
  mechanism of, 57
  therapies, 453
Benztropine, 454
Bertholite, 180
Berylliosis, 268
Beryllium, 267–269
Beta 2-adrenergic agonists, 58–59
Beta-adrenergic stimulation, 58
Beta-blockers, 15*t*, 39
  toxicity, 493
Betadine, 212
Betel nuts, 430
Bezoar, 537
Bicarbonate therapy, 456
Biguanides, 84
Biliary elimination, 291
Biogenic amines, 37
Biological warfare, 343
Bioterrorism weapons, 412
Bismuth, 269–270
  toxicity, 270
Bitter almond, 419
Biventricular tachycardia, 75
Black box warning, 33
Black henbane, 30
Black phosphorus, 237
Black widows, 367–369
  antivenom, 446
  spider bite, 369, 446
  venom, 368
Bleach, 176, 180
Body packers, 151, 532
Body stuffers, 151
Bone marrow suppression, 46, 125, 227
Bong, 146
Borane exposure, 166
Borates, 165–166
Boric acid, 165–166
Boron, 165–166

Botulin, 59–60
  in biological warfare, 343
Botulinum, 381
  antitoxin, 383, 456–457
  clostridium, 342, 381
  poisoning, 343
  toxicity mechanism of, 342
  toxin, 342–344
Botulism, 59
  acute, 382
  food-borne, 383
  infant, 383
  natural toxins, 381–385
  wound, 384
Bradycardia, 69, 97, 150, 510
Bradykinin, 26
Bretylium, 123
Bristleworm stings, 400
Bromates, 166–167
Bromides, 167–169
  poisoning, 221
  preparations, 220
Bromism, 168
Bromoderma, 168
Brompheniramine, 167
Bronchiolitis obliterans, 226
Bronchorrhea, 321
Bronchospasm, 171
Brown recluse spiders, 369–371, 538
  eye structure of, 370
  females, 369
Buck moth caterpillar, 541
Bufo toad venom, 366
Bufotenine, 143
Bulbar palsy, 3
Buspirone, 107, 113
Butyrophenones, 52

C. perfingens, 387
C. tetani, 439
Cadmium, 270–272
Caffeine, 60–62
  as stimulant, 61
  toxicity of, 62
Calcium, 4, 458–460
  disodium, 276
  gluconate, 200, 458

mechanism of, 459
oxalate crystals, 193, 194, 424, 550
Calcium channel blocker (CCB), 548
Calcium disodium ethylenediaminete-
traacetic acid (CaNa$_2$EDTA),
460–461
Camphor, 62–64, 169–170, 223
ingestion, 63
toxicity, 169, 386
uses of, 62, 169
Campylobacter, 387
CaNa$_2$EDTA. *See* Calcium disodium
ethylenediaminete-traacetic acid
Capsaicin, 432
Carbamates, 321–322
exposure, 322
poisoning, 450
Carbamazepine, 33, 64–65
Carbidopa, 292
Carbon disulfide, 76, 170–172
Carbon monoxide (CO), 172, 173, 222, 539
poisoning, 249
Carbon tetrachloride, 174–175
detection of, 175
metabolization of, 174
uses of, 174
Carbonic anhydrase, 32
Carboplatin, 298
Carboxyhemoglobin, 223, 466
Carcinogen, 274
copper as, 278
Carcinogenecity, 189
Cardiac dysrhythmias, 137, 196
Cardiac glycosides, 15*t,* 73, 417–418
Cardiac sodium channel blockade, 124
Cardiac tissue, 118
Cardiotoxicity, 36, 68
Carisoprodol, 114
Carnitine, 461
Carson, Rachel, 323
Carukia barnesi, 500
Cassava root, 418
Catecholamines, 175
excess, 109
Catechol-O-methyl transferase
(COMT), 37
Cathartics, 97
Cationic surfactants, 185
Caustics, 176–178
ingestion, 177

CBD. *See* Chronic beryllium disease
CCB poisoning, 482
Central Nervous System (CNS), 57, 107,
170, 175, 247
Centruroides, 371
Cephaeline, 89, 496
Cephalic tetanus, 441
Cephalosporins, 140
Cerebral ischemia, 134
CFC. *See* Chlorofluorocarbons
Chalcosis, 277
Charcoal, 462–464
activated, 13, 305, 463
hemoperfusion, 316
therapies, 462–464
Chelation, 276, 292
Chemical agents of terrorism, 342–365
botulinum toxin, 342–344
incapacitating agents, 344–345
incendiary agents, 345–346
nerve agents, 347–353
phosgene, 353–355
ricin, 356–359
3-Quinuclidinyl benzilate, 355–356
vesicants, 360–363
vomiting agents, 363–364
Chemical asphyxiants, 249
Chemical pneumonitis, 301
Chemotherapeutic agents, 65–67
Chewing tobacco, 149
Chironex fleckeri, 398
Chloracne, 189
Chloral hydrate, 113, 233
Chloramine fumes, 176
Chloramine gas, 156
Chlorates, 178–179
Chlordiazepoxide, 57
Chlorhexidine, 158
Chlorine, 179–180, 205
mechanism of, 180
Chlorine gas, 456
Chlorofluorocarbons (CFC), 202
Chloroform, 174, 181–182
exposure to, 182
uses for, 181
Chlorophenoxy, 313–316
Chlorophyllum molybdites, 406
Chloropicrin, 221
Chloroquine, 52
Chlorpromazine, 52

Chlorpropamide, 84
Cholecalciferol, 333–334
Cholelithiasis, 51
Cholestyramine, 50
Cholinergic excess, 510
Cholinesterase, 100
Chrome cleaning agents, 197
Chrome holes, 273
Chromium, 272–274
Chronic benzodiazepine, 479
Chronic beryllium disease (CBD), 268
Chronic dysphoria, 137
Chronic germanium exposure, 281
Chronic glycol toxicity, 206
Chronic lithium toxicity, 290
Chronic nickel exposure, 297
Chronic phenol toxicity, 235
Chronic phthalate poisoning, 239
Chronic selenium exposure, 301
Chronic thallium toxicity, 304
Chronic toluene abuse, 253
Chrysiasis, 282
Cicutoxin poisoning, 432
Cigarettes, 149
Ciguatera poisoning, 393
Ciguatoxin (CTX), 393
Cimetidine, 486
Cinchonism, 52
Citrate, 201
Claviceps purpurea, 78
Clitocybe mushrooms, 411
Clomipramine, 33
Clonidine, 68–69, 107
    related agents and, 68–69
Clonus, 38
Clostridium botulinum, 342, 381
Clostridium perfringens, 388
Clostridium tetani, 439
Clove oil, 63, 445
Clupeotoxism, 397
CN. *See* Cyanide
CNS. *See* Central Nervous System
CNS depression, 57, 175
CNS excitation, 107, 170
CNS/CV syndrome, 247
CO. *See* Carbon monoxide
Cobalt, 274–276
    medicinal uses of, 275
    skin exposure, 275
Cocaethylene, 134

Cocaine, 133–135, 250
    effects, 134
    freebasing, 133
    induced chest pain, 453, 508
    metabolization of, 134
    withdrawal, 457
Cock walk, 292
Cocoa, 60
Coffee, 60
Colchicine, 69–70, 431
Colesevelam, 50
Colestipol, 50
Colloidal silver, 302
Colorado tick fever (CTF), 377
Comfrey, 430
Common neuromuscular blockers, 503
Common rodenticide, 308
COMT. *See* Catechol-O-methyl transferase
Confusion, 77, 82
Conjunctivitis, 156
Contrast dye, 212
Co-oximeter, 219
Copper, 276–279
    as carcinogen, 278
Copperhead, 531
Coprine group, 402–403
Coral snake antivenom, 449
Corneal injury, 182
Cortinarius group, 403–404
Coumarin-derived rodenticides, 333
COX. *See* Cyclooxygenase enzymes
C-peptide, 83
Crotalid envenomation, 15*t*
Crotalidae polyvalent antivenom, 449
Crotalinae, 434
Crotalus scutulatus, 436
Crush injuries, 99
Cryptorchidism, 312
CTF. *See* Colorado tick fever
CTX. *See* Ciguatoxin
Cutaneous flushing, 128
Cyanide (CN), 15*t*, 102, 183–185, 210, 475
    antidote kit, 184
    antidote package, 465–466
    mechanism of, 183
    poisoning, 249
        Prussian blue and, 517
Cyanogenic glycosides, 418–419, 419
Cyanosis, 225
Cyclic antidepressants, 543

Cyclobenzaprine, 114
Cyclooxygenase enzymes (COX), 104
Cyclopeptide group, 404–406
Cyclophosphamide, 66
Cyproheptadine, 38, 43, 463–464, 464
Cystic acneiform lesions, 189
Cystinuria, 507
Cystosolic transformation, 222
Cytochrome oxidase, 172
Cytotoxic metabolites, 191

Dantrolene, 22, 467
Dapsone, 70–72
Date rape drug, 57
DCI. *See* Decompression illness
DDC. *See* Diethyldithiocarbamate
DDMA. *See* Digoxindicarboxymethoxy-
    lamine
DDT. *See* Dichlorodiphenyl-
    trichloroethane
Deadly nightshade, 30, 415
Death camases, 427
Decompression illness (DCI), 489
Decongestants, 72–73
Decontamination, 155
    dermal, 11
    external, 244
    gastrointestinal, 12–15
    of isocyanates, 214
    ocular, 11–12
DEET. *See* N,N-diethyltoluamide
Deferoxamine, 467–469
Delayed-onset pulmonary toxicity, 225
Delta-9-tetrahydrocannabinol (THC),
    146
Demeclocycline, 28
Depigmentation, 235
Depression, severe, 37
Dermacentor andersoni, 372
Dermacentor variabilis, 372
Dermal decontamination, 11
Dermal inhalation, 183
Dermatitis, 281, 313
    nickel, 296, 297
    plants producing, 420–422
    reversible, 313
Detergents, 185–187
Dexfenfluramine, 132
Dextroamphetamine, 132

Dextromethorphan, 38, 138–139, 167
    bromide, 139
    toxicity of, 139
DHFR. *See* Dihydrofolate reductase;
    Dihydrofolic acid reductase
Diabetes, Type 2, 87
Dialysis, 291, 469–470
    encephalopathy, 257
Diarrhea
    syndrome, 387
    traveler's, 388
Diazoxide, 85, 126, 530
DIC. *See* Disseminated intravascular
    coagulation
Dichlorodiphenyltrichloroethane
    (DDT), 322
Dichlorophenoxyacetic acid, 313
Dietary supplements, 295
Diethyldithiocarbamate (DDC), 297,
    471
Diethylene glycol, 206
Difenoxin, 44
Digifab, 473
Digitalis purpurea, 73
Digoxin, 73–76, 547
    elimination of, 74
    immune, 418
        fab, 471–473
        fragments, 472
    indications for, 74
    levels, 75
    mechanism action of, 74
Digoxindicarboxymethoxylamine
    (DDMA), 471
Dihydrofolate reductase (DHFR),
    479
Dihydrofolic acid reductase (DHFR),
    497
Diltiazem, 123
Dimercaprol (BAL), 260, 282
Dimercaptopropanesulfonic acid
    (DMPS), 470–471
Dimercaptosuccinic acid, 519
Dimethyl sulfoxide (DMSO), 187
Dimethyl-p-aminophenol (DMAP),
    474–476
Dinitrophenol (DNP), 231–232
    toxicity of, 232
Dioxins, 188–190
    disasters with, 188

poisoning, 190
toxicity, 189
Dipeptidyl peptidase-4, 87
Diphenhydramine use, 476
Diphenoxylate, 44
Diphenylhydramine, 53, 476
poisoning, 31
Diquat, 314–316
Direct-acting vasopressors, 25
Disease(s)
chronic beryllium, 268
lyme, 373, 374
Parkinson's, 37, 106, 110, 292
progressive pulmonary, 268
renal, 271, 281
Shaver's, 257
Wilson's, 278
wool-sorter's, 364
Disinfectants, 158–161
Disk batteries, 190–191
Disopyramide, 119
Disseminated intravascular coagulation
(DIC), 137
Disulfiram, 76–77, 402
Dithiocarbamates, 170, 311
Diuretics, 77–78, 289
Dizziness, 27, 139, 148, 253
DMPS. See Dimercaptopropanesulfonic
acid
DMSO. See Dimethyl sulfoxide
DNA synthesis, 67
DNP. See Dinitrophenol
Domoic acid, 396
Dopamine, 37, 44, 524
receptor antagonism, 53
Doxepin, 33
Doxycycline, 378
D-penicillamine, 506
Droperidol, 484–486
Drowsiness, 150
Drugs
of abuse, 132–153
amphetamines, 132–133
cocaine, 133–135
designer, 135–138
dextromethorphan, 138–139
ethanol, 139–141
gamma-hydroxybutyrate, 141–142
hallucinogens, 142–144, 407–408
inhalants, 144–145

marijuana, 146–147
mescaline, 147–148
nicotine, 149, 424
opioids, 150–152
phencyclidine, 152–153
date rape, 57
induced bradycardia, 451
induced hypoglycemia, 506
metabolites, 6
NSAIDs, 104–105
potassium efflux channel blocking, 9t
sodium channel blocking, 10t
urine, screening, 6–7
weight-loss, 77
Dry bite, 546
Dry mouth, 3
Dry mucous membranes, 48
Dysconjugate gaze, 550
Dysphagia, 395
Dysrhythmias
cardiac, 46, 137, 196
freon-induced, 203
Dystonic reactions, 44

Echinoderm envenomation, 399
Ecstasy, 544
EEG monitoring, 350
Elapidae envenomation, 433, 449
Electrocardiogram, 7–10
Electromagnetic radiation (EMR), 240
Electromyograph (EMG), 384
Elemental iron, 282
Elevated anion gap metabolic acidosis,
184
Elevated manganese levels, 292
Elevated osmolar gap, 214
Emergence reaction, 94
Emergent EEG monitoring, 350
Emergent endoscopic battery removal,
190
Emetine, 89, 496
EMG. See Electromyograph
EMR. See Electromagnetic radiation
Encainide, 121
Endocarditis, 544
Endoscopy, 155
Endrotracheal intubation, 1
Engine coolant, 192
Enterohepatic circulation, 13

Envenomations
  aquatic, 500
  crotalid, 15*t*
  echinoderm, 399
  elapidae, 433, 449
  human, 398
  sea snake, 401
  severe, 437
  stingray, 401
Environmental air pollution, 225
Environmental Protection Agency
    (EPA), 231
Environmental/industrial toxins,
    154–255. *See also* acids; Cyanide;
    Ethylene glycol
Eosinophilia-myalgia syndrome, 391
EPA. *See* Environmental Protection
    Agency
Epinephrine, 24, 492
EPS. *See* Extrapyramidal symptoms
Erethism, 294
Ergot derivatives, 78–80
Erythema multiforme, 470
Erythromycin, 378
Escherichia coli, 388
Esculoside, 432
Esophageal burns, 177
Essential oils, 63
  ingestion, 64
Ester-linked aminoesters, 23
Ethanol, 50, 136, 139–141, 477–478, 481
  absorption of, 139
Ethanol administration, 217
Ethanol dialyzable, 477
Ethanol intoxication, 140
Ethyl, 224
Ethylene dibromide, 191–192
Ethylene glycol, 15*t*, 192–195, 477, 480
  ingestion of, 192
  monobutyl ether, 206
  monomethyl, 206
  poisonings, 139, 193
Ethylene oxide, 195–197
  exposure to, 196, 199
Etomidate, 22
Eucalyptus oil, 64, 386
Euglycemia therapy, 122
Euphoria, 137
Europium, 300

Exacerbation, 41
Excessive methemoglobinemia, 475
Exocrine glands, 30
Exothermic neutralization, 177
Exotic scorpions, 372
External contamination, 244
Extrapyramidal reactions, 44
Extrapyramidal symptoms (EPS), 171
Ezetimibe, 50, 51

False hellebore, 536
Fast-acting sodium channels, 118
Fat solubility, 6
Fat-soluble vitamins, 126
Fenamic acids, 104
Fenfluramine, 132
Fetal hemoglobin, 173
Fibrates, 51
Fipronil, 330
Fire sponge, 400
Flecainide, 121
Fluconazole, 47
Flumazenil, 57, 114, 479
Flunitrazepam, 57
Fluorides, 197–200
Fluoroacetate, 200–201
Fluorouracil, 46
Flushed skin, 48
Flushing, 150, 225
Fly agaric mushroom, 30, 540
Folic acid, 479–480
Folinic acid, 218
Fomepizole (4-methylpyrazole, 4-MP),
    217, 480–481
Food poisoning, 386–389
Food-borne botulism, 383
Foreign bodies, 245
Formaldehyde, 201–202, 216
Foscarnet, 55
Fosphenytoin, 108, 508–509
Freons, 202–204
Fungicides, 311–313

G. esculenta, 409
G6PD Deficiency, 51
Gadolinium, 300
Gallium, 279–280

Gamma-hydroxybutyrate (GHB), 135, 141–142. *See also* Date rape drug; Rohypnol
  mechanism of, 142
  other chemicals converted to, 141
Gangrenous ergotism, 415
Garlic, 301
Gases
  chloramine, 156
  chlorine, 456
  environmental/industrial toxins, 204–205
  germane, 280
  high solubility of, 205
  highly soluble irritant, 347
  irritants, 204, 347
Gastric aspiration, 159
Gastric lavage, 12–13, 260
Gastrointestinal decontamination, 12–15
Gastrointestinal irritant group, 406–407, 422–423
Gastrointestinal syndrome, 246
G-CSF. *See* Granulocyte colony-stimulating factor
Gelled hydrocarbons, 345
Germane gas, 280
Germanium, 280–281
GI distress, 75, 167, 271
Gila Monster, 437
Gingivostomatitis, 294
Gingko biloba, 389
Glipizide, 84
Globus pallidus, 539
Glucagon, 122
  cardiac effects, 482
Glucocorticoids, 89, 269
Glufosinate toxicity, 320
Glutaraldehyde, 159
Glyburide, 84
Glycerol monoacetate, 201
Glycine receptor antagonism, 336
Glycoaldehyde, 193
Glycol. *See also* Ethylene glycol
  diethylene, 206
  ethers, 206–207
Glycol toxicity, 194
Glycolic acid, 193
Glycophosphate, 318
Glycopyrrolate, 450
Glycyrrhizin, 431

Glyoxylic acid, 193
Gold, 281–282
Gold sodium thiomalate, 281
Golden poison dart frog, 367
Gout, 69
Granulocyte colony-stimulating factor (G-CSF), 70
Gray baby syndrome, 29
Green tobacco illness, 424, 546
Gymnopilus, 407
Gyromitra species, 409
Gyromitra esculenta, 518

Hallucinogens, 142–144
  abuse of, 143
  group, 407–408
Halogenated hydrocarbon, 202, 204
Halons, 202–204
Haloperidol, 484–486
Halothane, 167
Hand washing, 389
Hapalochlaena, 400
HBO. *See* Hyperbaric oxygen
Hearing loss, 78
Heavy metals, 256–310
Hehnestritt, 292
Hellebore, 536
Hematopoietic syndrome, 246
Hemodialysis, 46, 84, 96, 195, 217, 261, 316
Hemoglobin
  fetal, 173
  level, 224
Hemolysis, 179
Hemolytic anemia, 128
Hemoperfusion, 164
Hemorrhagic cystitis, 66
Heparin, 80–81, 515
Heparin-induced thrombocytopenia (HIT), 81
Hepatic metabolism, 84, 106, 132
Hepatitis, 91
Hepatosplenomegaly, 312
Herbal products, 389–392
  hepatotoxicity associations, 390
Herbalist, 547
Herbicides, 178, 313–316, 407
Heroin, 250
Hexachlorobenzene, 312

HF. *See* Hydrofluoric acid
High anion gap metabolic acidosis, 193, 232
High osmol gap, 218
High solubility, 204
  gases, 205
  water, 304
High-dose barium ingestions, 266
High-dose IV penicillin, 28
Highly soluble irritant gas, 347
Highly volatile aromatic hydrocarbon, 252
Histamine-2 receptor antagonists, 486
HIT. *See* Heparin-induced thrombocytopenia
Hobo spiders, 379
Hoigne syndrome, 29
Hormone, polypeptide, 481
Hormones, thyroid, 117–118
Household bleach, 159
Huffing, 144
Human tetanus immune globulin, 442
Human-derived immune globulin, 384
Hydralazine, 126
Hydrocarbons, 207–210
  aryl, receptor, 189
  aspiration, 208, 209
  environmental/industrial toxins, 207–210
  gelled, 345
  halogenated, 202, 204
  highly volatile aromatic, 252
  ingestion, 209
  mechanisms of, 208
Hydrofluoric acid (HF), 155, 197
  burns, 458
  exposure, 459
Hydrogen peroxide, 159
Hydrogen sulfide, 210–211
Hydrogen sulfide concentrations, 211
Hydromorphone, 106
Hydrophobicity, 239
Hydroxocobalamin, 184, 487–488
Hydroxychloroquine, 52
Hydroxycoumarins, 526
Hyperammonemia, 125
Hyperbaric oxygen (HBO), 172, 488–490
Hyperbilirubinemia, 128
Hypercalcemia, 127, 333, 498
Hypercapnia, 99

Hyperchloremia, 212
Hyperglycemia, 58, 116, 124, 143, 548
Hyperinsulinemia, 122
Hyperinsulinemic-euglycemic therapy, 484, 493
Hyperkalemia, 25, 27, 49, 75, 81, 121, 122, 418, 550
Hypermagnesemia, 97
Hypernatremia states, 97
Hyperreflexia, 38, 116
Hypersalivation, 294
Hypersensitivity syndrome, 33
Hypersensitivity, type IV, 296
Hypertension, 27, 40, 68, 109, 123
Hyperthermia, 38, 137, 143
Hyperthyroidism, 212
Hypnotic toxidrome, 113
Hypocalcemia, 8, 186, 230, 238
Hypochlorite, 156
Hypochromic anemia, 256
Hypoglycemia, 122, 482, 484, 492, 505
  contribution of, 85
Hypoglycemic agents, 81–88
  insulin, 81–83
  sulfonylureas, 84–86
Hypokalemia, 8, 58, 68–69, 112, 116, 267, 456, 493–494
Hypomagnesemia, 8, 186, 266
Hyponatremia, 290
Hypophosphatemia, 116
Hypopituitarism, 82
Hyporeflexia, 129
Hypospadias, 312
Hypotension, 25, 54, 58, 69, 103, 150, 162, 466, 470, 508, 513, 521
  methylxanthine-induced, 514
  systemic, 515
Hypothermia, 8
Hypotonic lavage fluids, 13
Hypoventilation, 513
Hypoxia, 225, 321, 513

Iatrogenic benzodiazepine over-medication, 478
Ibotenic acid, 408–409
Ibuprofen, 104
Iliac crest bone biopsy, 258
Illnesses
  decompression, 489

green tobacco, 424, 546
  manifest, 247
Imidacloprid toxicity, 330
Imidazoline, 72
Imipramine, 33
Immediate pain, 156
Immune-mediated effects, 248
Inactivated sodium channels, 119
Inamrinone, 491
Incendiary agents, 345–346
Indomethacin, 515
Infant botulism, 383
INH. *See* Isoniazid
Inhalants, 144–145
  general classes of, 144
  long-term effects of, 145
Inhalation, 191
  acute, 253
  of ammonia, 157
  anthrax, 365
  of asbestos, 161
  dermal, 183
  gallium exposure, 279
  of iodine, 212
  large inhalation exposures, 230
  phosgene, 355
  smoke, 248–249
  tin, 305
Inhibitors
  angiotensin-coverting enzyme, 25–26,
    534
  monoamine oxidase, 37–39
  nonnucleoside reverse transcriptase, 54
  nucleoside reverse transcriptase, 54
  phosphodiesterase, 101
  selective serotonin reuptake, 39–41
  serotonin and norepinephrine
    reuptake, 41
Injuries
  from acids, 154
  acute lung, 249
  alkali acid, 154
  corneal, 182
  crush, 99
  lung, 98
  multi-system trauma/crush, 99
  ocular acid, 155
  stingray, 400
Inocybe mushrooms, 411
Insecticides, 321–331

carbamates, exposure, 322
  DDT, 322
  DEET, 329
  organochlorines, 322–323
  organophosphates, 324–327
  pyrethrins, 327–329
Insulin, 81–83, 492–494
  enteral administration of, 83
  history of, 82
Intermediate syndrome, 327
Internal contamination, 244
Intestinal absorption, 313
Intimacy, 137
Into the Wild (Krakauer), 428
Intoxication
  acute amphetamine, 133
  acute arsenic, 263–264
  amphetamine, 133
  arsine, 265
  barbiturates, 56
  chronic arsenic, 264
  concomitant ethanol, 194
  ethanol, 140
  ketamine, 93
  toxic alcohol, 4
Intracranial hemorrhage, 1
Intraluminal agents, 43
Intrathecal administration, 498
Intravascular hemolysis, 179
Invasive gastroenteritis, 388
Iodide, 494–495
Iodine, 211–213
  ingestion of, 212
  inhalation of, 212
  toxicity, 212
Ion flux, 32
Ionizing radiation, 241, 243
  sources, 241
Ipecac syrup, 89–90, 285, 495–496
Iron, 15*t*, 282–285
  absorption, 283
  poisoning, 467
Irritants, 346–347
  gas, 204, 347
  gastrointestinal, 406–407, 422–423
  mucosal, 311, 363
  poorly water-soluble, 354
  toxic, 204
Isocarboxazid, 37
Isocyanates, 213–214

Isoniazid, 15*t*
  mechanism action of, 91
  metabolism of, 91
Isoniazid (INH), 91, 410
  induced seizures, 452
Isopropanol, 214–215
Isoproterenol, 496–497
Ixodes scapularis, 373, 376

Jack-in-the-pulpit plant, 550
Jamestown, 416
Jarisch-Herxheimer reaction, 29
Jaundice, 128
Jellyfish, 537
Jequirity beans, 429
Jimson weed, 30, 416
Joint, 146

Karwinskia toxin, 432
KCN. *See* Potassium cyanide
Ketamine, 92–95
  antidote for, 94
  definition of, 92
  effects of, 93
  emergence reaction, 94
  recreational doses of, 92
  street names for, 92
Knock down phenomenon, 210
Komodo dragon, 438
Korsakoff's syndrome, 521
Krakauer, Jon, 428
Krebs cycle, 200, 303

Lacrimating agents, 347
Lactate dehydrogenase, 224
Lactic acidosis, 55, 84, 210
Laetrile, 418
Lamotrigine, 32, 33
Large bowel mucosa, 96
Large inhalation exposures, 230
Large tablet masses, 111
Latrodectus species, 367
Laudanosine, 100
Lavender, 64
Lead, 285–288, 534, 545
Leucovorin, 30, 66, 89

Leukocyte adherence, 173
Leukocytosis, 534
Leukopenia, 103
Lewisite, 262, 361
Licorice consumption, 391
Lidocaine, 25, 120, 498–499
Linamarin, 418
Lindane, 323
Linezolid, 30, 39
Lionfish, 542
Lipid solubility, 254
Lipodystrophy, 492
Liquid caustics, 177
Lithium, 95–96, 288–291
  carbonate, 288
  mechanism of action of, 289
  metabolism of, 95
  observing, 96
  toxicity, 95, 96
Liver, 77
Lobelia, 391
Lobelia inflata, 423
Local anesthetics, 23–25
Local irritation, 470
Local pain, 371
Lophophora williamsi, 147
Lorazepam, 453
Low acute toxicity, 147
Lung injury, 98
Lupus erythematosus, 67
Lyme disease, 373, 374
Lymphocyte count, 246
Lysergic acid, 345, 536

Macrophages, 161
Macrolides, 28
Magic mushrooms, 407
Magnesium, 4, 96–98, 499–500
  burns, 345
  dust, 98
  filtering of, 97
  medical preparation for, 96
Malaria, 51
Malignant hyperthermia (MH), 21, 467
Manganese madness, 292
Manganese toxicity, 159, 291–292
Manifest illness, 247
Mannitol, 527

Maprotiline, 33, 36
Marijuana, 146–147
Mark I kit, 352
Mastoparans, 379
MDMA. *See* 3,4-methylenedioxy-*N*-
    methylamphetamine
Medium-acting agents, 83
Mees lines, 535
Mefloquine, 52, 67
Megaloblastic anemia, 103
Meixner test, 405
Melaleuca oil, 386
Mentha pulegium, 385
Meperidine, 44, 106, 107
Mercury, 292–295
    absorption, 293
    elimination, 295
Mescaline, 143, 147–148
Metabolic acidosis, 112, 202, 207, 283
Metabolism
    anaerobic, 210
    hepatic, 84, 106, 132
    urea, 200
Metabolites
    acetaminophen, 17
    cytotoxic, 191
    drug, 6
Metal fume fever, 271, 308, 310–311
Metaldehyde, 215–216
    poisoning, 216
Metalloid, 258
Metformin, 84
Methadone, 107
Methanol, 15*t*, 480
    ingestions, 480
    intoxication, 216
Methcathinone, 138
Methemoglobin, 101
Methemoglobinemia, 24, 30, 52, 145,
        167, 218, 220, 223, 225, 410,
        475, 533
    inducers, 218–220
    symptomatic, 500
Methocarbamol, 528
Methotrexate poisoning
        and methotrexate toxicity,
        89, 497
1-methyl-4-phenyl-1,2,3,6-
        tetrahydropyridine (MPTP), 136

3,4-methylenedioxy-*N*-
        methylamphetamine (MDMA),
        132. *See also* Ecstasy
Methyl bromide, 220–221
Methyl salicylate, 63
Methylene blue, 71, 219
Methylene chloride, 145, 222–223
Methylphenidate, 132
Methylxanthine-induced dysrhythmias,
        514
Methylxanthine-induced hypotension, 514
Metoclopramide, 45, 527
Metronidazole, 28
Mexican beaded lizard, 437
Mexiletine, 120
Miglitol, 87
Minimally toxic household products,
        228–229
Mining, 271
Minoxidil, 126
Miosis, 54, 135
Mitral valve prolapse, 8
Molybdenum, 295–296
Monday morning fever, 310
Monoamine oxidase inhibitors, 37–39
Monomethylhydrazines group,
        409–410
Monoplace chambers, 490
Morchella esculenta, 410
Morphine, 106
Moscow Theater, 344
Mothballs, 223–224
MPTP. *See* 1-methyl-4-phenyl-1,2,3,6-
        tetrahydropyridine
Mucosal irritation, 203, 302, 311,
        363
    mucous membrane irritation, 165,
        176
Mucous membranes, 174
MUDILES mnemonic, 4
Munchausen's syndrome, 90
Muscarine group, 411–412
Muscimol group, 408–409
Muscle rigidity, 137
Muscle spasms, 540
Mushrooms
    Amanita, 445
    Clitocybe, 411
    coprine group, 402–403

cortinarius group, 403–404
cyclopeptide group, 404–406
fly agaric, 30, 540
gastrointestinal irritant group, 406–407
hallucinogen group, 407–408
Inocybe, 411
magic, 407
monomethylhydrazines group, 409–410
muscarine group, 411–412
muscimol group, 408–409
Mustard agent, 361
Mustard toxicity, 361
Myasthenia gravis, 28
Mycotoxins, 412–415
Mydriasis, 3, 48
Myeloneuropathy, 22
Myelosuppression, 298
Myocardial ischemia, 8
Myocardial repolarization, 7
Myocardium, 182
Myoglobin, 172
Myopathy, 49, 70
Myristicin, 64, 148

NAC. *See* *N*-acetylcysteine
N-acetylcysteine (NAC), 444
Nalmefene, 502–503
Naloxone, 44, 69, 106, 139
Naltrexone, 502–503
Napalm, 346
Naphthalene, 223
Nateglinide, 86
Nausea, 32, 148, 483
NDNMB. *See* Nondepolarizing
    neuromuscular blockers
Negative anion gap, 158
Nematocyst, 537
Neonatal tetanus, 441
Neonates, 445
Neostigmine, 505, 509–510
Nephrogenic diabetes insipidus, 96
Nephrogenic systemic fibrosis, 300
Nerium oleander, 73
Nerve agent exposure, 349, 351
Nerve agent poisoning, 349, 351
Neuroleptic malignant syndrome (NMS),
    20, 457
Neuromuscular blockers, 98–100,
    503–505

Neuromuscular hyperactivity, 40
Neuronal sodium channels, 107
Neuropsychiatric symptoms, 52
Niacin, 128
Nickel, 296–298
    carbonyl, 296
    dermatitis, 296, 297
Nicotine, 149. *See also* Chewing tobacco
    poisoning, 424
    replacement, 149
    tobacco and, 423
Nicotinics, 423–424
NIH. *See* Isoniazid
Nitrates, 100–101, 218
Nitric oxides (NO), 102
Nitrites, 101–102, 224–225
    administration, 466
Nitrofurantoin, 28
Nitrogen
    mustards, 66
    oxides, 225–228
Nitroprusside, 102
Nitrous oxides, 103–104
NMDA. *See* N-methyl-D-aspartate
    receptor
N-methyl-*D*-aspartate receptor
    (NMDA), 93
NMS. *See* Neuroleptic malignant
    syndrome
N,N-diethyltoluamide (DEET), 329
NNRTI. *See* Nonnucleoside reverse
    transcriptase inhibitors
NO. *See* Nitric oxide
Non-anion gap acidosis, 253
Noncardiogenic pulmonary edema,
    107, 214
Nondepolarizing neuromuscular blockers
    (NDNMB), 99, 326
Non-digoxin cardiac glycosides, 473
Nonnucleoside reverse transcriptase
    inhibitors (NNRTI), 54
Nonsteroidal anti-inflammatory drugs
    (NSAIDs), 104–105
Nontoxic household products, 228–229
Norepinephrine, 37, 522
Novichok nerve agents, 348
NRTI. *See* Nucleoside reverse
    transcriptase inhibitors
NSAIDs. *See* Nonsteroidal anti-
    inflammatory drugs

Nucleoside reverse transcriptase inhibitors (NRTI), 54
Nutmeg, 64, 143

Ochratoxins, 414
Ochronosis, 235
Octreotide, 505–506
Ocular acid injuries, 155
Ocular decontamination, 11–12
Olestra, 240
Oliguric renal insufficiency, 269
OP. *See* Organophosphates
OP exposure, 325
Opioids, 43, 105–107, 150–152
    opiates and, 106
    toxicity, 550
    ultra-potent, 344
Opisthotonus, 250
Opium poppy, 106
OP/nerve agent exposure, 350
Optic neuritis, 91
Oral calcium salts, 230
Oral glucose therapy, 83
Oral ricin poisoning, 357
Organic arsenic, 265
Organochlorine fungicides, 311
Organochlorines, 322–323, 323
Organophosphates (OP), 324–327, 347
Organophosphorus, 450
Organotins, 306
Oropharyngeal burning, 314
Oropharyngeal pain, 294
Osmolality, 5
Osmolar gap, 4–6, 194
    toxins elevating, 6t
Osmotic diuresis, 279, 298
Osteomalacic dialysis osteodystrophy, 257
Oxalates, 424–427
    crystals, 194
Oxalic acid, 229–230
Oxygen
    delivery, 218
    therapy, 269
Oxymetazoline, 68

Pain
    abdominal, 51, 148, 286
    cocaine-induced, 453, 508

immediate, 156
local, 371
oropharyngeal, 294
Palytoxin, 397
Panaeolus, 407
Pancreatitis, 91, 513
Pancuronium, 167
Paradichlorobenzene, 223
Paraquat, 316–318
Parkinsonian symptoms, 106
Parkinson's disease, 37, 110, 292
PCBS. *See* Polychlorinated biphenyls
PCP. *See* Pentachlorophenol;
        Phencyclidine
Peanut oil, 474
PEG-ES. *See* Polyethylene glycol-
        electrolyte solution
Penicillamine, 506–507
Penicillin G, 442
Pennyroyal oil, 63, 64, 385, 445
Pentachlorophenol (PCP), 231–232, 311
Perchloroethylene, 232–234
Peripheral alpha-1 receptors, 126
Peripheral neuritis, 91
Peripheral neuropathy, 103, 171
Peripheral vasoconstriction, 522
Peripheral vasodilation, 100
Personal protective equipment
        (PPE), 11
Pesticides, 165, 311–341, 407
    fungicides, 311–313
Peyote, 147
Phencyclidine (PCP), 152–153
Phenelzine, 37
Phenformin, 84
Phenobarbital, 33, 452
Phenol, 234–236
    marasmus, 235
    pharmacokinetics of, 235
    as preservative, 234
    toxicity mechanism of, 234
Phenothiazines, 52
Phentolamine, 507–508, 508
Phenylephrine, 72, 521
Phenylethylamine, 148
Phenytoin, 2, 33, 107–108, 120,
        508–509, 543
Phosgene, 204, 353–355
Phosphides, 236–237
Phosphine, 236–237

Phosphodiesterase inhibitors, 101
Phosphorus, 237–238
  black, 237
  burns, 346
  red, 237
  white, 237, 345
Phossy jaw, 238
Photosensitivity, 51
Phthalates, 238–239
Physostigmine, 32, 37, 48, 509–510
Phytophototoxic reactions, 422
Piperazine-based substances, 135
Plague, 364
Plants, 415–432
  anticholinergic, 415–416
  dermatitis-producing, 420–422
  gastrointestinal irritants, 422–423
  nicotinics, 423–424
  oxalates, 424–427
  sodium channel openers, 425–427
  solanine, 427–428
  toxalbumins, 428–429
  viperidae, 434–436
Plasma acetaminophen, 18
Platinum, 298–299
Pneumonitis, 176, 209
PNU. *See* Vacor
Podophyllin, 70, 431, 533
POEA. *See* Polyoxyethyleneamine
Poison dart frogs, 366
Poison hemlock, 546
Poison ivy, 549
Poisoning
  acetaminophen, 18
  acute arsenic, 264
  acute benzene, 164
  anticoagulants, 332
  antimony, 259
  arsenic, 264, 535
  bacterial food, 407
  barium, 267
  bromides, 221
  carbon monoxide, 249
  chronic phthalate, 239
  cicutoxin, 432
  ciguatera, 393
  dioxins, 190
  diphenylhydramine, 31
  diphydramine, 31
  diquat, 315
  ergot, 80
  ethylene glycol, 139, 193
  fluorides, 199
  food, 386–389
  glycol ether, 207
  metaldehyde, 216
  methotrexate, 89
  nerve, 349, 351, 353
  nicotine, 424
  oral ricin, 357
  palytoxin, 397
  phosgene, 355
  potential, 1
  scombroid, 392–393
  serious systemic, 388
  SMFA, 335
  strychnine, 337
  testing, 3–6
    anion gap, 3–4
    management, 10–15
    osmol gap, 4–6
  tetramine, 341
  vinca alkaloid, 431
  volatilized nerve agent, 349
  wintergreen, 386
Polar bear liver, 127
Polychlorinated biphenyls (PCBs),
    239–240
Polyclonal antibodies, 88
Polyethylene glycol-electrolyte solution
    (PEG-ES), 14
Polymorphic ventricular tachycardia, 7
Polyneuropathy, 70
Polyoxyethyleneamine (POEA), 318
Polypeptide hormone, 481
Polyvalent immune Fab therapy, 448
Poorly water-soluble irritants, 354
Portable recompression chambers, 490
Postsynaptic action, 32
Potassium, 4, 288
  bromate, 166
  chlorate, 178
  efflux channel blocking drugs, 9*t*
  influx, 58
  info cells, 483
Potassium cyanide (KCN), 183
Potential poisoning, 1
POW. *See* Powassan encephalitis

Powassan encephalitis (POW), 377
PPE. *See* Personal protective equipment
PR interval prolongation, 123
Pralidoxime, 326, 510–512
Pralidoxime chloride (2-PAM), 351
Priapism, 380
Primidone, 33
Procainamide, 119, 120
Procaine, 23
Procarbazine, 39
Progressive interstitial pulmonary
    fibrosis, 161
Propafenone, 121
Prophylactic antibiotics, 209
Prophylactic vitamin K therapy, 130
Prophylaxis, 51
Propofol, 22, 512–513
Propofol infusion, syndrome, 23, 513
Propoxyphene, 150
Propranolol, 514–515
Proserotonergic agents, 138
Prostaglandin D2, 128
Protamine, 515–516, 516
Prototypical chlorophenoxy herbicide, 313
Pruritus, 128, 150
Prussian blue, 3–5, 516–517
Pseudoephedrine, 72
Pseudohyperchloremia, 168
Psilocybin, 407
Psychedelic agent, 147
Pufferfish, 394
Pulegone, 385
Pulmonary edema, 162, 354
    freon and, 203
Pulmonary fibrosis, 123
    progressive interstitial, 161
Puncture wounds, 245
Puppy glove syndrome, 509
Pyraclostrobin, 313
Pyrazolones, 104
Pyrethrins, 327–329
Pyrethroids, 327–329
Pyridostigmine, 167
Pyridoxine, 30, 195
Pyrrolizidine alkaloid, 430

QRS prolongation, *34,* 52
QTc prolongation, 52

Quinidine, 119
    like effect, 8
Quinine, 52
    toxicity, 506
3-Quinuclidinyl benzilate, 355–356

Radiation, 240–248
    damage, 243
    dose, 242
    electromagnetic, 240
    equal absorbed doses of, 242
    measurement of, 242
Radioactivity, 242
Radioiodine, 494
Radiosensitive mammalian tissues, 243
Ragweed allergy, 328
Rare earths, 299–300
Rauwolfia alkaloids, 109–110
Recompression chambers, 490
Red man syndrome, 29
Red phosphorus, 237
Red pigmentation, 301
Red Squill, 338–339
Red tide, 397
Reflex tachycardia, 58, 126, 508
Renal cell carcinoma, 167
Renal disease, 271, 281
Renal dysfunction, 46
Renal elimination, 217
Renal failure, 151, 315
    acute, 179
Renal heparin, 80
Renal insufficiency, 83, 84, 102
Repaglinide, 86
Reptiles, 432–436
Respiratory depression, 135
Respiratory tract irritation, 171, 210
Reversible dermatitis, 313
Rhabdomyolysis, 49, 137, 153, 251, 540
Rheumatoid arthritis, 52
Ricin, 356–359, 531
    antidote, 358
    biological warfare, 358
Rifampin, 29
Right axis deviation, 35
Right bundle branch block, *354*
Risus sardonicus, 336
RNA synthesis, 67

Rocky Mountain Spotted Fever
   (RMSF), 374
Rocuronium, 505
Rodenticides, 129, 308, 331–341, 526
   anticoagulants, 331–333
   ANTU, 331
   cholecalciferol, 333–334
   pyrethrins, 327–329
   red squill, 338–339
   sodium monofluoroacetate, 334–335
   strychnine, 335–337
   Vacor, 337–338
Roentgen, 242
Rohypnol, 113
Rosiglitazone, 86
Roundup brand weed killer, 318
Rubbing alcohol, 214
Rubiacea, 495
Rumack-Matthew nomogram, 18

Salem witch trials, 79
Salicylates, 110–113, 455
   clinical presentation of, 111
   methyl, 63
Salmon sperm, 515
Salvinorin A, 143
Saxagliptin, 87
Saxitoxin (STX), 396
SCBA. *See* Self-contained breathing
   apparatus
Schizophrenia, 52, 153
Scombroid poisoning, 392–393
Scopolamine, 167, 532
Scorpions, 371–372, 447–448
   bark, 447
   exotic, 372
   natural toxins, 371–372
Sea bather's eruption, 399
Sea snake envenomation, 401
Sea snake venom, 402
Second-generation antihistamines, 47
Sedation, 109
Sedative-hypnotic agents, 113–114, 114
Seizures, 510
Selective serotonin reuptake inhibitors
   (SSRIs), 39–41
Selenious acid ingestion, 301
Selenium, 300–302

Self-contained breathing apparatus
   (SCBA), 196
Sensory neuropathies, 129
Serine hydroxyl residue, 347
Serious systemic poisoning, 388
Serotonergic neurons, 137
Serotonin, 37, 44, 109
   reuptake inhibition, 138
   syndrome, 38, 39, 42, 138, 289, 464
Serotonin and norepinephrine reuptake
   inhibitors (SNRIs), 41
Serum antimony levels, 260
Serum management, 97
Several hepatotoxicity, 50
Severe depression, 37
Severe envenomation, 437
Sewage treatment, 180
SIADH. *See* Syndrome of inappropriate
   anti-diuretic hormone
Silibinin/milk thistle, 518
Silver, 302–303
Simple asphyxiants, 248
Sinus tachycardia, 41
Sirolimus, 89
Sitagliptin, 87
Six-eyed crab spider, 380
Skeletal muscle relaxants, 30, 114–115
Skeletal muscle spasms, 250
Skin popping, 551
Slow infusion rate, 46
Smelting, 271
SMFA poisoning, 335
SMFA toxicity, 335
Smoke
   composition of, 248
   inhalation, 248–249, 249
Smoking, 162
Snakes, 432–436, 448–450
   Elapidae, 432–434
   Viperidae, 434–436
SNARE proteins, 382
Snowfield vision, 216
SNRIs. *See* Serotonin and norepinephrine
   reuptake inhibitors
Sodium, 288
   bicarbonate, 120, 454, 549
   channel blockade, 31, 455
   channel blocker toxicity, 455
   channel blocking drugs, 10*t*

channels, 426
chlorate, 178, 319
    ingestion, 320
hydroxide, 229
hypochlorite, 186
monofluoroacetate, 334–335
nitroprusside, 183
opener toxicity, 426
thiosulfate, 466, 475
Sodium polystyrene sulfonate (SPS), 529
Solanine, 427–428
    containing plants, 427
Soluble oxalates, 425
Soluble oxalic acid, 229
Somatostatin peptide, 505
Spanish fly, 381
Speedball, 133
Sphingomyelinase D, 370
Spiders
    Australian funnel-web, 380
    hobo, 379
    six-eyed crab, 380
    yellow sac, 379
SPS. *See* Sodium polystyrene sulfonate
SSDS. *See* Sudden sniffing death
        syndrome
SSRIs. *See* Selective serotonin reuptake
        inhibitors
St. Anthony's Fire, 79
Stannosis, 306
Stevens-Johnson syndrome, 543
Stibine, 261
Stinging nettle, 421
Stingray, 544
Stingray envenomations, 401
Stingray injury, 400
Stonefish, 401
Strength aspirin tablets, 111
Strobilurins, 313
Stropharia, 407
Strychnine, 249–251, 335–337
    lethal doses of, 250
Strychnos, 430
STX. *See* Saxitoxin
Succimer, 519
Succinylcholine, 99, 504, 505
Sudden sniffing death syndrome
        (SSDS), 145
Sulfhydryl groups, 293, 303

Sulfonamides, 29
Sulfonylureas, 84–86, 506
Sulfur dioxide, 251–252
Sunscreen, 314
Superwarfarins, 332
Supportive care, 271, 279, 428
Symmetric ascending paralysis, 207
Sympathetic adrenergic overstimulation,
        117
Sympathomimetic toxidrome, 31, 133
Sympathomimetics, 72
Symptomatic methemoglobinemia, 500
Syndrome of inappropriate anti-diuretic
        hormone (SIADH), 65
Syndromes
    acute radiation, 245
    Adams-Stokes, 498
    amotivational, 147
    CNS/CV, 247
    diarrhea, 387
    eosinophilia-myalgia, 391
    febrile, 308
    gastrointestinal, 246
    gray baby, 29
    hematopoietic, 246
    Hoigne, 29
    hypersensitivity, 33
    hypertoxic myopathic, 368
    intermediate, 327
    Irukandji, 399
    Korsakoff's, 521
    Munchausen's, 90
    neuroleptic malignant, 20, 457
    NMS, 20, 457
    propofol infusion, 23, 513
    puppy glove, 509
    red man, 29
    serotonin, 38, 39, 42, 138, 289, 464
    Stevens-Johnson, 543
    sudden sniffing death, 145
    withdrawal, 114
    Wolff-Parkinson-White, 498–499
Synergistic vasodilation, 101
Synthetic chlorinated organic
        compounds, 239
Systemic involvement, 438
Systemic loxoscelism, 370
Systemic oxalic acid toxicity, 230
Systemic oxygen utilization, 249

T-2 exposure, 413, 414
Tachycardia, 58, 73, 143, 352
  biventricular, 75
  polymorphic ventricular, 7
  QRS-complex, 119
  reflex, 58, 126, 508
  sinus, 41
Tachydysrhythmias, 120, 417, 523
TBE. See Tick-borne encephalitis
TBRF. See Tick-borne relapsing fever
Tea, 60
Terminal R wave, 35
Terrorism. See Chemical agents of
    terrorism
Tertiary amines, 31
Tetanus, 336, 439–442
  cephalic, 441
  immune globulin, 442, 443
  localized, 441
  natural toxins, 439–442
  neonatal, 441
  prophylaxis, 442
  toxoid, 443
Tetracaine, 23
Tetraethylthiuram disulfide, 76
Tetramine, 340, 341
Tetrodotoxin (TTX), 367, 392, 542
Thallium, 303–305
THC. See Delta-9-tetrahydrocannabinol
Theophylline, 115–116, 452
Therapies, 444–530
  acetylcysteine, 444–446
  antiemetics, 166
  antivenom, 446–447
  barbiturates, 451–452
  benzodiazepines, 453
  benztropine, 454
  bicarbonate, 454–456
  bromocriptine, 457–458
  calcium, 458–460
  calcium disodium ethylenediaminete-
      traacetic acid, 460–461
  charcoal, 462–464
  cyanide antidote package, 465–466
  cyproheptadine, 463–464
  dantrolene, 467
  deferoxamine, 467–469
  dialysis, 469–470
  diethyldithiocarbamate, 471

digoxin immune fab, 471–473
dimercaprol, 473–474
dimercaptopropanesulfonic acid,
    470–471
diphenhydramine, 476
ethanol, 477–478
euglycemia, 122
flumazenil, 478–479
folic acid, 479–480
fomepizole (4-methylpyrazole, 4-MP),
    480–481
glucagon, 481–483
haloperidol/droperidol, 484–486
histamine-2 receptor antagonists, 486
hydroxocobalamin, 487–488
hyperbaric oxygen, 488–490
hyperinsulinemic-euglycemic, 484,
    493
inamrinone, 491
insulin, 492–494
iodide, 494–495
isoproterenol, 496–497
leucovorin, 497–498
magnesium, 499
methylene blue, 500–501
NAC, 445
naloxone, 502–503
oral glucose, 83
oxygen, 269
phentolamine, 508
polyvalent immune Fab, 448
pralidoxime, 510–512
prophylactic vitamin K, 130
propofol, 512–513
propranolol, 514–515
protamine, 515–516
Prussian blue, 516–517
pyridoxine, 517–518
silibinin/milk thistle, 518
succimer, 519
thiamine (Vitamin B_1), 519–521
vasopressors, 521–525
vitamin K_1, 525–526
Thermite, 345
Thermometers, 293
Thiamine, 195, 520
Thiocyanate, 102
Thrombocytopenia, 103, 299, 448
Thyroid hormones, 117–118

Tiagabine, 33
TIBC. *See* Total iron-binding capacity
Tick-borne encephalitis (TBE), 376
Tick-borne relapsing fever (TBRF), 377
Ticks, 372–378
Tin, 305–306
  inhalation, 305
  toxicity, 306
Tissue preservatives, 158
Tissue toxicity, 199
Tocainamide, 120
Tocainide, 121
Toluene, 252–254
  intoxication levels of, 253
Topical analgesics, 63
Topical antifungal agents, 158
Topiramate, 33
Total iron-binding capacity (TIBC), 285
Toxalbumin exposure, 429
Toxalbumin-producing bean, 359
Toxic alcohol intoxication, 4, 140
Toxic alcohols, 5
Toxic effects, 73, 115
Toxic ingestion, 547
Toxic irritant gases, 204
Toxic psychosis, 152
Toxicities
  acetaminophen, 17
  acute, 159
  of arsine, 263
  of botulinum, 342
  of caffeine, 62
  camphor, 169, 386
  chronic, 116
  chronic glycol, 206
  chronic lithium, 290
  chronic phenol, 235
  copper, 277
  delayed-onset pulmonary, 225
  dermal, 169, 306
  of detergents, 185
  of dextromethorphan, 139
  digoxin, 459
  of dinitrophenol, 232
  dioxins, 189
  formaldehyde, 202
  of freons, 203

  glufosinate, 320
  glycol, 194
  gold, 281
  imidacloprid, 330
  lithium, 95, 96
  low acute, 147
  magnesium, 97
  manganese, 159, 291–292
  manifestations, 403
  methotrexate, 497
  mustard, 361
  opioids, 550
  pentachlorophenol, 232
  perchloroethylene, 233
  phthalates, 238, 239
  prolonged, 31
  SMFA, 335
  sodium, 426
  solanine, 428
  strychnine, 250
  systemic, 345, 368
  systemic oxalic acid, 230
  thallium, 304
  tissue, 199
  vitamin A, 127
  vitamin E, 127
  wintergreen cause, 386
Toxicologic emergencies, 1
Toxicology screen, 3
Toxicodenderon, 420
Toxidromes, 2–3, 2*t*
Toxin-induced agitation, 485
Track marks, 545
Traditional cyanide antidote kit, 488
Tramadol, 150
Transferrin, 283
Traveler's diarrhea, 388
Trialkyltin, 312
Tributyltin, 312
Trichloroethane, 254–255
Trichloroethanol, 233
Trichloroethylene, 254–255
Trichothecenes, 413
  mycotoxins, 359–360, 412
Tricyclic antidepressants, 64
Trifloxystrobin, 313
Tripping, 143
Trivalent, 259
Troglitazone, 86

TTX. *See* Tetrodotoxin
TTX poisoning, 395
Tularemia, 375
Type 2 diabetes, 87
Type I antidysrhythmic agents, 118–121
Type II antidysrhythmic agents, 121–122
Type III antidysrhythmic agents, 122–123
Type IV antidysrhythmic agents, 123–124
Type IV hypersensitivity, 296
Typical antipsychotics, 52
Tyramine, 37

Ultra-potent opioids, 344
Unbound toxin, 442
Union Carbide Plant, 214
Urea metabolism, 200
Urinary alkalinization, 456
Urine drug screening, 6–7
Urticaria, 470

Vacor (PNU), 337–338
Valproic acid, 124–125
Vanadium
    excretion of, 307
    pentoxide, 306
Vancomycin, 28
Vasoconstriction, 73
Vasodilation, 225
    peripheral, 100
    synergistic, 101
Vasodilators, 125–126
Vasopressors, 26, 521–525
Vecuronium, 505
Venlafaxine, 42
Venom
    black widows, 368
    Bufo toad, 366
    components, 370
    crotalid, 435
    sea snake, 402
    vespid wasp, 379
Venomous lizards, 437
Ventricular tachydysrhythmias, 120
Verapamil, 123

Veratrum, 427
Vertebrates, 400–402
Vesicants, 360–363
Vespid wasp venom, 379
Vibrio parahemolyticus, 388
Vietnam War, 314
Vildagliptin, 87
Vinclozolin, 312
Vinca alkaloid poisoning, 431
Vineyard sprayer's lung, 278
Viperidae, 434–436
Vitamin A toxicity, 127
Vitamin E toxicity, 127
Vitamin K_1, 130, 525–526
Vitamins, 126–130, 519–521, 525–526
Volatilized nerve agent poisoning, 349
Vomiting, 32, 77, 148, 483
    agents, 363–364

Warfarins, 51, 129–131
    metabolism of, 130
    skin necrosis, 130
    super, 332
    toxicity, 526
Warm water immersion, 542
Warning property, 205
Wasps, 378, 379
WBI. *See* Whole bowel irrigation
Weakness, 32
Weight-loss drugs, 77
Wernicke's encephalopathy, 520
Whippets, 227
White phosphorus, 237, 345
Whole bowel irrigation (WBI), 14
Wilson's disease, 278
Wintergreen poisoning, 386
Withdrawal syndrome, 114
Wolff-Parkinson-White syndrome, 498–499
Wool-sorter's disease, 364
Wound botulism, 384

Xanthine dehydrogenase, 295
Xanthine oxidase, 295
Xerostomia, 40

Yellow oleander, 418
Yellow rain, 413
Yellow sac spider, 379
Yersinia enterocolitica, 468
Yohimbine, 391
Ytterbium, 300

Zinc, 307–309
   chloride, 307
   oxide, 307
   phosphide, 308
Zolpidem, 113
Zygomycetes, 468